OPERATIVE SURGERY

Fundamental International Techniques

Orthopaedics

Part I

OPERATIVE SURGERY

Fundamental International Techniques

Third Edition

Under the General Editorship of

Charles Rob
M.C., M.D., M.Chir., F.R.C.S.

Professor and Chairman of the Department of Surgery,
University of Rochester School of Medicine and Dentistry,
Rochester, New York

and

Rodney Smith (Lord Smith of Marlow)
K.B.E., Hon.D.Sc., M.S., F.R.C.S., Hon.F.R.A.C.S.,
Hon.F.R.C.S.(Ed.), Hon. F.A.C.S., Hon. F.R.C.S.(Can.),
Hon.F.R.C.S.(I.), Hon.F.D.S.

Associate Editor

Hugh Dudley
Ch.M., F.R.C.S., F.R.C.S.(Ed.), F.R.A.C.S.

Professor of Surgery,
St. Mary's Hospital, London

OPERATIVE SURGERY

Fundamental International Techniques

Orthopaedics
Part I

Edited by

George Bentley
Ch.M., F.R.C.S.

Professor of Orthopaedic Surgery, University of Liverpool;
Honorary Consultant Orthopaedic Surgeon, Royal Liverpool Hospital,
Broadgreen Hospital and the Royal Liverpool Children's Hospital

BUTTERWORTHS
LONDON · BOSTON
Sydney · Wellington · Durban · Toronto

THE BUTTERWORTH GROUP

ENGLAND

Butterworth & Co (Publishers) Ltd
London: 88 Kingsway, WC2B 6AB

AUSTRALIA

Butterworths Pty Ltd
Sydney: 586 Pacific Highway, Chatswood, NSW 2067
Also at Melbourne, Brisbane, Adelaide and Perth

SOUTH AFRICA

Butterworth & Co (South Africa) (Pty) Ltd
Durban: 152–154 Gale Street

NEW ZEALAND

Butterworths of New Zealand Ltd
Wellington: T & W Young Building,
77–85 Customhouse Quay 1, CPO Box 472

CANADA

Butterworth & Co (Canada) Ltd
Toronto: 2265 Midland Avenue, Scarborough, Ontario M1P 4S1

USA

Butterworths (Publishers) Inc
Boston: 10 Tower Office Park, Woburn, Mass. 01801

First Edition Published in Eight Volumes, 1956–1958
Second Edition Published in Fourteen Volumes, 1968–1971
Third Edition published in Nineteen Volumes, 1976–1979
This Volume First Published 1979
This Volume Reprinted 1980

©
Butterworth & Co (Publishers) Ltd
1979

Part I: ISBN 0 407 00630 3
Part II: ISBN 0 407 00631 1
Set: ISBN 0 407 00632 X

British Library Cataloguing in Publication Data

Operative Surgery. – 3rd ed.
   Orthopaedics
   1. Surgery, Operative
   I. Rob, Charles II. Smith, Rodney, *Baron Smith, b.1914* III. Dudley, Hugh Arnold Freeman
   IV. Bentley, George
617′.91   RD32   79-40020

ISBN 0-407-00632-X (Set)
ISBN 0-407-00630-3 (Part 1)
ISBN 0-407-00631-1 (Part 2)

Typeset by Butterworths Litho Preparation Department
Printed in England by The Whitefriars Press Ltd., London and Tonbridge
Bound by the Newdigate Press Ltd., Dorking, Surrey

OPERATIVE SURGERY

Volumes and Editors

ABDOMEN	Hugh Dudley, Ch.M., F.R.C.S., F.R.C.S.(Ed.), F.R.A.C.S. Charles Rob, *M.C.,* M.D., M.Chir., F.R.C.S. Rodney Smith (Lord Smith of Marlow), K.B.E., M.S., F.R.C.S.
ACCIDENT SURGERY	P. S. London, M.B.E., F.R.C.S.
CARDIOTHORACIC SURGERY	John W. Jackson, M.Ch., F.R.C.S.
COLON, RECTUM AND ANUS	Ian P. Todd, M.S., M.D.(Tor.), F.R.C.S.
EAR	John Ballantyne, F.R.C.S., Hon.F.R.C.S.(I.)
EYES	Stephen J. H. Miller, M.D., F.R.C.S.
GENERAL PRINCIPLES, BREAST AND HERNIA	Hugh Dudley, Ch.M., F.R.C.S., F.R.C.S.(Ed.), F.R.A.C.S. Charles Rob, *M.C.,* M.D., M.Chir., F.R.C.S. Rodney Smith (Lord Smith of Marlow), K.B.E., M.S., F.R.C.S.
GYNAECOLOGY AND OBSTETRICS	D. W. T. Roberts, M.Chir., F.R.C.S., F.R.C.O.G.

THE HAND	R. Guy Pulvertaft, C.B.E., Hon.M.D., M.Chir., F.R.C.S.
HEAD AND NECK *[in 2 volumes]*	John S. P. Wilson, F.R.C.S.(Eng.), F.R.C.S.(Ed.)
NEUROSURGERY	Lindsay Symon, T.D., F.R.C.S.
NOSE AND THROAT	John Ballantyne, F.R.C.S., Hon.F.R.C.S.(I.)
ORTHOPAEDICS *[in 2 volumes]*	George Bentley, Ch.M., F.R.C.S.
PAEDIATRIC SURGERY	H. H. Nixon, F.R.C.S., Hon.F.A.A.P.
PLASTIC SURGERY	Robert M. McCormack, M.D. John Watson, F.R.C.S.
UROLOGY	D. Innes Williams, M.D., M.Chir., F.R.C.S.
VASCULAR SURGERY	Charles Rob, *M.C.,* M.D., M.Chir., F.R.C.S.

OPERATIVE SURGERY

Contributors to these Volumes

CHRISTOPHER E. ACKROYD
M.A., F.R.C.S.

Clinical Reader, Nuffield Department of Orthopaedic Surgery, University of Oxford

J. R. ADDISON
F.R.C.S.

Consultant Orthopaedic Surgeon, Worthing Hospital, Southlands Hospital, Shoreham-by-Sea and Royal West Sussex and St. Richard's Hospitals, Chichester

E. W. O. ADKINS
F.R.C.S.

Consultant Orthopaedic Surgeon, Derbyshire Royal Infirmary and Derby City Hospital

PAUL AICHROTH
M.S., F.R.C.S.

Consultant Orthopaedic Surgeon, Westminster Hospital, London, Westminster Children's Hospital, London and Queen Mary's Hospital, Roehampton; Honorary Consultant Orthopaedic Surgeon, The Hospital for Sick Children, Great Ormond Street, London

J. C. ANGEL
F.R.C.S.

Consultant Orthopaedic Surgeon, Royal National Orthopaedic Hospital, Stanmore, Middlesex

R. L. BATTEN
F.R.C.S.

Consultant Orthopaedic Surgeon, General Hospital, Birmingham and Royal Orthopaedic Hospital, Birmingham

GEORGE BENTLEY
Ch.M., F.R.C.S.

Professor of Orthopaedic Surgery, University of Liverpool; Honorary Consultant Orthopaedic Surgeon, Royal Liverpool Hospital, Broadgreen Hospital and the Royal Liverpool Children's Hospital

SIR GEORGE M. BEDBROOK
O.B.E., Hon.M.D.(W.A.), M.S.(Melb.), D.P.R.M., F.R.C.S., F.R.A.C.S.

Chairman, Department of Orthopaedic Surgery and Senior Spinal Surgeon, Royal Perth (Rehabilitation) Hospital, Western Australia

MARTIN BIRNSTINGL
M.S., F.R.C.S.

Consultant Surgeon, St. Bartholomew's Hospital, London

N. J. BLOCKEY
M.Ch.(Orth.), F.R.C.S.(Eng.), F.R.C.S.(Glas.)

Consultant Orthopaedic Surgeon, Royal Hospital for Sick Children, Glasgow and Western Infirmary, Glasgow

H. BOLTON
Ch.M., F.R.C.S.

Consultant Orthopaedic and Accident Surgeon to the Stockport Group of Hospitals

DONAL BROOKS
M.A., F.R.C.S.(I.), F.R.C.S.

Consultant Orthopaedic Surgeon, University College Hospital and Royal National Orthopaedic Hospital, London; Civilian Consultant in Hand Surgery to the Royal Navy and Royal Air Force

J. E. BUCK
F.R.C.S.(Eng.), F.R.C.S.(Ed.)

Consultant Orthopaedic Surgeon, Greenwich and Bexley Area Health Authority

A. CATTERALL
M.Chir., F.R.C.S.

Consultant Orthopaedic Surgeon, Royal National Orthopaedic Hospital, London and Charing Cross Hospital Group

J. CHALMERS
M.D., F.R.C.S.(Eng.),
F.R.C.S.(Ed.)

*Consultant Orthopaedic Surgeon, Royal Infirmary
and Princess Margaret Rose Orthopaedic Hospital, Edinburgh*

SIR JOHN CHARNLEY
C.B.E., F.R.S., F.R.C.S.,
F.A.C.S.

*Emeritus Professor of Orthopaedic Surgery, University of Manchester;
Honorary Orthopaedic Surgeon, Centre for Hip Surgery, Wrightington
Hospital, Wigan; Consultant Orthopaedic Surgeon, King Edward VII
Hospital, Midhurst, Sussex*

S. C. CHEN
F.R.C.S.

Consultant Orthopaedic Surgeon, Enfield Group of Hospitals

HENRY V. CROCK
M.D., M.S., F.R.C.S., F.R.A.C.S.

*Senior Orthopaedic Surgeon, St. Vincent's Hospital,
University of Melbourne*

ROGER DEE
F.R.C.S.(Eng.)

*Chairman, Department of Orthopedic Surgery, State University of
New York at Stony Brook and Nassau County Medical Center;
Chief of Orthopedics, Veterans Administration Hospital, Northport,
New York*

ROBERT A. DICKSON
Ch.M., F.R.C.S.

*Clinical Reader, Nuffield Department of Orthopaedic Surgery,
University of Oxford;
Consultant Orthopaedic Surgeon, Nuffield Orthopaedic Centre, Oxford*

DENIS M. DUNN
F.R.C.S.(Ed.), F.R.C.S.(Eng.)

*Consultant Orthopaedic Surgeon, Black Notley Hospital
and The London Hospital*

R. B. DUTHIE
M.A., Ch.M., F.R.C.S.

*Nuffield Professor of Orthopaedic Surgery,
Nuffield Department of Orthopaedic Surgery, University of Oxford*

M. A. EDGAR
M.Chir., F.R.C.S.

*Consultant Orthopaedic Surgeon, The Middlesex Hospital, London
and Royal National Orthopaedic Hospital, London*

G. R. FISK
F.R.C.S.(Ed.), F.R.C.S.(Eng.)

*Orthopaedic Surgeon, St. Margaret's Hospital, Epping and
Princess Alexandra Hospital, Harlow*

J. A. FIXSEN
M.Chir., F.R.C.S.(Eng.)

*Consultant Orthopaedic Surgeon, The Hospital for Sick Children,
Great Ormond Street, London and St. Bartholomew's Hospital, London*

ADRIAN E. FLATT
M.D., M.Chir., F.R.C.S.

*Professor of Orthopedics, University of Iowa Hospitals, Iowa City;
formerly First Assistant, Orthopaedic and Accident Department,
The London Hospital*

DOUGLAS FREEBODY
M.B., B.S., F.R.C.S.(Eng.).
F.R.C.S.(Ed.)

Consultant Orthopaedic Surgeon, Kingston Group of Hospitals

D. J. FULLER
M.S., F.R.C.S.

*Consultant Orthopaedic Surgeon,
Nuffield Orthopaedic Centre and Radcliffe Infirmary, Oxford*

E. H. GUSTAVSON
M.B., F.R.C.S.

Consultant Plastic Surgeon, University College Hospital,
The Hospital for Sick Children, Great Ormond Street and
Royal Masonic Hospital, London

DAVID L. HAMBLEN
Ph.D., F.R.C.S.

Professor of Orthopaedic Surgery, Western Infirmary, Glasgow

B. HELAL
M.Ch.(Orth.), F.R.C.S.

Consultant Orthopaedic Surgeon, The London Hospital
and Enfield Group of Hospitals

ADRIAN N. HENRY
M.Ch., F.R.C.S.

Senior Consultant Orthopaedic Surgeon, Guy's Hospital, London

R. C. HOWARD
F.R.C.S.(Ed.)

Consultant Orthopaedic Surgeon, Norfolk and Norwich Hospital

JAMES M. HUNTER
M.D.

Associate Professor of Orthopedic Surgery, Jefferson Medical College;
Chief of Hand Surgery, Thomas Jefferson University Hospital, Philadelphia

J. P. JACKSON
F.R.C.S.

Consultant Orthopaedic Surgeon, Harlow Wood Orthopaedic Hospital
and Mansfield and Nottingham Children's Hospitals

LIPMANN KESSEL
M.B.E., M.C., F.R.C.S.

Professor of Orthopaedics, Institute of Orthopaedics;
Honorary Consultant Orthopaedic Surgeon,
Royal National Orthopaedic Hospital, London

KEVIN F. KING
F.R.C.S., F.R.A.C.S.

Senior Orthopaedic Surgeon, Western General Hospital, Melbourne;
Orthopaedic Surgeon, St. Vincent's Hospital, Melbourne

E. O'GORMAN KIRWAN
F.R.C.S.(Eng.), F.R.C.S.(Ed.)

Consultant Orthopaedic Surgeon, University College Hospital and
Royal National Orthopaedic Hospital, London

W. ALEXANDER LAW
O.B.E., M.D., F.R.C.S.

Consultant Orthopaedic Surgeon, The London Hospital,
Royal Masonic Hospital, London and
Robert Jones and Agnes Hunt Orthopaedic Hospital, Oswestry

IAN J. LESLIE
F.R.C.S.(Ed.)

Lecturer in Orthopaedic Surgery, University of Liverpool;
Honorary Senior Registrar, Liverpool AHA (T)

ALAN LETTIN
M.S., M.B., B.Sc., F.R.C.S.

Consultant Orthopaedic Surgeon, St. Bartholomew's Hospital, London
and Royal National Orthopaedic Hospital, London

E. LETOURNEL
M.D.

Professor of Orthopaedic Surgery and Traumatology,
Centre Medico-Chirurgical de la Porte de Choisy, Paris

P. S. LONDON
M.B.E., F.R.C.S.

Surgeon, Birmingham Accident Hospital

CHARLES MANNING
F.R.C.S.

Surgeon, Royal National Orthopaedic Hospital, London;
Consultant Orthopaedic Surgeon, St. Bartholomew's Hospital, London

R. H. MAUDSLEY
F.R.C.S.(Eng.)

Consultant Accident and Orthopaedic Surgeon, King Edward VII Hospital, Windsor, Maidenhead General Hospital, Wexham Park Hospital, Slough and Heatherwood Orthopaedic Hospital, Ascot

SIR HENRY
OSMOND-CLARKE
K.C.V.O., C.B.E., F.R.C.S.(I),
F.R.C.S.(Eng.)

Former Orthopaedic Surgeon to her Majesty Queen Elizabeth II; Consulting Orthopaedic Surgeon, The London Hospital and Robert Jones and Agnes Hunt Orthopaedic Hospital, Oswestry; Honorary Civilian Consultant in Orthopaedics, The Royal Air Force; Consultant in Orthopaedic Surgery, King Edward VII's Hospital for Officers; Chairman of Consultants at Osborne House

H. PIGGOTT
M.B., B.Chir., F.R.C.S.(Eng.)

Consultant Orthopaedic Surgeon, United Birmingham Hospitals, Royal Orthopaedic and Warwickshire Orthopaedic Hospital, Coleshill

A. G. POLLEN
F.R.C.S.

Consultant Orthopaedic and Traumatic Surgeon, Bedford General Hospital

R. GUY PULVERTAFT
C.B.E., Hon.M.D., M.Chir.,
F.R.C.S.

Emeritus Orthopaedic Surgeon, Derbyshire Royal Infirmary; Honorary Civil Consultant, Royal Air Force

D. A. CAMPBELL REID
M.B., B.S.(Lond.), F.R.C.S.

Consultant Plastic Surgeon, Sheffield Royal Hospital, Sheffield Royal Infirmary, Sheffield Children's Hospital, Hallamshire Hospital and Chesterfield Royal Hospital; Honorary Clinical Lecturer, University of Sheffield

ROBERT ROAF
M.Ch.(Orth.), F.R.C.S.(Ed.),
F.R.C.S.(Eng.)

Emeritus Professor of Orthopaedic Surgery, University of Liverpool; Consultant Orthopaedic Surgeon, United Liverpool Hospitals and Robert Jones and Agnes Hunt Orthopaedic Hospital, Oswestry

G. K. ROSE
F.R.C.S.

Consultant Surgeon (Paediatric Orthopaedics) and Director of Orthoptic Research and Locomotor Assessment, Robert Jones and Agnes Hunt Orthopaedic Hospital, Oswestry

W. J. W. SHARRARD
M.D., Ch.M., F.R.C.S.(Eng.)

Consultant Orthopaedic Surgeon, Sheffield Royal Infirmary and Children's Hospital, Sheffield

E. W. SOMERVILLE
F.R.C.S.(Ed.), F.R.C.S.(Eng.)

Consultant Orthopaedic Surgeon, Nuffield Orthopaedic Centre, Oxford

JOHN D. M. STEWART
F.R.C.S.(Eng.)

Consultant Orthopaedic Surgeon, Chichester and Graylingwell, and Worthing, Southlands and District Group of Hospitals

J. G. TAYLOR
V.R.D., M.B., B.S.(Lond.),
F.R.C.S.(Eng.)

Consultant Orthopaedic Surgeon, Norfolk and Norwich Hospital

JOHN TRICKER
M.B., B.S., F.R.C.S.

Lecturer, Nuffield Department of Orthopaedic Surgery, University of Oxford

E. L. TRICKEY
F.R.C.S.

Consultant Orthopaedic Surgeon,
Royal National Orthopaedic Hospital, London

J. WATSON-FARRAR
F.R.C.S.(Eng.)

Consultant Orthopaedic Surgeon, Norfolk and Norwich Hospital

W. WAUGH
M.Chir., F.R.C.S.

Professor of Orthopaedic and Accident Surgery,
University of Nottingham

PAUL C. WEAVER
M.D., F.R.C.S., F.R.C.S.(Ed.)

Consultant Surgeon, Portsmouth and South East Hampshire
Group of Hospitals; Clinical Teacher, University of Southampton

J. N. WILSON
Ch.M., F.R.C.S.(Eng.)

Consultant Orthopaedic Surgeon,
Royal National Orthopaedic Hospital, London and
The National Hospital for Nervous Diseases, London

OPERATIVE SURGERY

Contents of Part I

OPERATIVE SURGERY

Contents of Part II

Thigh and Knee

Introduction

The principle aim in this Third Edition of *Orthopaedics* is to reflect the expansion in orthopaedic surgical procedures as the emphasis has shifted from pure surgical craft to applied science. Hence, although several classic procedures are retained, chapters on corrective spinal surgery in children, total joint replacement, treatment of fractures by internal and external fixation, knee ligament injuries, hand injuries and arthroscopy feature, together with updated chapters on important standard procedures. The chapters dealing with principles of repair and replacement of injured musculoskeletal tissues, spinal injuries and treatment of orthopaedic diseases illustrate the multidisciplinary background which forms an integral part of modern orthopaedics.

Individuality is a traditional strength of orthopaedic surgery. The authors have described their methods in their own style within the overall framework. No attempt has been made to be totally comprehensive but the conditions and procedures described are those likely to be encountered in most units. Overlap has been inevitable and accepted especially where necessary to emphasize important points.

Throughout, the needs of the orthopaedic trainee and training programme have been kept in mind particularly since postgraduate programmes are now relatively short. To this end the traditional emphasis on diagrammatic illustrations has been blended with authoritative discussion and bibliography where necessary.

I am greatly indebted to all the authors who, despite their busy lives, have kept to deadlines. I am especially indebted to Charles Manning who laid the foundations of these volumes. My particular thanks are due to the editorial staff of Butterworths for their special and essential skills.

GEORGE BENTLEY

Emergency Skin Cover in Orthopaedics

E. H. Gustavson, M.B., F.R.C.S.
Consultant Plastic Surgeon, University College Hospital,
The Hospital for Sick Children, Great Ormond Street and
Royal Masonic Hospital, London

Indications

Emergency skin cover is necessary for the following reasons.
(*1*) Prevention of infection.
(*2*) Covering of vital structures.
(*3*) Decrease in healing time and scar formation.
Wound closure or skin cover should be performed within 6 hr of injury when possible. This time limit can be extended to 12 hr for the head and neck.

In heavily contaminated wounds debridement should be meticulously performed and then the wound packed lightly open. Tetanus prophylaxis should be given in all wounds.

Debridement

The purpose of debridement is to remove all foreign bodies and all devitalized tissue. As far as the skin and subcutaneous tissues are concerned, any doubtfully viable skin edges or flaps should be excised back to bleeding tissue and then a further 2 cm excised. If the viability of the tissue is in doubt, then it must be excised. This is the opposite rule to the head where tissue which may possibly be viable should be preserved.

PRIMARY SKIN CLOSURE

1

More skin is lost because of suturing under tension, either at the time of surgery or because of subsequent massive oedema, than for any other surgical reason. For this reason it is important to assess the degree of soft tissue contusion and, therefore, the likely post-operative oedema and also whether any actual skin loss occurred at the time of the accident.

If no skin loss has occurred, and there is little contusion, then the wound may be closed with drainage. A well-padded pressure dressing should be applied and the injured part elevated for 5 days postoperatively. Stitches should be evenly spaced at equal distances from the edge and should not be tied tightly.

If, on closure, there is tension, or if there has been tissue lost, the skin edges should not be approximated but allowed to lie where they are. The resultant defect can be filled with a split-thickness skin graft. This will provide primary healing and the skin graft will subsequently contract and, if necessary, can be excised 6 months later.

Extensive undermining, suturing under tension and severe postoperative oedema may produce extensive skin necrosis in otherwise viable tissue.

The use of relieving incisions is not to be recommended.

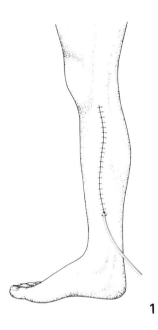

1

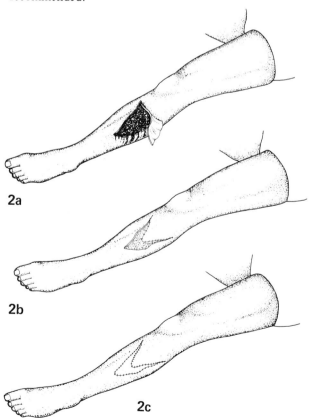

2a

2b

2c

AVULSION FLAPS

2 a, b & c

These flaps (*a*) should not be stitched back into position. After debridement they should be allowed to lie in their contracted state and lightly stitched down to deeper structures (*b*). The resultant defect should be closed, where applicable, with a split-thickness skin graft (*c*).

In patients over the age of 50 and those who have been on steroids for a long time, the flap rarely survives and should be excised as a primary procedure, *in toto*, and the areas skin-grafted.

FREE SKIN GRAFTS

Free skin grafts can be of variable thickness, from very thin to full-thickness skin. As an emergency procedure the thinner the graft the better. Full-thickness grafts should only be used on surgically produced defects.

Being free skin grafts, they need to be placed on a vascular bed in order to obtain a blood supply. They will therefore not take in the following conditions.

(1) Bare cortical bone without periosteum.

(2) Tendon without paratenon.

(3) Cartilage without perichondrium.

(4) There is a reduced chance of take if the area has had previous radiotherapy.

Contrary to popular belief, free skin grafts take well on deep fascia, periosteum and cancellous bone provided that this tissue has not been allowed to dry.

Properties of skin grafts

A thin skin graft:

(1) will take more readily than a thick split-thickness skin graft if the wound is contaminated;

(2) having taken, it will contract quite markedly;

(3) it will not stand up to wear and tear readily;

(4) it will not look like normal skin.

A thick split-thickness skin graft or full-thickness skin graft will:

(1) only take if there is no infection;

(2) having taken, will not contract appreciably;

(3) will appear more like normal skin;

(4) will stand up to wear and tear more readily.

For this reason, in contaminated fields, a thin split-thickness skin graft is better than a thick or full-thickness skin graft.

SPLIT-THICKNESS SKIN GRAFTS

Donor area

The thinner a split-thickness graft the quicker the donor area heals and the less the residual scarring.

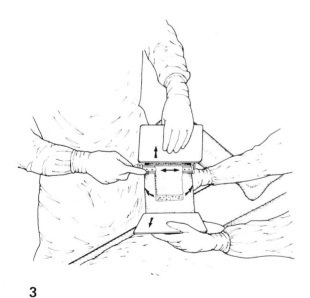

3

Taking a split-thickness skin graft

The thigh is the commonest donor site but the buttock may be preferred in women. The arm is best avoided for functional and cosmetic reasons.

The donor area, skin graft knife and surgeon's board are lubricated with sterile liquid paraffin.

The assistant places his right hand beneath the thigh to produce as flat a surface as possible and to tighten the skin of the thigh circumferentially. With his left hand holding a skin graft board, he stretches the skin cephalad. He should not move either hand whilst the graft is being cut unless instructed by the surgeon. The surgeon holds the skin graft knife with his index finger pointing along its long axis. The graft knife is drawn backwards and forwards in the same plane, not in a yawing motion. The left hand, holding the skin board, stretches the skin caudally. The graft knife should be flat on the skin and follows as the surgeon's board is slowly moved caudally. The skin graft knife should not be pushed forwards consciously.

When taken, the skin graft is spread on paraffin gauze, raw surfaces upwards, and moistened immediately with saline. If not to be used immediately, it should be folded, raw surface to raw surface, and covered with a saline swab.

The donor area is covered initially with a saline swab and, when the surgeon is certain that no more skin is required, it can be dressed with paraffin gauze, dressing gauze, wool and a crêpe bandage.

Application of a split-thickness skin graft

A split-thickness skin graft will not take if there is:
(*1*) infection, particularly with haemolytic streptococcus;
(*2*) haematoma;
(*3*) seroma;
(*4*) a shearing strain between the graft and its bed.

4

After meticulous haemostasis, the skin graft is applied and stitched to the edges of the defect. Stitches should be through the graft and the bottom edge of the defect in order to 'snug' the graft to the edge. On convex surfaces, the graft can then be covered with paraffin gauze, flavine wool, dressing gauze, cotton wool and a crêpe bandage.

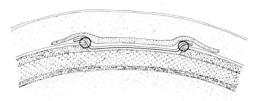

4

5

On the concave surfaces, one end of each suture is left long and these are tied over a large pad of flavine wool to similar long ends at the opposite side of the graft. This is a tie-over dressing and whilst it does not itself apply pressure, it does hold the dressing in place, allowing the pressure dressing on top to apply pressure on the exact place of the graft.

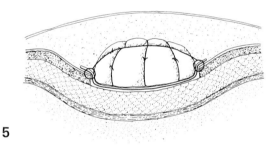

5

6

Shearing strains between the graft and its bed will prevent the revascularization of the graft. In those areas which are difficult to immobilize completely, the dressing may act as a shearing force. In this case the wound should be dressed with paraffin gauze and saline soaked gauze, stored in a refrigerator and, when the patient has fully recovered from the anaesthetic and is co-operative, the graft can be laid on the wound in the ward, without stitching, and left exposed. This is an excellent method for all areas except the limbs.

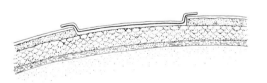

6

SKIN FLAPS

Unlike free skin grafts, skin flaps are never completely detached from the body and have their own blood supply. They can, therefore, be used to cover avascular vital structures and fractures.

They are not without their hazards and should not be used by the inexperienced. All too often there is only one ideal flap on the limbs and if this is lost subsequent repair can be lengthy.

Skin flaps may be local or distal. They may have a known blood vessel running throughout their length, and are then known as axial pattern flaps, or they may be supplied by the subdermal plexus with no specific artery of supply. These latter flaps are the more common and are called random pattern flaps. Their length should never be more than their breadth, with the possible exception of those around the knee joint where there is a richer cutaneous blood supply.

Basic rules for skin flaps

The following are basic rules for most forms of skin flaps.

(*1*) Plan before cutting the flap. The use of a paper pattern will show whether the flap will cover the defect or not. Similarly, the use of a swab along the length of the flap can show whether it will transpose and reach its object.

(*2*) Make all dimensions larger than you think necessary. On the whole a large flap is much safer than a small one.

(*3*) It is essential to make the skin defect fit the flap and not vice versa. This may involve removing relatively large areas of normal skin around the original defect, but it must be done in order to allow a flap of safe dimensions to be used.

(*4*) The flap is raised just superficial to the deep fascia.

(*5*) It should have a length to breadth ratio of 1:1.

(*6*) All tension should be avoided.

(*7*) Haemostasis should be meticulous.

(*8*) Careful suturing is essential to prevent local lines of tension.

(*9*) Usually drainage beneath the flap should be provided.

(*10*) The secondary defect from whence the flap has been raised will usually require a skin graft.

(*11*) The flap should not be covered with a dressing or plaster-of-Paris splint. Close postoperative inspection is necessary in order to check the position of the flap and to ensure that no haematoma is occurring. It will also enable the early detection of infection.

(*12*) Most distal flaps are divided 3 weeks after the initial operation.

(*13*) At the time of division, the remaining raw edge on the flap should be lightly inset. If this cannot be done without tension, then a thin split-thickness skin graft should be applied to the raw edge. Tension can cause death of skin over quite a considerable area in the flap. Failure to close the raw edge may predispose to infection and massive fat necrosis beneath the flap.

Relieving incisions

Relieving incisions should, in general, not be used. While occasionally effective, the bridge of skin between the wound and the relieving incision which is, in effect, a long narrow flap, frequently dies, making the problem even larger. A relieving incision parallel to the wound still places the maximum tension at the suture line.

7a

Should a relieving incision be used, it should be curved toward the wound, shifting the axis of the skin bridge in that direction and relieving tension when sutured. This is still a risky procedure.

7b

A better method, particularly for the calf, is the sliding transposition flap. There is no tension at the suture line and the secondary defect is grafted. The 'dog-ear' may require trimming at a later date.

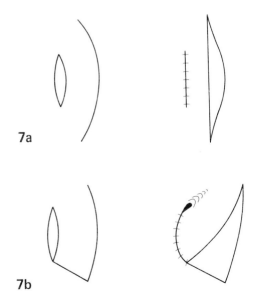

7a

7b

DISTANT FLAPS

Distant flaps, e.g. cross-thigh flaps, cross-leg flaps and abdominal flaps, will require some form of fixation in order to hold the flap against the recipient area for a period of 3 weeks. This may be done with Elastoplast fixation in the case of abdominal flaps going to the forearm or hand, or with plaster-of-Paris fixation in the case of the cross-leg or cross-thigh flap. As with all fixation, care must be taken to avoid pressure over bony prominences and subcutaneous nerves.

8

Cross-thigh flap

This flap should, ideally, be reserved for children. It requires suppleness on the part of the patient, and in adults the weight of the limb can cause pressure necrosis over the fibula of the recipient leg or over the quadriceps of the donor leg. Fixation is by plaster-of-Paris splinting.

9, 10 & 11

Cross-leg flap

The cross-leg flap may be used to cover vital structures and fractures in the lower limb and ankle. It is a flap *par excellence* where the basic rules of flap transfer must be followed; otherwise partial necrosis will occur.

The use of a pattern is essential in order to provide a flap of safe dimensions, and the flap should be of sufficient length, not only to cover the defect but to provide a bridge of skin to the donor leg. Not only must the dimensions of the flap be planned, but positions of both legs should be confirmed in order to see that the proposed side-by-side or cross-leg position is, in fact, feasible.

The flap is raised just superficial to the deep fascia and the base of the flap should not divide the long saphenous vein; otherwise impaired venous drainage will result, with partial or complete necrosis of the flap.

The secondary defect and the under-surface of the flap bridge are skin-grafted. The flap is sutured with no tension and drainage may be needed.

Fixation is with plaster-of-Paris splintage, holding the legs together above and below the flap and joining the upper and lower plaster-of-Paris segments together with metal or wooden longitudinal struts (not illustrated here).

The plaster is allowed to harden for 48 hr postoperatively, and then both legs are placed in high elevation with slings.

The flap is divided at 3 weeks.

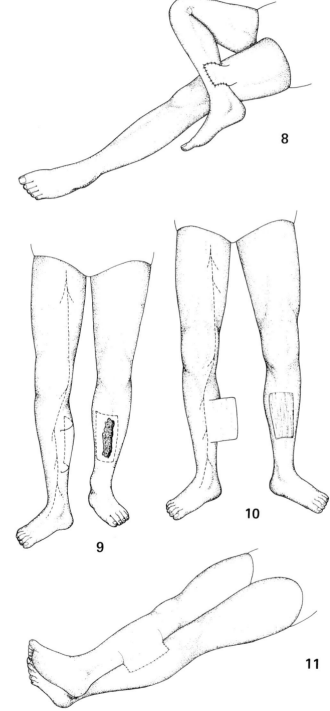

8

9

10

11

12 & 13

Abdominal flaps

These are useful flaps for covering defects of the fore-arm and hand. Their base may be either superior or inferior, depending on the area to be covered. The basic rules of flap procedure should be followed.

There is little vascular cross-over in the mid-line and, for this reason, abdominal flaps should never be raised across the mid-line.

In order to aid fixation, it is better for the upper arm to be held firmly against the lateral chest wall. As a general rule, for defects involving the hand, the flap should be raised on the other side of the body whereas for defects involving the forearm, the flap should be raised on the same side of the body. This will of course vary depending on the build of the patient.

Fixation is usually by one-way stretch Elastoplast, one piece encircling the upper arm and fixing it to the chest with appropriate padding to protect the radial nerve. Another piece runs along the undamaged surface of the forearm, closely applied to the abdomen. A third piece passes around the forearm or wrist and over the shoulder to prevent downward movement and a fourth piece passes around the limb and downwards to prevent upward movement.

Depending on the patient, the transverse fixation can usually be removed after a few days, leaving only the superior sling of Elastoplast to maintain position. This allows inspection of the grafted secondary defect and cleaning of the under-surface of the arm and hand to prevent maceration.

The flap is divided at between 2 and 3 weeks.

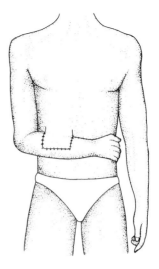

12

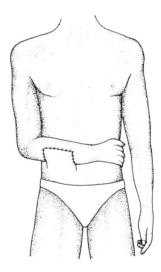

13

14

PEDICLE MUSCLE FLAPS

In relatively small but vital defects, a pedicle muscle flap can be mobilized and swung to cover the defect. Having done this, a split-thickness skin graft may then be applied to the transposed muscle, resulting in primary healing. This procedure may avoid the use of some of the larger flaps.

The medial head of the gastrocnemius is supplied solely by a large branch from the popliteal artery entering the muscle in the popliteal fossa 2 cm medial to the mid-line. The muscle may therefore be detached from the tendo Achillis below and mobilized up to this vascular attachment. It can cover the upper one-fifth of the anterior surface of the tibia or the medial aspect of the knee joint.

The lateral head of the gastrocnemius is smaller than the medial head and is supplied by a single branch from the popliteal artery entering high in the mid-line. The muscle is also closely related to the peroneal nerve proximally. It may be freed from the tendo Achillis below and will cover the lateral tibial condyle or the lateral aspect of the knee joint.

The medial component of the soleus arises from the soleal line and the middle third of the medial border of the tibia. It lies over the upper part of the flexor digitorum longus and is covered posteriorly and medially by the large medial head of the gastrocnemius. The blood supply is from the posterior tibial artery which enters via two or three branches on the deep surface of the muscle, 1—2 cm from its attachment to the medial border of the tibia. Separation of the medial and lateral constituents of the soleus allows the whole medial component of the muscle to be swung medially without detachment below to cover an area approximately 4 cm by 8 cm between the upper and middle fifths of the anterior aspect of the tibia.

The flexor digitorum longus is supplied from the posterior tibial artery by four arteries. The first artery enters 5 cm distal to the proximal origin of the muscle and the vessels enter at approximately 3 cm intervals. These branches enter on the posterolateral aspect of the muscle proximally, but on the anterior aspect distally. Mobilization of the muscle, with sharp dissection of the muscle from its tibial attachment and blunt dissection from its deep fascial attachment will cover an area approximately 5 cm by 5 cm between the distal and middle fifths of the anterior surface of the tibia.

The extensor hallucis longus has a blood supply from the anterior tibial artery via four or five small

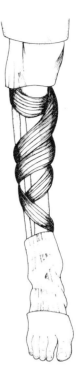

14

branches which enter on its tibial aspect at approximately 4 cm intervals and 1 cm behind the tendon. The muscle is mobilized by freeing it distally from the deep attachments, but proximally, where it is covered by tibialis anterior, it cannot be mobilized. The anterior aspect of the tibia between its distal and middle fifths may be covered.

The abductor hallucis has a single arterial supply which enters on the deep surface of the muscle, two fingers' breadth distal to its calcaneal origin. It may be mobilized freely in its distal half but proximally, where it is blended with flexor digitorum brevis, it must be separated by sharp dissection. The mobilized muscle will cover the medial aspect of the heel or the medial malleolus.

FREE FLAP TRANSFER

It is now possible, using the operating microscope, to anastomose arteries with a diameter of 0·5 mm and veins with a diameter of 1 mm successfully. This allows the free transfer of axial pattern flaps as a one-stage procedure. These flaps may be of the maximum dimension of 16 cm by 10 cm and allow immediate full-thickness skin cover with subcutaneous fat. This is highly specialized surgery and should not be attempted by anyone inexperienced in this field. It also has a tremendous application in the replantation of multiple traumatic digital amputations.

[The illustrations for this Chapter on Emergency Skin Cover in Orthopaedics were drawn by Mr. J. M. P. Booth.]

The Principles of Tendon Repair, Replacement and Re-adjustment

B. Helal, M.Ch.(Orth.), F.R.C.S.
Consultant Orthopaedic Surgeon, The London Hospital
and Enfield Group of Hospitals

and

S. C. Chen, F.R.C.S.
Consultant Orthopaedic Surgeon, Enfield Group of Hospitals

PRE-OPERATIVE

History

Damage to a tendon may be localized or extend over a distance. Apart from mechanical injury, the tendon can be injured from within by sharp fragments of bone or by avulsion, or from without by thermal agents such as severe burns or frostbite, by chemical agents and disease processes or radiation. When treating hand injuries it is important to know the occupation and hobbies of the patient, which hand is dominant and the time lapse since the injury.

Examination

A careful clinical examination should be made of every open wound, being constantly aware of the possibility of tendon injury. A tendon may appear to be intact in the depth of the wound, but it may be cut some distance away depending on whether the nearby joint or joints were flexed or extended at the time of injury. When in doubt, the wound should always be explored under regional or general anaesthesia.

Wound toilet

Preparation of the wound is important if primary healing is to take place. Dead and crushed tissues must be excised. Use of cleansing agents such as surgical spirits or iodine on exposed tendons can cause extensive chemical damage. Even a small puncture wound can take in fluid due to capillary action and involve, for instance, the whole flexor apparatus in a hand. Bland agents like Savlon should be used. Physical scrubbing or jet lavage is necessary if the wound is grossly contaminated with dirt or mud.

Use of antibiotics

In contaminated wounds it is a wise precaution to use bactericidal antibiotics in adequate dosage. A carefully planned and executed surgical operation can be ruined by infection.

Appropriate tetanus prophylaxis should be given in such cases.

Primary tendon repair

Primary repair is the treatment of choice if:
   (1) damage to the tendon is localized;
   (2) there is good quality soft tissue cover;
   (3) the associated joints are mobile;
   (4) adequate surgical and anaesthetic skills; and
   (5) good theatre facilities are available.

It is permissible in certain situations to carry out a primary repair in the presence of more extensive damage to the tendon. The tendon can be lengthened locally by Z-shaped incisions or by advancement using this technique more proximally, e.g. extensor tendons of the hand and the tendon of the flexor pollicis longus. Conditions 2, 3 and 4 must be fulfilled.

Associated injuries

Fractures underlying tendon damage should be stabilized beforehand.

Other soft tissue injuries, for example to vessels and nerves damaged at the same level, may be repaired simultaneously. Cross-adhesions to nerves can be prevented by isolating the nerve and wrapping it in silicone rubber membrane.

It must be emphasized that unless these criteria are adhered to, not only is the repair likely to fail, but the outcome of reconstructive measures at a later date will be prejudiced.

Contra-indications to primary tendon repair

(1) Extensive tendon damage.
   (2) Damage to overlying soft tissues.
   (3) Severe contamination of the wound.
   (4) Underlying fractures which cannot be stabilized because of the nature of the fracture or due to contamination.
   (5) Damage to joints resulting in stiffness.
   (6) Lack of available surgical skill and operating facilities are contra-indications to primary repair.

Primary repair is best carried out with a minimum of delay but, under certain circumstances, it may be postponed for 2 or 3 days for certain tendon repairs, for example the flexor apparatus of the hand, and for up to 2 weeks in other situations. After this period, there may be permanent retraction of the muscle belly.

Closure of the skin is mandatory if delay is anticipated.

In primary tendon repair, the tendon sheath should be preserved and if possible repaired, as this reduces adhesion formation.

Tendon replacement

This is indicated if the above criteria listed for primary repair cannot be met, or if there is paralysis of the muscle belly. There are situations when even tendon replacement is neither possible nor advisable, for instance if there is extensive damage to other structures such as joints, nerves or vessels, when amputation might be the treatment of choice, or in the presence of extensive joint damage, when arthrodesis or tenodesis may be indicated.

Tendons may be replaced by:
   (1) transposition of a suitable tendon;
   (2) free tendon autografts;
   (3) fascial autografts;
   (4) muscle advancement techniques;
   (5) two-stage tendon replacement by a temporary silicone rubber spacer followed by an autograft;
   (6) an autograft of tendons and sheath (whole flexor apparatus of a toe);
   (7) cadaver material — either free grafts or whole flexor apparatus; and
   (8) artificial tendons.

GENERAL PRINCIPLES OF SURGICAL TECHNIQUE

Suture materials

These should not cause any tissue reaction as adhesions may form. Stainless steel wire or monofilament nylon are suitable materials. Prolene or Mersilene sutures can also be used.

Suture technique

Many techniques have been described for attaching tendon to tendon. The handling must be gentle to cause the minimum trauma. There are four methods for end-to-end anastomosis of tendons of equal girth.

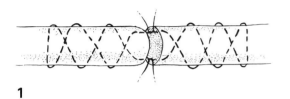

1

1

The classic Bunnell criss-cross suture tends to damage the tendons by a concertina action.

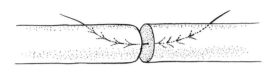

2

2

The Shaw barbed wire stitch tends to fragment.

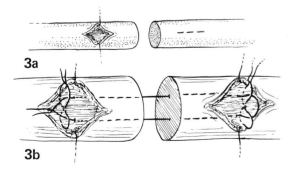

3a

3b

3 a & b

The Tsuge, Ikuta, Matsuishi intratendinous stitches are technically more demanding and in unskilled hands create more damage to the tendons.

4 & 5

The Kessler grasping stitch is preferable to the others as it is strong and simple. It is possible to insert this with one knot, which can be tied in the gap between the tendon ends. To join two tendons of unequal girth the following method is used. The smaller tendon is woven into the larger tendon through several stab incisions and these are anchored together with several sutures. The end of the larger tendon is split to enclose the smaller tendon like a 'fish-mouth'.

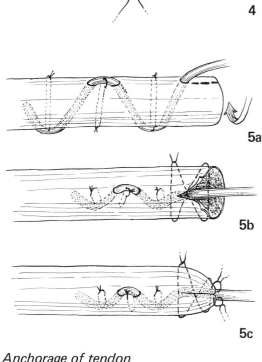

4

5a

5b

5c

Anchorage of tendon

6

To bone

A drill hole is made in the bone to which the tendon is to be attached. The tendon is drawn into the hole by a pull-out stitch. The stitch is then tied over a button on the skin. After 3 weeks the pull-out stitch is removed.

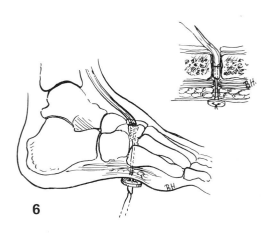

6

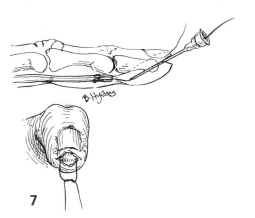

7

7

Apical suture

Many techniques have been described for the distal attachment of the profundus tendon to the terminal phalanx. For ease of insertion and the least soft tissue disturbance, the best technique is the apical suture on the palmar aspect of the terminal joint of the finger. The suture can be fed accurately into place by passing a hollow needle on either side of the tuft of the distal phalanx to the base of the phalanx and then passing the sutures through these hollow needles. A groove is made across the tuft of the distal phalanx through a transverse apical incision. The suture is tied across this groove and the skin incision closed.

Principles of tendon transfer

There are certain basic principles to be observed if a tendon transfer is to be successful.

Power

The muscle to be used for a tendon transfer should have normal power, i.e. MRC Grade V. It should have as much power as the original muscle before injury.

Line of pull

The tendon used for the transfer should act efficiently as near as possible to the line of pull of the tendon of the non-functioning muscle.

Synergism

The muscle used for the tendon transfer should be in the same synergistic group as the non-functioning muscle it replaces.

Attachment

The tendon should be attached as distally as possible on the bone it has to move.

Tendon can be spared

The tendon to be used can be spared, i.e. there is another muscle or muscles which has (have) the same action as the muscle whose tendon is to be used for transfer.

Protection of the repaired tendon

A repaired tendon takes about 3 weeks to heal. During the first week there is very little reaction. During the second week the repaired tendon is oedematous and weak and any tension during this stage will result in dehiscence of the tendon ends. During the third week the repaired tendon starts to heal by fibrous tissue crossing the approximated tendon ends. During the first 3 weeks of a tendon repair tension must be taken off the repair.

Protecting the suture line can be carried out by:

Plaster immobilization

This is preferred in hand injuries in children because it is the most immune to interference. The wrist and metacarpophalangeal joints are held in flexion, the plaster extending to the finger tips over the dorsal surface with the fingers kept straight.

After tendon repairs in other parts of the upper limb and in the lower limb, plaster immobilization for 3 − 6 weeks is essential.

8

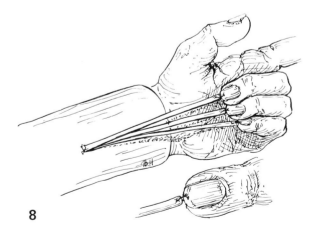

8

Flexor tendon repair using the Kleinert technique

This allows for early mobilization of the injured finger after a flexor tendon repair, thus avoiding the complication of joint stiffness. This method relies on the muscle actively relaxing when its antagonistic muscle is actively contracting. After the flexor tendon is repaired, a rubber band is attached from the finger nail by a suture to a plaster splint on the forearm. Limited extension against the elastic band is allowed from the start. It is important to include the other two unaffected ulnar digits when one of the three ulnar profundi have been repaired because this section of the muscle acts *en masse*.

*Extensor tendon repair using the dynamic radial
nerve palsy splint*

When extensor tendons are repaired the same principle
of reflex inhibition of antagonist muscles can be
applied by the use of a dynamic radial nerve palsy
splint.

Protection of the repaired extensor tendons is
necessary for only 10 days when injured in the triangular expansion but requires 3 weeks at other sites
(Stuart, 1965).

Immobilizing the motor tendon

This can be achieved by:

9

(*1*) A pull-out wire suture into the tendon proximal
to the suture line. The wire is anchored over a button
on the skin.

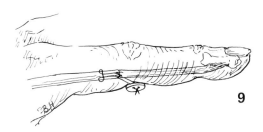

9

10

(*2*) Transfixing the tendon proximal to the suture with
a thin Kirschner wire and bringing it out through the
skin for ease of removal at the end of the third week.

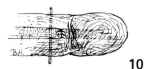

10

Tension of tendon repair

It is important to judge the tension of tendon repair
correctly. If the repair is too tight the joint under the
influence of the repaired tendon cannot extend fully.
If the repair is too lax, the muscle contractions cannot
be fully transmitted to the tendon and therefore the
joint will not have its full range of movement. Correct
tension of tendon repair is very critical in flexor tendon
injuries of the hand. Too lax a tendon repair distally
will produce relatively increased lumbrical tension on
the extensor, and paradoxical extension of the finger
will occur when flexion is attempted (Athol Parkes).
Division of the lumbrical tendon will abolish this.

Complications

Wrong tension of repair

Too tight or too loose a repair, unless very gross, can be compensated for by the muscle actively lengthening or shortening. If there is gross error in the tension, then the correct tension has to be achieved by lengthening or shortening the tendon surgically.

Adhesions

These may occur between tendon and sheath or skin. It is best to wait for about 6 months before a tenolysis is carried out. This is because an early tenolysis may give rise to further adhesions. Adhesions may also occur between a tendon and the overlying skin. Likewise it is best to wait for about the same period of 6 months before a dermolysis is carried out.

Bowstringing

It is important to leave pulleys particularly the finger flexor pulleys, the extensor retinaculum of the wrist, and the superior extensor retinaculum of the ankle, to prevent bowstringing of tendons. Sometimes their removal is unavoidable and such structures may have to be sacrificed or they may have been damaged. Severe bowstringing can affect the efficiency of tendon function especially in the hand, and reconstruction of missing pulleys has to be undertaken.

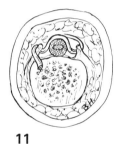 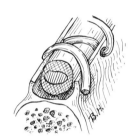

11

11

Technique of pulley reconstruction

Either a strip of fascia lata or the palmaris longus tendon can be used. It is woven through the sides of the gutter in the proximal phalanx from side to side like a shoe lace, over the flexor tendon or a Silastic rod. The ends are anchored with non-absorbable sutures.

References

Bunnell, S. (1956). *Surgery of the Hand*. Third Edition. Philadelphia: Lippincott
Kessler, I. (1973). ' "Grasping" technique for tendon repair.' *The Hand* **5,** 177
Kleinert, H. E., Kutz, J. E., Atasoy, E. and Stormo, A. (1973). 'Primary repair of flexor tendons.' *Orthop. Clins N. Am.* **4,** 865
Parkes, A. R. (1970). 'The "Lumbrical plus" finger.' *J. Bone Jt Surg.* **52B,** 236
Shaw, P. C. (1968). 'A method of flexor tendon suture.' *J. Bone Jt Surg.* **50B,** 578
Stuart, D. (1965). 'Duration of splinting after repair of extensor tendons in the hand.' *J. Bone Jt Surg.* **47B,** 72
Tsuge, K. Ikuta, Y. and Matsuishi, Y. (1975). 'Intratendinous tendon suture.' *The Hand* **7,** 250

[The illustrations for this Chapter on The Principles of Tendon Repair, Replacement and Re-adjustment were drawn by Miss B. Hyams.]

Nerve Repair and Grafting

Robert A. Dickson, Ch.M., F.R.C.S.
Clinical Reader, Nuffield Department of Orthopaedic Surgery, University of Oxford;
Consultant Orthopaedic Surgeon, Nuffield Orthopaedic Centre, Oxford

INTRODUCTION

The first surgeon to resuture divided nerves was a Professor of Surgery at Bologna in the thirteenth century, William of Saliceto, but it took 700 years and two world wars before peripheral nerve repair became an established surgical technique. Publications based on the experience gained in the Second World War came from both the British and American governments (Seddon, 1954; Woodhall and Bebe, 1956). Although 300 years ago the great Dutch microscopy and Italian naturalist schools demonstrated the detailed anatomy of the peripheral nerve it is only in the last 15 years since the advent of the operating microscope that this information could be utilized for nerve repair. The present increased interest in peripheral nerve repair is therefore attributable to the application of microsurgical principles.

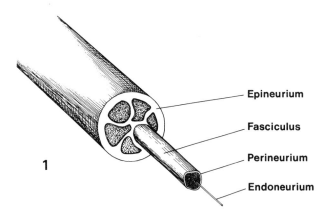

1

1

Surgical anatomy

The peripheral nerve is surrounded by an outer tube of connective tissue, the *epineurium,* which also forms the internal framework of the nerve. Within this tissue axons are grouped into bundles, *fasciculi,* surrounded by *perineurium.* Each individual axon is surrounded by an even more delicate sheath, the *endoneurium.* In the proximal course of the nerve, fasciculi interchange in their pattern and in some anatomical sites the nerve-to-connective tissue ratio of the peripheral nerve may be only of the order of one to five or six. Methods of repair based upon the approximation of the epineurium do not seek to restore fascicular alignment and a few degrees of malrotation may lead to a complete loss of nerve tissue continuity. Epineurial repair therefore achieves useful functional recovery in only a small proportion of patients (Saunders and Young, 1942; Seddon, 1954, 1963). With the introduction of the operating microscope it has become technically feasible to repair fasciculus to fasciculus and the results show a considerable improvement over past methods of repair (Owen, 1976). It should be remembered that there never is a perfect result from peripheral nerve repair nor will there ever be since it is quite impossible to restore the ultrastructure to normality.

Epineurium

Fasciculus

Perineurium

Endoneurium

Mechanical properties of mammalian peripheral nerve

Knowledge of the mechanical properties of nerve tissue is also important. When a nerve is divided the cut ends retract and, if then approximated, some degree of tension must result. Furthermore it has been shown that the perineurium contains contractile elements (Ross and Reith, 1960) and this is particularly evident when the fasciculi are dissected from the surrounding epineurium. This resultant tension at the suture site has been suggested as one of the most important local factors encouraging the formation of a gap and enhancing connective tissue proliferation. If there is significant tension at the anastomosis then a better result may be achieved when the deficit is bridged by interfascicular nerve grafts even though the regenerating axons have to cross two anastomoses (Millesi, Meissl and Berger, 1972). What precise tension is required to damage a nerve is a source of debate. Liu, Benda and Lewey (1948) claimed that the perineurium was destroyed by an elongation of 6 per cent while Hoen and Brackett (1956) found little evidence of damage with a permanent elongation of 100 per cent. The vast experience of Millesi (1977) suggests that a nerve graft should be used if the defect cannot be closed when the nearby joints are in neutral position. This usually corresponds with defects of 0·5 cm or more.

Evolution of present day methods of nerve repair

Early attempts at restoring the continuity of the divided peripheral nerve were based on accurate coaptation of the epineurium. To minimize fibrosis and neuroma formation, various materials were used as barriers or tubes around the site of repair. Tantalum tubes were used but initial promise was followed by secondary fragmentation, scar tissue formation, and reduction of function (Weiss, 1944). Millipore was found to calcify *in vivo* leading to increased scarring (Bassett and Campbell, 1960). A cuff of silicone rubber proved better in the experimental animal than millipore (Campbell and Luzio, 1964). The great im-

portance of tension, however, was demonstrated over 30 years ago when secondary Wallerian degeneration was noted following extension of joints previously held flexed to facilitate nerve mobilization (Highet and Holmes, 1943). The late nineteenth century saw the introduction of grafts to bridge deficits in peripheral nerves. Phillipeaux and Vulpian (1870) demonstrated that fibres would go through a graft and Albert (1885) first used a nerve homograft to bridge a deficit in a median nerve. Immunological problems have, however, plagued the use of homografts since that time. Irradiating the homograft was considered a feasible method (Marmor, 1963) but only 4 of 25 cases so treated showed any sign of recovery (Marmor, 1967). Although immunosuppressive agents were recommended (Pollard, Gye and Macleod, 1966), cortisone had previously been shown to inhibit myelin deposition by Schwann cells (Lytton and Murray, 1954). Furthermore Ochs, Sabri and Ranish (1970) showed that protein transport in nerve was strongly inhibited by immunosuppressive treatment and felt that this was a high price to pay for preserving graft morphology. To avoid immunological problems, autografts were introduced (Ballance and Duel, 1932). The classic technique of cable grafting was initially used in which several pieces of cutaneous nerve are used to form a cable of the same diameter as the divided nerve. No attention was paid to fascicular coaptation and the central grafts in the cable, having lost contact with nourishing tissue fluid, necrosed. Although the controversy of macroneurorrhaphy versus microneurorrhaphy has never been resolved by a prospective trial there is little doubt that microneurorrhaphy has improved the results of nerve repair. Nonetheless impeccable surgical technique is the key to successful nerve repair (Van Beek and Kleinert, 1977). This includes elimination of tension, the use of an atraumatic technique, proper mapping and aligning of fasciculi, prevention of gaps, avoidance of lengthy nerve mobilization with its devascularizing effect, the use of meticulous intraneural haemostasis and the minimization of foreign body reaction. An interfascicular technique, approximating groups of fascicles, is technically feasible with the operating microscope and conforms to these principles.

INTERFASCICULAR NERVE REPAIR

With a wound that is favourable and with no significant loss of nerve substance primary interfascicular nerve repair is the treatment of choice for cleanly-incised, fresh nerve injuries. These conditions are most commonly fulfilled in incised wounds of the upper extremity distal to the elbow. The patient's upper extremity is prepared and draped in the usual fashion. A tourniquet is not used in peripheral nerve surgery because it is important to ensure haemostasis by bipolar coagulation in the vicinity of the nerve. The wound will almost certainly require elongation in the appropriate direction to expose the ends of the divided nerve. This part of the operation and the subsequent wound excision and closure are performed using standard hand surgery instruments. The microsurgery instruments are used for microsurgery only.

It is important at this stage to 'get set' for micro-surgery. The microscope is introduced and there are three horizontal levels requiring adjustment. These are the heights of the eye pieces, the operating field, and the surgeon's seat. These should be adjusted appropriately at the start lest fatigue or discomfort impairs performance. Only three microsurgical instruments are necessary to perform an interfascicular nerve repair. These are a pair of straight microsurgical forceps, a pair of curved microsurgical forceps, and a pair of gently curved microsurgical scissors. At all times the straight microsurgical forceps are held in the left hand and the curved microsurgical forceps (which will also be the future needle holders) or the scissors in the right hand. The entire operation is performed under the lowest resolution of the microscope with one exception and that is the piercing of the microneedle through the perineurium of the fasciculus which is performed under the highest resolution in order to avoid the incorporation of neurological tissue in the knot.

2

The first stage in peripheral nerve repair is to identify the fascicular patterns in the proximal and distal cut ends. In some areas (the median and ulnar nerves in the forearm) the corresponding fascicular groups can be readily identified. Rotational orientation can be checked by alignment of the longitudinally running blood vessels. Motor fasciculi tend to be larger than sensory fasciculi which latter are sometimes grouped into 'macrobundles'. Electrostimulation may be necessary to identify a motor fasciculus but in a distal lesion the fasciculi of the distal stump can be traced from their final branches minimizing the possibility of mismatching. In this manner correct fascicular alignment is achieved in 90 per cent of cases (Millesi, 1977).

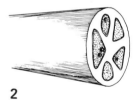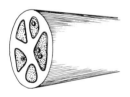

2

3

It is always preferable to attempt to suture macro-bundles rather than subdivide them into their intrinsic fasciculi which, individually, would be too small to tolerate the microneedle. The interfascicular repair technique of Acland (1976) or Millesi (1977) is recommended. The epineurium is removed from the cut surfaces until the perineurium of the fasciculi is visualized. The perineurium can be identified by its white transverse striations. When the fasciculi have been cleared of epineurial tissue the perineurium is held gently by the straight microsurgical forceps held in the left hand while the microneedle pierces the perineurium. This is performed under the high resolution of the operating microscope.

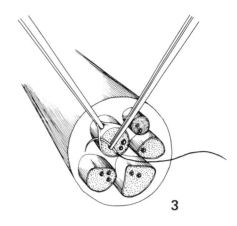

3

4

As soon as the needle has pierced the perineurium low power again is used to draw the remainder of the needle and the suture material (10/0 or 11/0 nylon) through the perineurium. The knot is then tied and this procedure is repeated for the other anastomoses. It has been suggested that a posterior stay suture placed in the epineurium facilitates the placement of interfascicular sutures without the danger of tension or tearing (Van Beek and Kleinert, 1977).

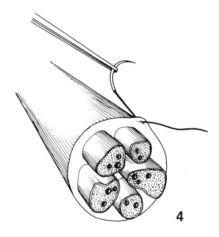

4

However, tension should not be a problem in a fresh wound as the initial portion of the force-displacement characteristic of the mammalian peripheral nerve is almost horizontal, significant displacement being achieved with minimal or zero force. If a portion of the circumference of the anastomosis gapes when the knot is tied then there is too much tension and interfascicular nerve grafting is indicated. After each fascicle has been coapted to its appropriate counterpart the microscope is set aside and the wound is closed with hand instruments. The postoperative course is in the nature of 3 weeks' immobilization in a wool and crêpe bandage supported by a volar plaster slab after which time all dressings and support are removed. Clinical and electrophysiological assessments are performed regularly to document recovery.

INTERFASCICULAR NERVE GRAFTING

When there has been delay between injury and repair or significant loss of nerve substance interfascicular nerve grafting is indicated. A defect of greater than 0·5 cm is considered an indication for grafting (Millesi, 1977), but experience and skill are necessary in the absence of reliable data to judge when a defect can be closed by primary repair or when a graft would be more appropriate.

Nerve grafting is also indicated when primary neurorrhaphy has failed and there is no function or minimal function 6 months after neve repair associated with a neuroma-in-continuity. In the absence of a neuroma-in-continuity the nerve ends are prepared in a similar fashion to that for primary interfascicular nerve repair. If a non-functional neuroma-in-continuity is present then the technique of Millesi (1977) is recommended. The nerve proximal to the neuroma is entered and fasciculi identified by removing the epineurium. After dissection these can be identified as they merge with fibrous tissue in the region of the neuroma.

5

At the termination of normal nerve tissue each fascicular group is transected and this should be at different levels so that the cut end comprises fasciculi protruding with different lengths from the cut surface. Matching fasciculi is performed as for interfascicular nerve repair.

6

At this point the wound should be covered with swabs impregnated with Ringer's solution and attention turned to obtaining a nerve autograft. The sural nerve is the most useful donor nerve being almost 40 cm long, having a distinct fascicular pattern, and having no branches in the calf. Furthermore, removal of the sural nerve only gives rise to a mild hypo-aesthesia in a small area behind the lateral malleolus. While the nerve can be removed in its entirety from one incision using a nerve stripper, it is preferable to use four horizontal incisions commencing behind the lateral malleolus where the nerve is located adjacent to the small saphenous vein. Serial incisions are made up the calf until the nerve is delivered from the popliteal fossa.

In the great majority of cases of peripheral nerve injury only one sural nerve is required to provide donor material. Occasionally as with brachial plexus injuries a great deal of donor nerve tissue is required and in these cases the lateral cutaneous nerve of the thigh, the posterior cutaneous nerve of the forearm and the superficial radial nerve may require to be removed. The graft is soaked in Ringer's solution until used. In estimating the required length of nerve autograft a significantly greater length of graft is required than the defect it has to bridge in order to counter retraction. This is particularly important if the bed is unfavourable when a bigger length of graft can be used to reroute the course of the nerve appropriately. Twenty per cent should, therefore, be added to the length of the deficit in order to calculate the length of graft required. The graft is prepared as in the preparation of the nerve ends by removing the epineurium so that the perineurium projects.

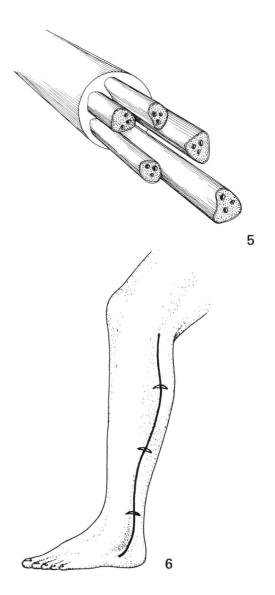

5

6

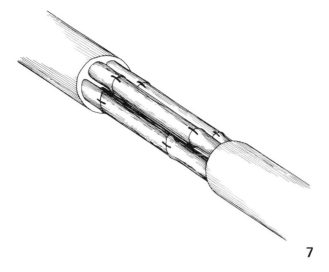

7

The two anastomoses, proximal fasciculus to graft and graft to distal fasciculus, are fashioned in the same way as for interfascicular nerve repair. The postoperative management is exactly the same as interfascicular nerve repair.

7

References

Acland, R. (1976). Personal communication.

Albert, E. (1885). 'Einige Operationem an Nerven.' *Weiner Medizinsche Presse* **26**, 1285

Ballance, C. and Duel, A. B. (1932). 'The operative treatment of facial palsy by the introduction of nerve grafts in the fallopian canal and by other intratemporal methods.' *Archs Otolar.* **15**, 1

Bassett, C. A. L. and Campbell, J. B. (1960). 'Calcification of millipore *in vivo.*' *Transplant. Bull.* **26**, 132

Campbell, J. B. and Luzio, J. (1964). 'Facial nerve repair: new surgical techniques.' *Trans. Am. Acad. Ophthal. Otolar.* **68**, 1068

Highet, N. B. and Holmes, W. (1943). 'Traction injuries to the lateral popliteal nerve and traction injuries to peripheral nerves after suture.' *Br. J. Surg.* **30**, 212

Hoen, T. L. and Brackett, C. E. (1956). 'Peripheral nerve lengthening: experimental.' *J. Neurosurg.* **13**, 43

Liu, C. T., Benda, C. E. and Lewey, F. H. (1948). 'Tensile strength of human nerves.' *Archs Neurol. Psychiat.* **59**, 322

Lytton, B. and Murray, J. G. (1954). 'Effects of the peripheral pathway on the regeneration of nerve fibres.' *J. Physiol.* **126**, 627

Marmor, L. (1963). 'Regeneration of peripheral nerve defects by irradiated homografts.' *Lancet* **1**, 1191

Marmor, L. (1967). *Peripheral Nerve Regeneration using Nerve Grafts.* Springfield, Illinois: Charles C. Thomas

Millesi, H. (1977). 'Interfascicular grafts for repair of peripheral nerves of the upper extremity.' *Orthop. Clins N. Am.* **8**, 387

Millesi, H., Meissl, G. and Berger, A. (1972). 'The interfascicular grafting of the median and ulnar nerves.' *J. Bone Jt Surg.* **54A**, 727

Ochs, S., Sabri, M. L. and Ranish, N. (1970). 'Somal site of synthesis of fast transport materials in mammalian nerve fibres.' *J. Neurobiol.* **1**, 329

Owen, E. (1976). 'Editorial'. *J. Bone Jt Surg.* **58B**, 397

Phillipeaux, J. M. and Vulpian, A. (1870). 'Note sur des essais de greffe d'un troncon de nef lingual entre les deux bouts nerf hypoglasse, après excision d'un segment de ce dernier nerf.' *Archs Physiol. normal Pathol.* **3**, 618

Pollard, J., Gye, R. S. and Macleod, G. J. (1966). 'An assessment of immunosuppressive agents in experimental peripheral nerve transplantation.' *Surgery Gynec. Obstet.* **132**, 839

Ross, M. H. and Reith, E. J. (1960). 'Perineurium: evidence for contractile elements.' *Science* **165**, 604

Saunders, F. K. and Young, J. E. (1942). 'The degeneration and reinnervation of grafted nerves.' *J. Anat.* **76**, 143

Seddon, H. J. (1954). *Peripheral Nerve Injuries.* London, HMSO (Medical Research Council Special Report Series 282)

Seddon, H. J. (1963). 'Nerve grafting.' *J. Bone Jt Surg.* **45B**, 447

Van Beek, A. and Kleinert, H. E. (1977). 'Practical microneurorrhapy.' *Orthop. Clins N. Am.* **8**, 377

Woodhall, B. and Bebe, G. W. (1956). 'Peripheral nerve regeneration. A follow-up study of 3,656 World War II Injuries.' Veterans Administration Medical Monograph, Washington, D. C. United States Government Printing Office

Weiss, P. (1944). 'The technology of nerve regeneration: A review. Sutureless tubulation and related methods of repair.' *J. Neurosurg.* **1**, 400

[The illustrations for this Chapter on Nerve Repair and Grafting were drawn by Mr. J. M. P. Booth.]

Artery Repair

Martin Birnstingl, M.S., F.R.C.S.
Consultant Surgeon, St. Bartholomew's Hospital, London

OPEN ARTERIAL INJURIES

1

Control of bleeding (e.g. in a groin wound)

Direct clamping may add to the vessel damage and bleeding should, if possible, be controlled by local swab pressure. The uninjured artery proximal to the wound should then be exposed, either by extending the wound proximally or through a separate incision. The proximal artery is surrounded with a light rubber sling, avoiding its accompanying vein. The ends of this sling may be passed through a short length of wide-bore rubber tubing to provide a controlled tourniquet, or if necessary the artery clamped with an Atraugrip vascular clamp. Venous bleeding is controlled by local swab pressure.

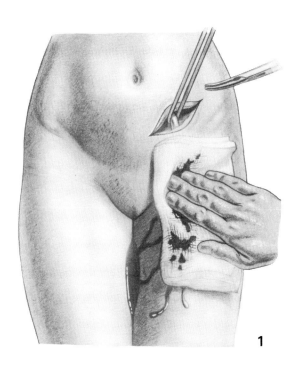

1

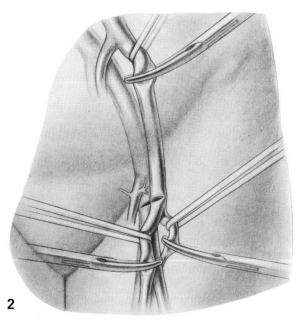

2

2

Preparation for repair

In a groin wound the next step is control of the distal arteries to prevent back-bleeding. The deep femoral artery arises from the back of the common femoral trunk. Before clamping this artery, it is necessary to lift the parent trunk forwards by rubber slings placed immediately above and below the origin of the deep branch (proximal femoral sling not shown).

Vascular repair

3

Artery

The arterial supply to the limb must be preserved, either by repair of the vascular laceration or by ligation of the vessel followed by an immediate bypass bridging procedure. Lateral suture of arteries is seldom satisfactory and, to avoid narrowing the vessel, a patch repair is usually needed. Autogenous vein provides the most reliable material and is taken from long or short saphenous or from an arm vein, as convenient. Leg veins are better than arm. Dacron fabric is disastrous in the presence of infection.

The surgeon must ensure that the distal vessel is patent before undertaking any repair.

Vein

Ligation of large veins should be avoided where lateral suture is a feasible alternative. Certain veins are expendable and patching or bridging is only necessary in crucial sites such as the popliteal vein and where extensive soft tissue loss has destroyed the collateral drainage from a limb.

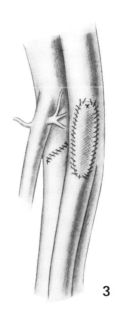

3

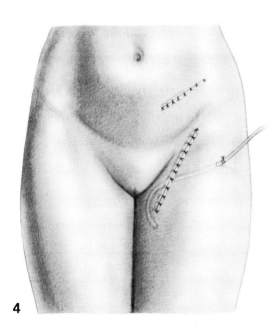

4

4

Wound closure

Contaminated and high velocity missile wounds must be treated by delayed primary closure. Such wounds include all rifle bullet and bomb blast injuries. The repaired blood vessels can sometimes be partly covered by available soft tissue, but immediate cover is not essential and the aim should be secondary suture after 5–8 days.

In stab wounds and other low velocity injuries (e.g. shot-gun or pistol), excision of non-viable tissue and vascular repair are followed by primary skin closure as far as possible. Suction drainage should be used.

Anticoagulants are not necessary. Distal fasciotomy must be considered where major veins have been ligated or marked swelling is expected. Prophylactic antibiotics are useful.

CLOSED ARTERIAL INJURIES

The crux of closed arterial injuries is the problem of ischaemia. This may be *early* as a result of the actual vessel injury (compression, angulation, disruption or lesion in continuity) or *late* from changes within the closed fascial compartments in the distal part of the limb. Such subfascial compression may be due to a local haematoma or muscle damage, or the result of secondary ischaemic muscle swelling.

In the presence of overt ischaemia the damaged artery must be explored urgently and repaired where possible. The popliteal and brachial arteries are particularly vital in this respect. Irreversible changes occur within 6 hr of injury. Repair may not be possible in the smaller vessels in the leg or arm, in which case distal fasciotomy may be sufficient to restore the circulation.

The arterial lesion in continuity

The site of arterial damage usually corresponds to the level of any co-existent fracture. Arteriography may be useful, but must never occasion delay. The outside appearance of the artery may give no indication of extent of internal damage apart from diminished or absent pulsation.

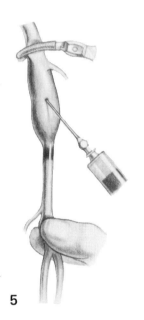

5

5

Distension of the vessel with saline injected into the lumen reveals the precise site of internal damage. This segment must be opened longitudinally.

The commonest lesion is an intimal tear, with a variable degree of local dissection and superadded thrombosis. Closed arterial lesions in continuity are a common complication of wounds due to high velocity missiles, in which they may easily be missed unless the surgeon is vigilant.

Arterial spasm

A contracted, pulseless, string-like vessel is usually either the result of compression by haematoma or muscle swelling, or due to elastic recoil of the wall in the segment distal to an obstructive lesion in continuity. Therefore spasm must not be assumed unless these causes have been excluded with certainty. This requires exposure of the injured part of the vessel. Traumatic arterial spasm is very rare.

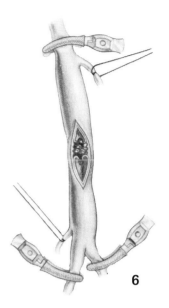

6

Repair of intimal tear

6 & 7

Good local haemostasis is necessary. The main trunk can be controlled without damage by slings and bull-dog clamps. Branches should be surrounded with double-looped lengths of silk for traction control. Arterial branches must not be sacrificed.

Damaged or detached intima is carefully trimmed away. The distal intimal tube may need pinning down with fine (6/0) interrupted arterial sutures, placed with the knots outside. Make sure that the distal vessels are patent by a back-bleed test, saline injection or after removal of distal clot using a balloon-tipped catheter.

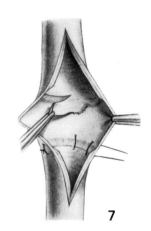

7

8

The opening in the artery is repaired with an oval autogenous vein patch (5/0 arterial suture). The double-needle suture starts above. The needle is always passed *in* through the edge of the patch and *out* through the host artery, in order to pin back any remaining intima. Care must be taken to avoid narrowing at the ends of the oval, which are cut fairly square.

Where a local patch repair is not feasible, a bypass graft must be constructed. Patch repair is not suitable for high velocity missile wounds.

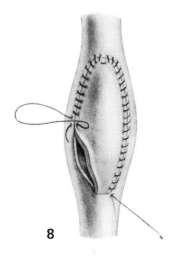

8

9

Leakage at suture lines

Leaks are the result of poor suture technique. Here the individual sutures have been placed too widely and tension is insufficient.

Sutures should be about 1 mm apart and 1 mm from the edge of the vessel. The surgeon's assistant must maintain traction on each individual stitch, while the next is being placed. This is essential when multifilament material is used (e.g. Mersilene or silk), but less important when a smooth monofilament is used (e.g. Ethiflex or Prolene). Both types have their advantages and disadvantages.

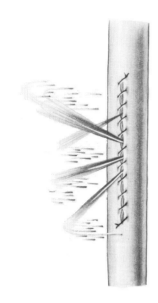

9

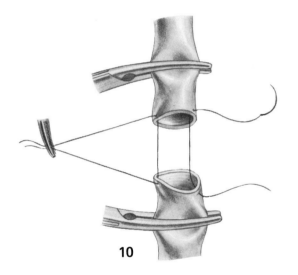

10

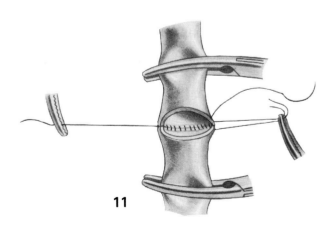

11

10 & 11

End-to-end anastomosis

(Terminal anastomosis is seldom possible in arterial trauma, since the vessel must be trimmed back beyond the damaged zone and the suture line must be free from tension.)

One stitch is used as a stay suture. Another stitch is started opposite this and continued across the front of the anastomosis. Finally both clamps are rotated 180° and the same suture continued around the circumference of the anastomosis to meet its original end, to which it is tied. (4/0 or 5/0 is used.)

In small arteries (radial, ulnar, popliteal) it is easier to insert two stay sutures and then use interrupted sutures. (6/0 or 7/0 is satisfactory.)

BYPASS BRIDGING PROCEDURES

Where several centimetres of artery are damaged or lost, a bridging procedure is needed. This is likely to be the case in most high velocity wounds, where the actual vascular damage is always more extensive than might first be apparent. The anastomoses should there-fore be made to accessible, healthy segments of artery well away from the original wound. The ends of the graft or prosthesis are sectioned obliquely and then anastomosed to the side of the host artery at each end. A pair of technically sound anastomoses is more important than the actual route of the bypass graft.

Autogenous vein

Long saphenous vein is the most useful. This is exposed by a long incision and removed by careful sharp dissection, ligating branches as they are encountered.

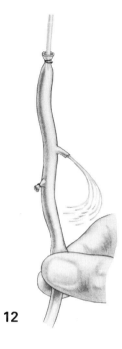

12

12

After removal the vein is distended with saline and further tributaries tied.

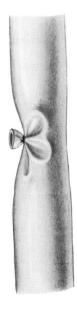

13

13

When tying branches, one should avoid narrowing the vein graft.

Anastomosis of vein graft

14

The ends of the vein are reversed to avoid the action of its valves. Each end is prepared by clean transection, a vertical slit (slightly longer than the longitudinal slit in the artery) is made and finally the two corners excised. This provides an oblique oval end.

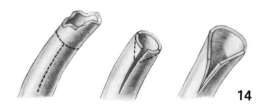

14

15

Two double-needle sutures are used. (In the drawing these are made by tying two sutures together.) The end sutures are then pulled up and tied, before making a continuous suture along each side in turn.

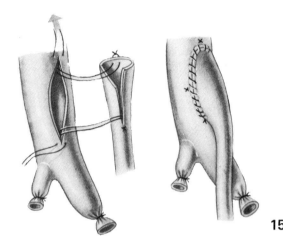

15

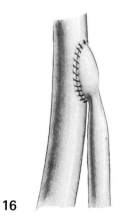

16

Common mishaps

16

Narrowing of the vein should be avoided at the lower end of the suture line, where minimal bites of vein wall must be taken.

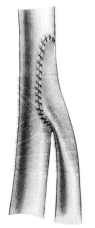

17

17

A tight drum-head effect, with consequent flattening and compression of the lumen of the vein must also be avoided. This result is inevitable if too much artery is excised and it is sufficient to incise the host artery without cutting away any of its wall before anastomosis. The cowl of the vein should bulge up like a cobra's head.

Dacron bypass prosthesis

Dacron should not be used if possible in open and high velocity injuries or where any possibility of contamination exists. In all other cases a prosthesis is best when replacing large vessels of the calibre of external iliac (shown) or subclavian.

18

Two double-needle sutures (3/0 or 4/0) and the basic technique is similar to that used in a vein graft. The end of the Dacron prosthesis is transected obliquely at about 30° and the artery slit longitudinally to match its rigid oval circumference. Woven Dacron 8–10 mm diameter with or without velour is satisfactory.

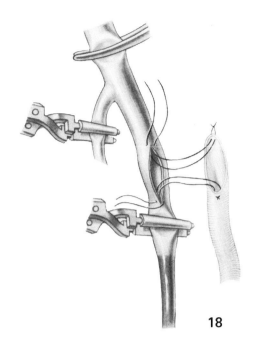

18

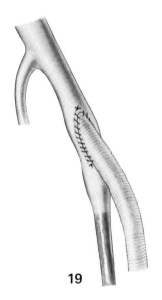

19

19

The continuous suture passes *in* through the stiff Dacron and *out* through the host artery.

Haematomas carry a high risk of infection and suction drainage to the region of both anastomoses is advisable.

Care is necessary to avoid fraying the cut ends during suturing and kinking if the bypass is a long one.

Local or systemic heparinization is advisable when using Dacron. It need not be continued postoperatively.

Patency of the distal arterial bed

When arterial repair is delayed for several hours, the distal arteries become obstructed by clot which must be removed at the time of the repair. Patency in the run-off area must always be assured before repairing or bridging damaged vessels. A free back-bleed indicates patency.

20, 21 & 22

In the absence of a copious back-bleed, it is essential to pass a Fogarty-type balloon-tipped catheter down into the narrow distal vessels. The balloon is then lightly inflated with water (0·5–1 ml) and the catheter gently withdrawn to extract the clot, followed by the balloon. Two or three such extractions are usually needed, followed by injection of saline or heparinized saline (1000 units of heparin per 500 ml normal saline).

Systemic heparinization after operation is unwise in the presence of soft tissue wounds or arterial repair, owing to the likelihood of serious bleeding.

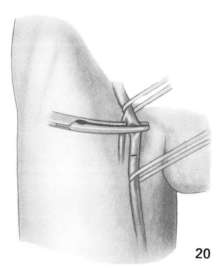

20

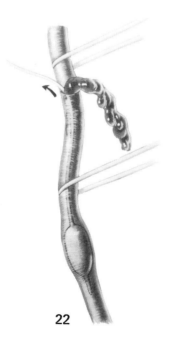

22

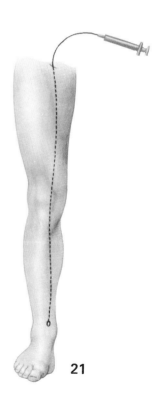

21

FASCIOTOMY PROCEDURES

23

A vascular injury which causes unrelieved ischaemia for several hours results in marked swelling of the distal muscle bellies, after the circulation has been restored. Such swelling will again compromise the distal limb circulation, particularly since the arteries and veins lie deeply within closed fascial compartments.

A subfascial fracture haematoma can also occlude the vessels, as can prolonged external pressure on the calf, as seen in coma.

An adequate fasciotomy in the lower limb must decompress the deep posterior and anterior tibial compartments, and two incisions are necessary.

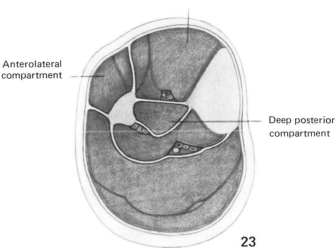

Anterior tibial compartment

Anterolateral compartment

Deep posterior compartment

23

Indications for fasciotomy

(*1*) Subfascial haematoma due to injury or primary bleeding (haemophilia).

(*2*) Vascular repair carried out after more than 6 hr of ischaemia.

(*3*) Extensive soft tissue injury, crushing or high velocity damage, liable to subsequent swelling even after debridement.

(*4*) Ligation of major veins (e.g. iliac or femoral).

Standard fasciotomy

24

In most cases it is sufficient to slit the investing deep fascia with scissors, through limited skin incisions. One fasciotomy is on the medial side of the leg and the other over the anterior tibial compartment.

When marked swelling is present, or likely to be present, the skin as well as the fascia should be cut in the upper two-thirds of the limb. The raw area is later skin-grafted after disappearance of all swelling.

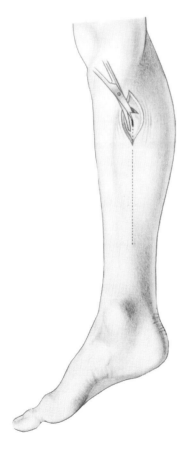

24

Fibulectomy fasciotomy

25

In the presence of extensive deep damage or where vascular repair has been delayed for many hours, a thorough decompression can be achieved through the bed of the fibula.

The middle two quarters are resected subperiosteally, avoiding the lateral popliteal nerve above and the syndesmosis below. The deep layer of periosteum is then incised vertically to enter the individual fascial compartments, which are separately decompressed. The partial loss of the fibula has no effect upon subsequent function of the limb.

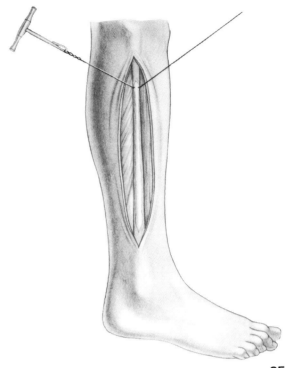

25

SUMMARY

The essentials of management of vascular injuries are as follows.

(*1*) Early exploration when haemorrhage or ischaemia is evident.

(*2*) Repair or reconstruction instead of ligation in all major vessel injuries.

(*3*) Preservation of patency of the distal vascular bed by removal of intravascular clot and decompression by generous fasciotomy. High velocity missile wounds are a frequent source of vascular injury and require, in addition, delayed primary wound closure.

Sympathetic block or sympathectomy has no place in the management of traumatic arterial ischaemia.

Reference

Ernst, C. B. and Kaufer, H. (1971). *J. Trauma* **11**, 365

[*The illustrations for this Chapter on Artery Repair were drawn by Mr. P. Jack.*]

Principles of Fracture Treatment

P. S. London, M.B.E., F.R.C.S.
Surgeon, Birmingham Accident Hospital

With so many methods of treatment available and a number of apparently irreconcilable opinions it is important to consider first, the surgeon's objective when he is treating fractures and second, how fractures heal, including the difficulties and complications. It is then possible to decide, at least in principle, how a particular fracture might best be treated. This will depend also on the predilections of the surgeon and should take into consideration the personality and the requirements of the patient. The statement that the man with a method is the most dangerous man in surgery should be kept prominently in mind.

Objective

This is to achieve bony union with no more than acceptable deformity and maximum strength and range of movement.

Deformity

Acceptable deformity varies with the part affected, the nature of the deformity and the age of the patient. It is most objectionable in the face and jaws, in the forearms of adults and with some fractures of the hands and feet and into joints. It is least troublesome with fractures near the epiphyses of bones with more than a year or two of further growth, during which even severe deformity can be obliterated.

Types of fracture

Fractures may be divided into two types: the easy and the difficult. This may seem too simple but there are few surgeons that have not misinterpreted fractures and rued the day.

Easy fractures

The favourable characteristics are that a good position is easily achieved and maintained and that bony union occurs rapidly. This behaviour is characteristic of most fractures in children and of fractures with a large proportion of cancellous bone in large apposing surfaces with little displacement. Such fractures have a good blood supply and little tendency to continuing movement.

Stability. Following fracture the fragments of bone can become steady at rest in a position that varies from perfect to unacceptable. Easy fractures are stable in good position, but if difficult fractures have any stability it is likely to be in a position of unacceptable deformity.

Difficult fractures

The apposing surfaces are small and largely cortical with a poor blood supply, perhaps because of comminution, which also compromises stability. Also there are complicating injuries.

DEFORMING FORCES AND PATTERNS OF FRACTURE

There are four causes of deformity: the injuring force, muscular action, gravity and the bony hinge of a greenstick fracture. Their effects depend mainly on the extent and severity of damage to the soft tissues surrounding the fracture. The correction of deformity requires the reversal of the deforming forces and the corrective influence must be maintained until the healing process enables the fragments to withstand the residual deforming forces.

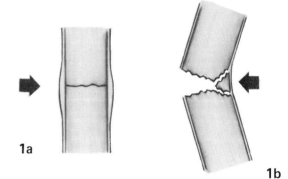

1a

1b

The injuring force

1 a-i

Bones are broken by being (*a*) struck sharply, (*b*) bent, (*c*) twisted, (*d*) pulled or (*e–i*) pushed. Some of these are easy fractures, others less so.

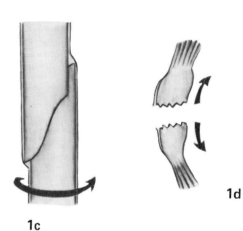

1c

1d

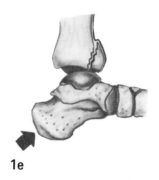

1e

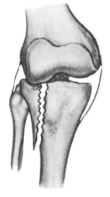

1f

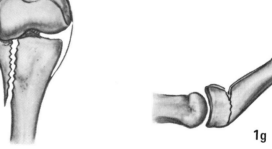

1g

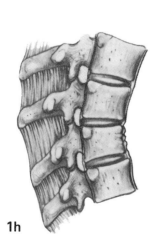

1h

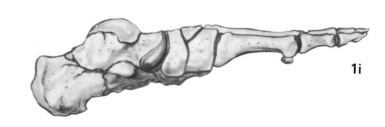

1i

2

Simple transverse or short oblique fractures of the tibia can give rise to objectionable bowing of the shapely leg of a woman. If the fibula is intact, it may be regarded as a splint and therefore an ally, but it provides pivots at the tibiofibular joints at which the muscles spanning the gap between the tibia and fibula can, and do, move the fragments of tibia and bring them to rest against the fibula.

In the forearm, too, fracture of one bone renders it liable to deformity for a similar reason.

The simple patterns shown in *Illustration 1* become complicated by irregularities of the bones themselves and by the fact that the injurious force can continue to act on bones that have broken and can superimpose a second pattern of fracture upon the first.

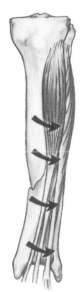

2

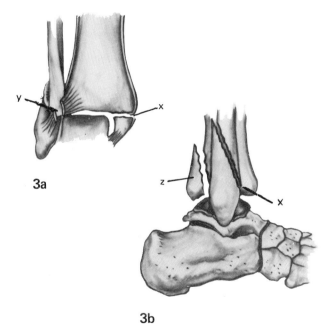

3a

3b

3a & b

Fracture-subluxation of the ankle is a well-known example of the combination of avulsion (x), twisting (y) and crushing force (z), with also an element of translation, or sliding.

4 a-d

Illustration 4 shows how an initial spiral fracture (*a*) can acquire a bending component (*b*) that may give the impression that the cause was bending alone (*c*) unless it is remembered that bending a bone breaks it obliquely (*d*) whereas twisting it causes a spiral fracture.

Muscular action

This usually makes fragments overlap, and it often bends and sometimes twists the part.

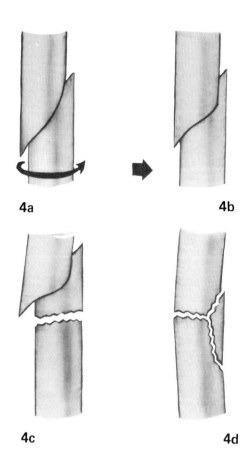

4a   4b

4c   4d

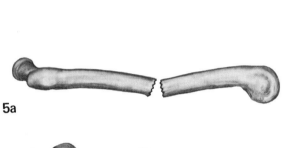

5a

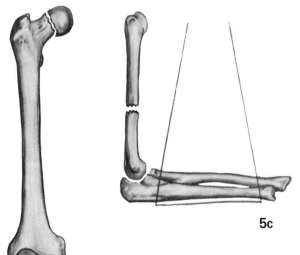

5b   5c

5 a, b & c

Gravity

The force of gravity can (*a*) bend, (*b*) twist or (*c*) separate fragments according to their disposition.

THE SOFT TISSUES

The need to treat the soft tissues in all cases and the bones in most cases of fracture is generally accepted but the contribution that the soft tissues can make to the treatment of a fracture is not well understood.

6 a, b & c

The concept of a hinge of soft tissue (*a*) or of bone (*b*) in the case of greenstick fractures is widely accepted, as is the place of 'three-point fixation' (*c*) in the treatment of such fractures.

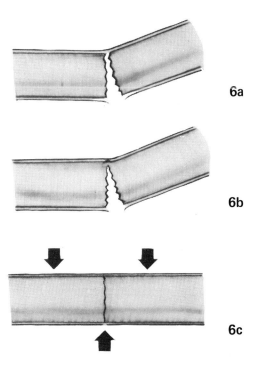

6a

6b

6c

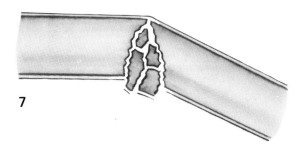

7

7

The existence of a hinge, at least of soft tissue, offers no assurance that the fracture will be stable in a good position, particularly when the fracture is oblique or comminuted.

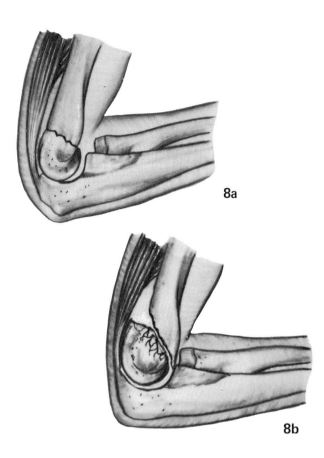

8a

8b

8 a&b

Thus the belief that the tension of the triceps will hold a supracondylar fracture of the humerus securely in place (*a*) may prove to be unfounded because as the muscle is rendered taut it can cause the fracture to shorten (*b*).

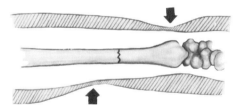

9a

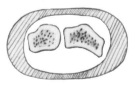

9b

9 a&b

The springiness of the bony hinge of a greenstick fracture is still regarded by some surgeons as an impediment to complete correction of deformity, with the result that they advise that it be deliberately broken. This is as ill-advised as breaking the hinges on a door that can be closed but repeatedly springs open. The surgical equivalent of a chair under the handle or a lock or a bolt on the door is a carefully moulded plaster-of-Paris cast that will keep the hinge taut. The secret of success is thick padding, which provides adequate room to accommodate any swelling within the plaster, the moulding of which nevertheless enables it to grip the fracture.

MANIPULATION AS A DIAGNOSTIC TOOL

As well as its familiar therapeutic role manipulation has a valuable diagnostic role. Traction is the best known and most used method of reducing deformity and once an acceptable position is achieved the part is encased in plaster-of-Paris and the traction may then cease. It is customary to describe such a procedure as immobilization in plaster, regardless of the fact that the fragments often become displaced within a day or two. Nevertheless, the consequent deformity may still be acceptable. If it is, one may reasonably ask if there is any purpose in achieving no more than temporary improvement of the position.

One may further ask if there is any means of knowing that the best position that can be achieved by manipulation may not be one that can be maintained by external splintage. Diagnostic manipulation can provide answers that will cause some to decide to operate on the fracture, others perhaps to maintain traction and still others to manipulate again, use wedge plasters and otherwise try to keep deformity within acceptable limits. Diagnostic manipulation can also reduce exposure to x-rays by enabling the manipulator to distinguish between acceptable and unacceptable degrees of deformity so that radiography is needed only to confirm that an acceptable position in plaster has been achieved.

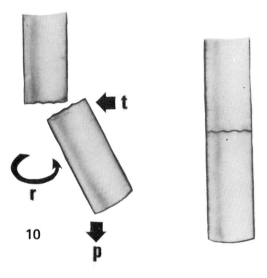

10

The diagnostic use of manipulation requires that first the deformity be reduced as far as possible. This is usually accomplished by traction (p), which may have to be accompanied by twisting (r) and translation (t).

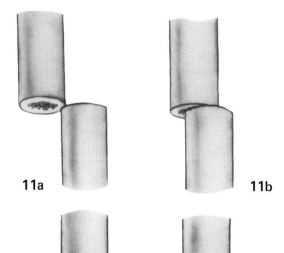

11 a-d

Then the part is subjected to longitudinal compression. In the case of flat, transverse bony surfaces the fracture will not shorten unless the contact is (a) precarious because of being little more than edge-to-edge. The greater the area of contact the less the ease with which the fragments can be rocked, and if the rocking movement is carried out in two directions at right angles it is possible to identify the direction in which deformity needs to be further reduced. (b) Shows anteroposterior stability, with lateral mobility; (c) the opposite; and (d) neither.

12 a & b

When a fracture is oblique, spiral or comminuted, testing in compression shows not only how easily but how far it can be displaced. (*a*) Shows the restraint imposed by an intact hinge of soft tissue and (*b*) that without such a hinge the deformity is unacceptable.

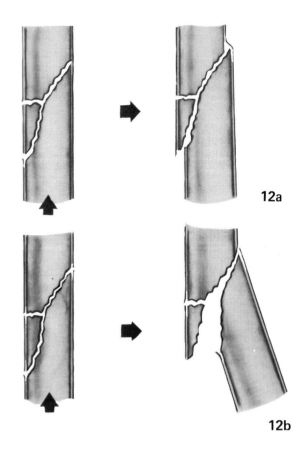

12a

12b

13

A special case

When a transverse fracture is overlapped it is not usually possible to bring the fragments end-to-end simply by pulling because the length of hinge available as the hypotenuse (h) of a right-angled triangle with a base (b) should be the base (b^1) of a longer right-angled triangle. The problem can usually be solved by bending the fracture by as much as 60° or 70° and then sliding the distal fragment distally on the proximal fragment until it is clear of it and able to come into line with it. The area of end-to-end contact is then estimated by pushing and rocking the fragments.

It should be noted that this manipulation is particularly useful for a child's forearm, even when only one bone is broken and overlapped and that the bending carried out by the surgeon is certainly less forcible and very likely less severe than that caused by the original violence. Such accentuation of the 'resting' deformity might be dangerous (it would certainly be difficult) if much swelling had occurred and particularly if there were signs of ischaemia beyond the fracture.

Successful manipulation requires an understanding of what it can be expected to achieve, the ability to interpret the evidence that it is capable of providing and the ability to make good use of that evidence. A good manipulator will prove what x-ray appearances may merely suggest.

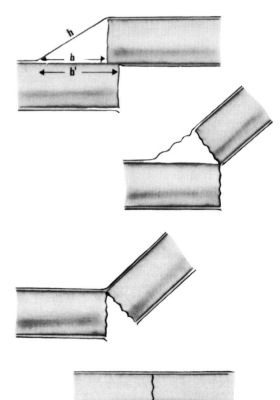

13

'IMMOBILIZATION' OF FRACTURES

Self-splintage of fractures

14 a&b

Under the combined influences of the injuring force, muscular tone and gravity, the broken fragments displace to the position at which the deforming forces are opposed by the restraining forces of soft tissues. With mild, spiral fractures the sleeve of soft tissue is not widely torn and neither widely nor extensively stripped from the bone; as a result the sleeve fits fairly snugly, which means that such displacement as does occur produces only a little shortening with a little twisting. As one fragment slides on the other it is brought to rest by the tension in the sleeve of soft tissues, and if there is unacceptable angulation this can be corrected by wedging.

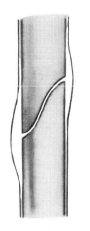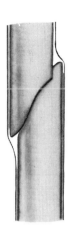

14a   14b

15 a-d

Other fragments are driven into stable positions; common examples occur on the 1st (*a*) and 5th (*b*) metacarpal bones, at the bases of phalanges (*c*) and sometimes in the neck of the femur (*d*).

Encasing such fractures in plaster-of-Paris, for example, undoubtedly protects them and it may support them but it can hardly be expected to immobilize them. Immobilization of a fracture by plaster-of-Paris is not to be expected unless the fracture has a hinge and the hinge is kept taut by a suitably applied cast.

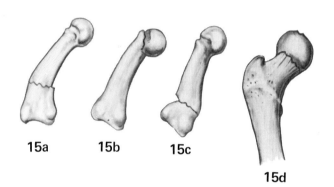

15a   15b   15c

15d

16a&b

The role of most plaster casts is to prevent bending and twisting and in the case of the casts used by Sarmiento and others the plaster has no immobilizing function except that it limits the amount of shortening to the increase in diameter of the limb that can be accommodated within the plaster. Such a plaster cast may permit less movement when the fracture can shorten than when it remains capable of rocking movement (*b*).

When simple external splintage will not maintain an acceptable position of the fracture it may be necessary to use other methods.

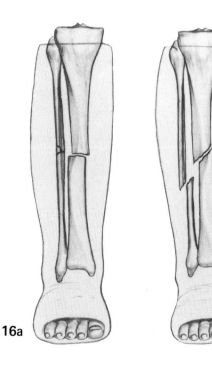

16a   16b

TRACTION

Skin traction

Surgeons should know how this should be applied and maintained and should be acutely aware of its shortcomings and possible dangers.

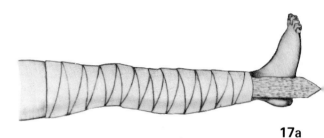

17a

17 a-e

(*a*) Shows that the adhesive strips should be taken well above the fracture and that the turns of bandage should be close together. The malleoli should be protected from pressure by passing the traction cords round the sidebars of the splint (*b*) by the use of a spreader (*c*) (those supplied with ready-made traction kits are not wide enough) or by suitable pads around but not over the malleoli (*d*).

Too short a length of adhesive plaster and too few or too loose turns of bandage lead to wrinkling or constriction at the ankle (*e*). Ventfoam requires more care and more frequent attention if it is to remain effective.

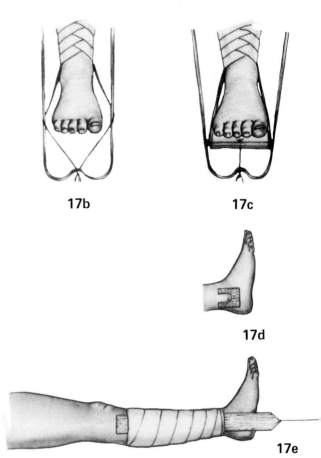

17b   **17c**

17d

17e

Skeletal traction

18 a,b&c

Skeletal traction should be used on adults when more than about 10 lb (22 kg) pull is required for more than a week or so. Denham's pin (*a*) has the advantage over Steinmann's pin (*b*) and Kirschner's wire (*c*) in that its thread grips the bone and is therefore less likely to work loose and promote infection.

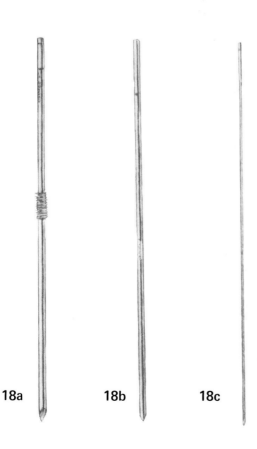

18a   **18b**   **18c**

19

In young adults the best place for insertion is the slight hollow just behind the tibial tuberosity. Here the bone is firm enough to grip well but not so thick or hard enough to make that penetration difficult. With old persons or those with Paget's disease it is a useful precaution to radiograph the tibia to see where it will be strong enough to grip the pin firmly – this may be more than half-way down the leg. If traction is to be applied to the lower end of the tibia the place chosen should enable the pin to have a good grip on the tibia without going through the fibula as well; that is 2–3 inches (5–7 cm) above the tip of the lateral malleolus.

Calcanean traction should be used only when it is undesirable to transfix the tibia and the pin should be in line with the tibia. It should not be used when there is an unstable fracture of the tibia, because in this case having the pin through the broken bone enables it to be used to 'steer' the lower fragment.

Skeletal traction is occasionally applied to the olecranon, the lower end of the femur and, directed more laterally, to the greater trochanter.

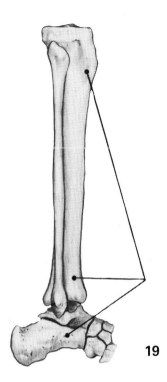

19

Inserting the pin

20

If local anaesthetic is used one must remember that the periosteum must be anaesthetized and that the marrow is also sensitive but cannot be anaesthetized. The pin should not be driven through an actual or imminent haematoma and if the skin is not cut, no leakage occurs in most cases, no dressing is needed and infection is less likely to occur. The pin is most likely to be inserted in the right line if the lower limb is left exposed and the foot is brought up to a right angle. The pin should be inserted at right angles to the line of the tibia and roughly parallel with the floor so as to allow for the fact that the limb lies slightly on its outer side.

Particularly in the conscious patient, the operator should support the limb with his other hand, taking care to keep his fingers out of the line of the pin. The usual T-shaped handle is tiring to use with Steinmann's or Denham's pin, especially if they are blunt, and an airdrill is preferable.

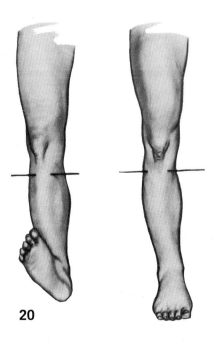

20

21

Kirschner's wires require a telescopic guide to fit into the drill.

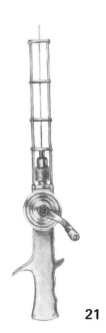

21

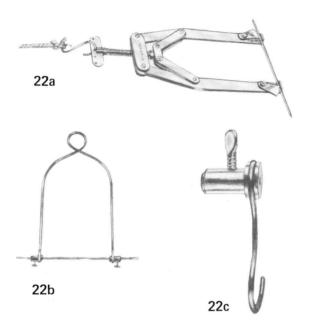

22a

22b

22c

22 a, b & c

The various stretchers (*a*), stirrups (*b*) and swivel hooks (*c*) that are available are satisfactory if used correctly.

External skeletal fixation

This has become increasingly popular for difficult fractures, particularly when the soft tissues have been badly damaged, and some use it as a method of choice. To be effective it must remain firmly fixed in the bone and it must fix the fracture securely.

23

Hoffmann's device is the most reliable.

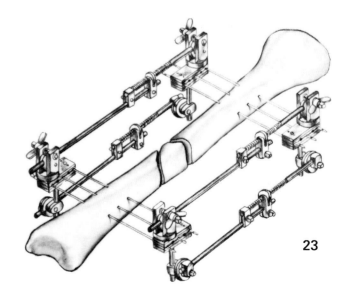

23

24

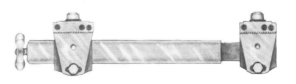

However, there are many who are satisfied with one-sided appliances such as Wagner's.

In spite of being cumbersome these appliances enable the patient to be mobile without harming the injured limb.

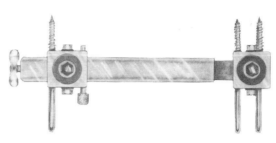

24

INTERNAL FIXATION

The indications for internal fixation of fractures are likely to remain controversial for a very long time but the following degrees of necessity may be accepted.

Absolutely necessary

(*1*) When accurate restoration of shape is necessary for the sake of appearance, as with the face and jaws, or for the sake of function, as with some fractures of the adult forearm, and of the hand and foot.

(*2*) When one component is avascular, most often with fractures of the neck of the femur.

(*3*) When a severed part is to be re-attached.

Highly desirable

(1) Fractures into joints should be fixed if this can be done accurately and securely enough to allow early movement of the joint. This applies most often to the ankle but also to the knee, hip, elbow and to Bennett's fracture of the first metacarpal bone.

(*2*) With complicated injuries in which the restoration of skeletal security is a necessary preliminary to repairing the soft tissues.

(*3*) When there are multiple injuries and the fixation of some fractures will facilitate both nursing and rehabilitation of the patient; examples include the tetra- or paraplegic patient with fractures of limbs, and a restless person with a head injury.

(*4*) Old persons may benefit from internal fixation when it accelerates their return to activity.

(*5*) With pathological fractures fixation may restore comfort and stability even though, as with cancer fractures, union may not take place.

(*6*) Fixed joints in the broken limb may concentrate movement at the fracture.

(*7*) Non-union and delayed union may require fixation, with or without bone grafting.

(*8*) Social reasons sometimes lead to a request for whatever treatment will allow the earliest discharge from hospital.

METHODS OF INTERNAL FIXATION

Plates

These fall into two categories, those that fix fractures rigidly and those that do not.

25

Plates and rigidity

Hicks sought rigidity by making strong plates that also prevent rotation.

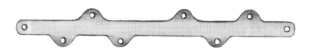

25

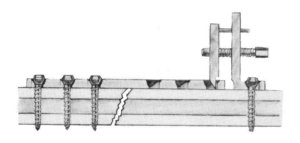

26a

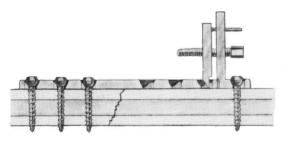

26b

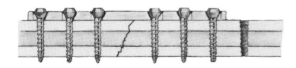

26c

26a-f

The A.O. have achieved rigidity by compression, which may be applied by a special tool or by the design of the plate, the holes in which cause the plate to be displaced by the first screw's head as it is driven home.

Strong plates are bulky and if they are near the surface may make it difficult to close the skin.

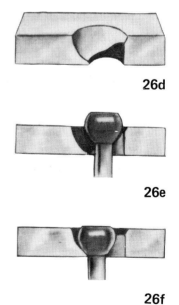

26d

26e

26f

27

Thick plates are likely to allow blood to accumulate in the angle between plate, bone and overlying tissues.

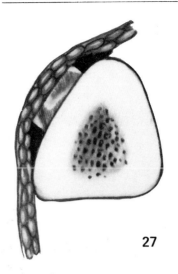

27

28

The standard cortical screws designed by A.O. are large enough to occupy a fairly large proportion of a small bone such as the radius or the ulna and may so weaken the bone as to cause fracture.

Plates near the surface may be laid bare if the wound breaks down, preventing healing until they are removed, which may not be until the fractures have healed.

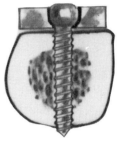

28

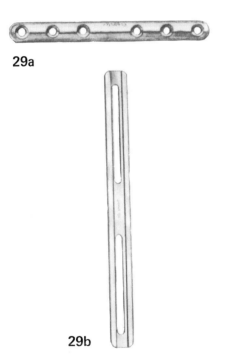

29a

29b

29 a, b & c

The older designs of plate do not provide rigid fixation.

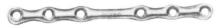

29c

30-33

Medullary nails

When used for the long bones such as the femur or humerus, these are most successful when they fit the marrow snugly for some distance on either side of the fracture (*Illustration 31*), which may require that the marrow be reamed to quite a large bore. They can be used for fractures at two levels and for spiral fractures if they are supplemented by wire loops binding the fracture or by a small plate with short screws.

The single, strong nails may be inserted at the fracture by opening it and driving the nail first up the proximal fragment and then down across the fracture after the fragments have been placed end to end, or they may be inserted through a small incision in the buttock or at the knee. Open nailing is generally quick, easier and technically less demanding than closed nailing, but it carries a greater risk of infection and should be employed with caution.

When nails can be used they do not complicate closure of the skin nor promote haematomas. The fact that they often require smaller incisions may be advantageous when the skin has been damaged; and if the skin does break down they may, unlike plates, remain unexposed.

Rush's nails (*Illustrations 30 and 32*) cannot be relied upon to give rigidity and when used singly they do not prevent rotation. In the hand (*Illustration 32c*) this does not matter.

Kirschner's wires (*Illustration 33*) are particularly useful in the hands and feet, where they can be used singly or in groups.

Smith-Petersen's and similar nails are more likely to slide out of the femur than are nail-plates.

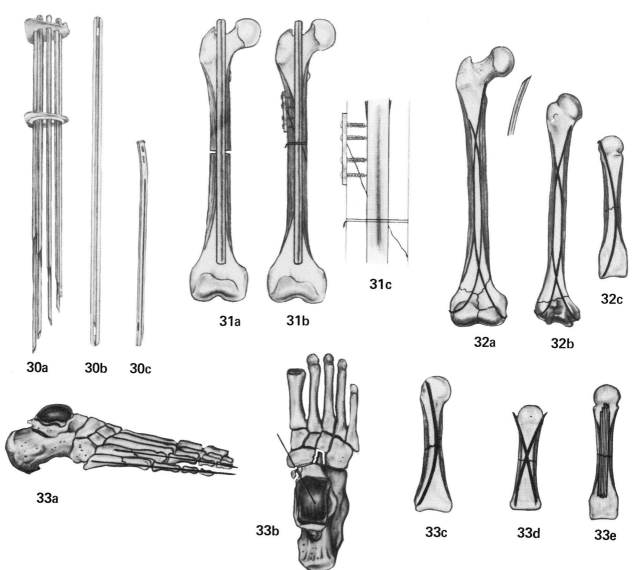

30a   30b   30c

31a   31b

31c

32a   32b

32c

33a

33b

33c   33d   33e

34 a,b &c

Nail-plates

McLaughlin's (*a*) are the easiest to use because the angle is adjustable but they can be uncomfortably prominent, especially in thin persons, and the nut works loose. Capener-Neufeld's (*b*) and Jewett's (*c*), nail-plates are less bulky but not quite so easy to use.

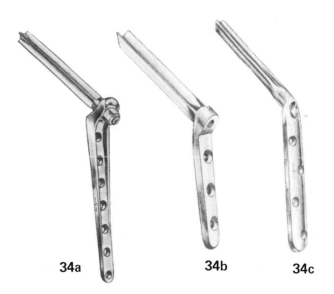

34a   34b   34c

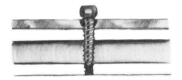

35a

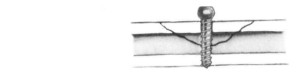

35b

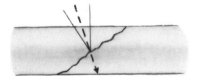

35c

35 a-d

Screws

These are used either to hold plates on the bones (*a*) or to hold pieces of bone together. When used in cortical bones they are most effective when the hole is tapped as well as drilled but if they are to press fragments together they must slide through the proximal one and grip the other (*b*). Screws used to draw oblique or spiral fracture surfaces together should cross the fracture at an angle half-way between the perpendicular to the fracture and the perpendicular to the surface of the bone (*c*). Screws may also be used to hold subsidiary fragments in place before the main fracture is nailed or plated (*d*).

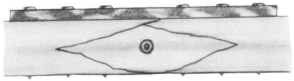

35d

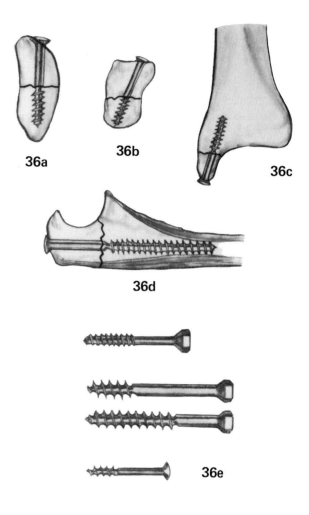

36a   **36b**   **36c**

36d

36e

36 a-e

Screws engaging cancellous bone should be large and have coarse threads; if they are only partly threaded it is not necessary to drill holes of different sizes but the threaded section must be entirely within the distal segment.

The use of screws to draw or press two pieces of bone together is widely referred to as the lag effect but the derivation of this term is not clear, whereas the meaning of the term 'draw-screw' is less open to objection. A danger that exists whenever screws are used in this way is that one or other piece of bone may be split.

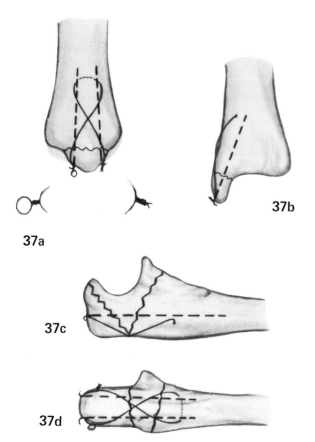

37a   **37b**

37c

37d

37 a-d

Compression wiring

This has the advantage that it can be used both safely and successfully with much smaller pieces of bone than screws can.

Cerclage or wire binding

This method has a bad reputation. However, this should belong to those who mis-apply the method and not to the method itself. It is a useful way of holding pieces of bone temporarily in place while screws are inserted or a plate applied — in this case a single loop suffices.

38 a & b

If it is to be left in place, as with a spiral fracture (*see also Illustration 31*) double loops are preferable because at least one of them will be tight. If the method is to succeed the loops must be tight and must remain so, which means that they must be hard up against bone all the way round.

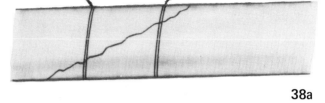

38a

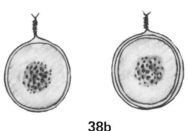

38b

39

If they are applied to tapering bone this should be notched to prevent them from slipping.

Loose wires allow the fracture to move and can then erode the bone and cause a fracture at that level.

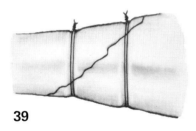

39

40 a & b

Cerclage is best used to supplement other methods of fixation (*see also Illustration 31*), and in the writer's experience, if used correctly it is very successful.

The choice of method of treatment

This can be made only by the surgeon concerned. A wise choice is most likely to be made by a surgeon who has had experience of all the methods available and has gained this experience in both secondary operations and emergency cases.

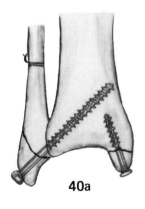

40a

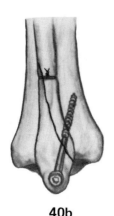

40b

OPEN FRACTURES

These are better regarded as wounds complicated by loss of the usual skeletal support than as fractures complicated by a wound and consequently at risk from infection. The first concept emphasizes repair, security and function whereas the latter enjoins caution and acceptance of a rather slow timetable and a poor functional result. There is no doubt that primary internal fixation of open fractures, combined with suitable repair of soft tissues, can yield a quality of result that cannot be attained by other methods, but there is equally no doubt that disaster can follow such treatment and end in amputation. The arguments for and against primary internal fixation have become tedious and uninformative, but there is no doubt that some surgeons will continue to practise and advocate it whereas others will continue to shun and condemn it. Against this background of disagreement the following statements are accepted.

(*1*) Primary internal fixation of open fractures requires skill and judgement.

(*2*) It does not mean that the whole operation has to be completed on one occasion. Delayed primary closure of the wound, delayed primary repair of special tissues and delayed primary fixation of the fracture may all be desirable.

(*3*) Internal fixation of the fracture does not in any way reduce the importance of thorough exploration, toilet and decompression of the wound.

(*4*) Antibiotics are best regarded as possible safeguards when used to supplement skilled tissue-craft.

(*5*) Internal fixation that requires much additional damage to soft tissues is particularly difficult to justify.

(*6*) Any surgeon who undertakes primary internal fixation of open fractures should not only be aware of the dangers but should be competent to deal with the complications.

(*7*) External skeletal fixation is a particularly useful method of dealing with severe open fractures.

(*8*) Any serious open fracture can safely be dealt with by:

  (*a*) exploration, decompression and surgical toilet;
  (*b*) loosely filling the wound with gauze and applying a firm, bulky dressing;

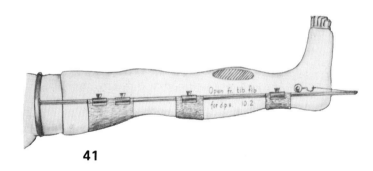

41

41

(*c*) applying skeletal traction to the lower limb and supporting the limb in a suitable plaster cast.

DELAYED UNION AND NON-UNION

Delayed union is easier to define than non-union but in practice delayed union is what makes a surgeon think he is going to have to operate on a fracture whereas non-union is what persuades him that he must.

TYPES OF UNION

Union with callus

42

Typically, union occurs with more or less visible callus.

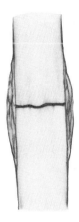

42

Union without visible callus

43a, b & c

After primary and particularly after rigid fixation callus may not appear and bony union may be very difficult to determine unless the fracture can be seen to disappear gradually.

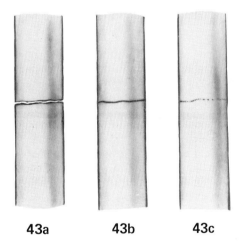

43a   43b   43c

TYPES OF NON-UNION

Non-union with callus

44

The well-known appearance of dense and enlarged bone-ends with a persistent gap between them is evidence that the bone has the ability to produce callus but not in sufficient amount to heal the fracture.

Movement is now recognized as being responsible for the failure of bony union in such cases and rigid fixation is the logical method of dealing with this condition.

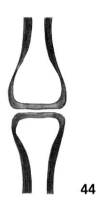

44

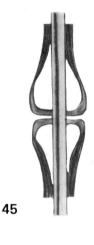

45

45 & 46

Unless the position of the fracture is not acceptable the fracture should not be disturbed except to enable a medullary nail to pass it or a plate to rest on it, and there need be no hesitation in adapting a plate to fit acceptable mal-union. In such a case it may be convenient to use bone removed from one side of the fracture to supplement the other (*Illustration 46c*).

Non-union with no callus

The bone's ends are dead, and rigid fixation needs to be supplemented by bone grafts. It is now generally accepted that fresh, autogenous, cancellous bone (e.g. from the iliac crest) is best for this purpose because it may remain to some extent osteogenic and because it provides a permeable trellis — an important and potentially viable callus — to extend to living bone on each side of the fracture. Cortical bone possesses some strength but lacks permeability and is rarely employed.

CONCLUSIONS

Fractures treated according to the above principles will in many cases do well. With a clear understanding of the biological as well as the mechanical aspects of the healing of fractures and a good practical training the surgeon should be able to increase the proportion of good results and reduce both the number and severity of complications.

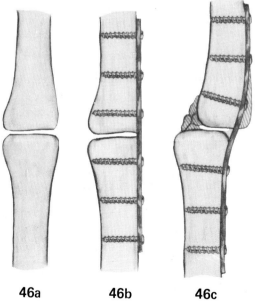

46a   **46b**   **46c**

[*The illustrations for this Chapter on Principles of Fracture Treatment were drawn by Mr. G. Lyth.*]

General Techniques of Internal Fixation of Fractures

R. L. Batten, F.R.C.S.
Consultant Orthopaedic Surgeon, General Hospital, Birmingham
and Royal Orthopaedic Hospital, Birmingham

PRE-OPERATIVE

Indications

One important indication for internal fixation of a fracture is to enable a patient to get out of bed soon and so to avoid the complications of long recumbency; this is especially indicated with fractures of the neck of the femur in the elderly. A second important indication is a fracture that enters or is near to a joint; it is then desirable to restore the shape of the articular surfaces in an attempt to reduce the degree of degenerative change. A third indication is that more than one segment of the same limb is involved and a fourth occurs with multiple injuries, when it is important to neutralize as many fractures of long bones as possible so as to make nursing easier. Internal fixation also plays a major part in the management of non-union, whether this has followed conservatively treated fractures or those which have been operated upon primarily. Other indications are pathological fractures and the restoration of the shape of bones where this is necessary for the sake of function or appearance, as for example, in the face, the forearm of adults, the hand and the foot and the protection of soft tissues that need repair. The ultimate example of this is the re-attachment of a severed part, but there are many severe injuries for which the risks of internal fixation are less than those of leaving fractures movable.

In general, the techniques of internal fixation require the use of wires, nails and screws either independently or in combination with metal plates. None of these implants should be used unless the conditions for internal fixation are all suitable. These conditions include satisfactory sterility of the theatre, the instruments and the implants themselves. The surgeon must make sure that he has the full complement of equipment necessary to undertake this sort of work and he should also possess the necessary judgement and skill. *Internal fixation of fractures is a potentially dangerous procedure and can produce very bad results unless high standards of aseptic technique can be ensured.*

Although a sterile air enclosure in the operating theatre may reduce the dangers of infection, these expensive devices are not widely available; safe operations can be carried on in normal theatres, as long as they are not also used for treating surgically dirty cases of any kind. The preparation of the patient's skin and the surgeon's hands is most safely done by the application of 0·5 per cent chlorhexidine in 95 per cent alcohol with 2 minutes' scrubbing of the surgeon's hands, and rubbing this solution into the patient's skin with the gloved hand as a separate procedure (Lowbury and Lilley, 1975). It is important to isolate the area of operation as far as possible from the anaesthetist and the rest of the patient's body and the movement of persons inside the operating theatre should be reduced to a minimum. Whenever possible, it is desirable to use a bloodless field by applying a pneumatic tourniquet above the site of operation; it is probably better not to exsanguinate the limb, but simply to elevate it before the tourniquet is inflated.

KÜNTSCHER NAILING

The open method of Küntscher nailing is preferred by many surgeons on the grounds that a really accurate reduction of the fracture is more quickly and easily achieved, and one can be sure that no soft tissue is present between the bone ends. The other advantages are that x-ray control is not necessary during the operation, and that the large haematoma which is always present at the site of a fracture of the shaft of the femur can be evacuated and suction drains inserted. The chief disadvantage is the increased risk of infection compared with closed methods.

Before engaging in medullary fixation, the full armamentarium must be available. There must be a full set of nails of all diameters and lengths, and each nail should be sharpened and slotted at both ends. A full set of reamers should be provided and the best are those in which there is a hole in the handle of the same diameter as the cutting end. This will ensure that the nail will not be too wide for the reamed-out channel.

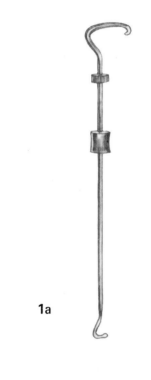

1a

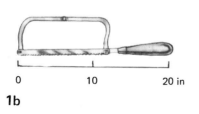

0   10   20 in

1b

1 & 2

Extractors are long rods with a hook at the end and the best design has a sliding cylindrical hammer on the rod. It is important to have two of these, lest the hook break off one. To avoid the predicament in which a nail becomes jammed because of an error in technique, it is wise to have a blacksmith's hacksaw with a high-speed steel blade in the operating set, so that the nail may be sawn off short if it cannot be driven down fully. A selection of reamers and nails is illustrated.

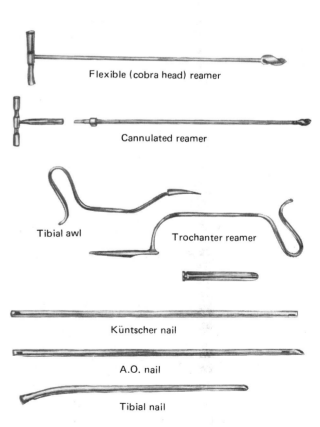

Flexible (cobra head) reamer

Cannulated reamer

Tibial awl   Trochanter reamer

Küntscher nail

A.O. nail

Tibial nail

2

TECHNIQUE FOR THE FEMUR

Intramedullary nailing may be employed for transverse or short oblique fractures of the mid-shaft of the femur. It is seldom possible to employ this method of treatment on the femur with the help of a tourniquet, so it is important to have enough blood available and an intravenous infusion running before beginning the operation. Diathermy and suction apparatus must also be arranged.

3, 4 & 5

The patient should be lying on the unaffected side with the injured thigh extended and separated from the underlying flexed limb by a macintosh-covered pillow. The limb should be securely towelled distal to the fracture so that it can be manipulated to help in the reduction of the fracture. A lateral longitudinal incision is made and the fascia lata is divided in the line of the incision. Using rake retractors the vastus lateralis is then split and retracted backwards and forwards to expose the shaft of the femur and the fracture. A number of perforating vessels must be picked up and coagulated, and good haemostasis must be secured before the fracture is approached.

The lower end of the upper fragment is caught with a bone clamp and brought out into the wound, care being taken not to retract or damage the periosteum around its end. A hook should not be used for this purpose because if, as is not unusual, there are cracks leading away from the main fracture, the hook may pull off another piece of bone.

6

Haematoma and small bone fragments are removed before a reamer is passed into the open end of the upper fragment. The size of the reamer is judged according to the appearance on the x-ray films and should be the largest size that will be accommodated by the narrowest part of the medullary canal.

The canal is reamed up to the greater trochanter and the cortex perforated here, after which the reamer can be removed. If it passes very easily, the next size of nail should be chosen, because it must be the thickest that can be firmly gripped in the medullary canal. The reamer is then withdrawn and a guide wire passed proximally through the hole in the trochanter and out through the skin of the buttock. This guide wire must not be too thick for the size of the nail that has been chosen for the fixation. A transverse incision 1·25 inches long is made over the buttock at

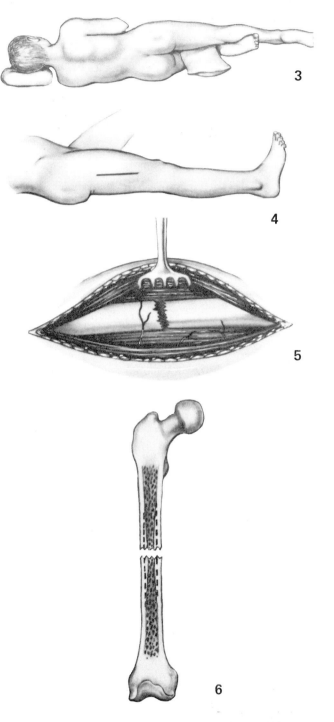

3

4

5

6

the point of exit of the guide wire, and the chosen nail is passed into the femur along the guide wire. The length of nail may be estimated by passing a guide wire down to the knee from the fracture and measuring the length of this segment, as well as passing the same guide wire up to the trochanter and measuring that length. The sum of the two lengths with an addition of 0·5 inches is the right length to choose for the fixation of a straightforward transverse or short oblique fracture.

7, 8 & 9

However, if the shaft of the femur is more than slightly bowed, a nail of this length may jam or it may perforate the cortex. It is desirable that whenever possible the nail should be long enough to get a purchase in the firm cancellous bone above the intercondylar notch. The nail is hammered down the medullary canal, directed by the guide wire, until it projects about 0·5 inches from the lower end of the upper fragment. The guide wire should then be removed, and using suitable bone-holding forceps of the Hey Groves type, the bone ends can be manipulated so that the lower end of the nail is engaged in the distal fragment. This may be most easily effected by flexing the femur so that the fragments are edge to edge and the projecting end of the nail engages in the open end of the lower fragment, after which the femur can be straightened again and the position held while the nail is driven finally home. When the upper end of the nail reaches the skin of the buttock, a cylindrical punch must be applied to it, so as to drive it down to the trochanter while protecting the skin. Half an inch of the nail should be left projecting because this has the slot that facilitates removal of the nail. At this point it is sensible to have an anteroposterior x-ray film taken of the knee to ensure that the nail is far enough down and not too far. A nail which ends 4 inches short of the knee joint gets an indifferent hold in the lower fragment, and the required degree of rigidity cannot be obtained. If the x-ray appearance is satisfactory, it must now be decided whether the fracture itself has enough resistance to rotational displacement to be left, or whether an additional antirotational measure is needed.

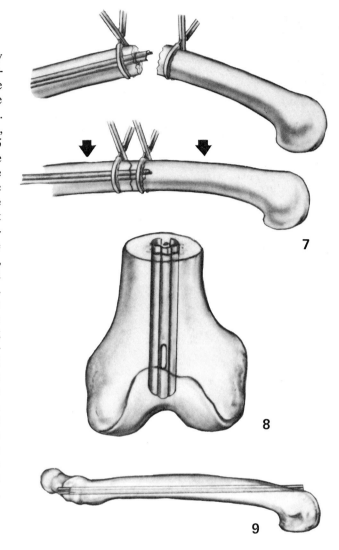

7

8

9

Supplementary fixation. Plating

10

If there are strong bony irregularities on a fracture of the shaft of the femur these can prevent rotation at the fracture but with oblique fractures and smooth transverse ones a simple medullary nail cannot be expected to do this. In this case it is a useful practice to apply a short stainless steel plate on the lateral side of the femur to span the fracture, and the A.O. (Arbeitsgemeinschaft für Osteosynthesefragen) dynamic compression plate is admirably suited to this. It does not require any further division of muscles to apply it, and being of a self-compressing type, the fracture gap itself can be snugly closed by its use. Single-cortex screws are adequate if they are of the A.O. type, for which the thread is tapped, using the appropriate tap before they are inserted. It is important not to damage the nail with either the drill or the tap while inserting this plate.

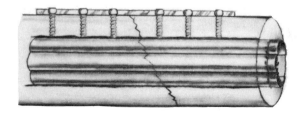

10

11 & 12

In a fracture with a third fragment or of a long oblique type, it may still be possible to get adequate fixation with a medullary nail, but an additional step will be required. This can be either to apply one or two cerclage wires, or to include the third fragment under the antirotation plate applied laterally. Cerclage wires are best passed subperiosteally, using a special curved tubular wire-passer. Having passed this device round the shaft of the bone, a length of stainless steel wire of 1·2 mm diameter can be inserted into the open end of the tube. When the device is removed it leaves the wire encircling the bone. It is often better to pass this same wire round a second time, using the same device and then to twist the ends up firmly with one of the several forms of wire-twister which are available.

The wire should then be cut off short, leaving two or three turns at the most, bent over and hammered home with a punch so that the movement of muscle over it is not disturbed. It may be necessary to put two separate cerclage wires round to hold a long oblique fracture. There is no place for Parham bands, which are often made of indifferent metal and certainly disturb the periosteal blood supply quite markedly.

Before closing the wound, haemostasis must be secured as far as possible, a suction drain should be inserted down to the fracture, and except in very thin young subjects, it is wise to insert another one in the

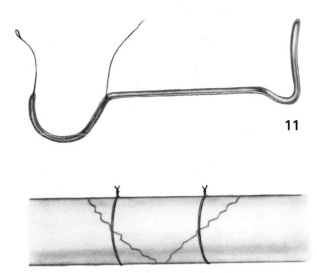

11

12

subcutaneous layer. The wound is then closed in layers with careful suturing of the skin and it is good practice, especially in females, to use a subcuticular prolene stitch in the skin. It is important to secure the exit points of the drains with a small length of strapping lest they become displaced while the patient is turned and lifted on to the trolley.

Postoperative care

13

The injured leg should be placed on a specially high Braun's frame with the knee well flexed for at least 48 hr.

The intravenous infusion can be taken down when it is certain that the blood lost has been fully replaced, though it must be expected that some loss from the suction drains will continue for 10 hr or so. To make sure that the drains are working efficiently, they should be withdrawn 0·5 inches in each hour because otherwise they may be blocked by soft tissue sucked into the holes. When each tube has been shortened so that the holes appear at the skin, the drains can be removed. Active exercises of the knee and foot can begin on the second postoperative day and the patient is often able to leave hospital within a week, walking on the good leg with crutches, and swinging the injured one. Comminuted fractures of the femur at whatever level are seldom suitable for medullary nailing and are better treated by applying a dynamic compression plate of suitable size.

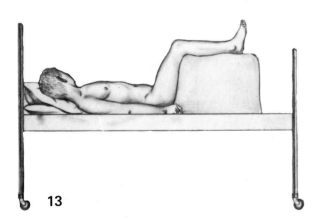

13

TIBIAL NAILING

14 & 15

Medullary nailing has a place with fractures of the tibia, but it is not so often indicated as in the femur. Here again, the selection of the case is important and nailing should be considered for transverse or short oblique fractures of the shaft without comminution; the open method is the safest. The first step is to arrange the leg so that the knee is flexed with the foot held on the table by a sandbag to provide resistance to the hammering when the nail is driven home. A vertical incision is made alongside the patellar tendon and then in the mid-line through the tendon to reach the anterior edge of the upper end of the tibia, just in front of the articular surface. The medullary canal is then entered with a special triangular-pointed awl, opening up a hole wide enough for the passage of the appropriate guide wire. The fracture is then exposed by a longitudinal incision over the tibial crest and the guide wire passed down and directed into the lower fragment, holding the position either with a bone clamp alone or with a small plate held to each fragment with a pair of clamps. The guide wire is passed down until it reaches the level of the medial malleolus, when it is safer to confirm its position by a radiograph. A nail of this length is selected.

The medullary nail for the tibia has a curve at the upper end adapted to the shape of the tibia, and it is driven down the guide wire by gentle blows of the hammer, making sure that it goes across the fracture and does not impinge on the cortex of the lower fragment. When it is completely home, it should be almost flush with the cortex in the upper end but a small length must be left projecting to facilitate its removal.

Both incisions are then closed using suction drains. Active movements can be begun on the first day after operation. With a transverse fracture and good alignment is often possible to allow weight-bearing within the first 6 or 8 weeks.

A.O. advocate reaming out the medullary canal of both tibia and femur to a wide enough diameter to allow the passage of a very large nail to give full rigidity. This technique needs special instruments, including a flexible, powered reamer with increasing diameters of cutting head, and it gives excellent results in their hands. Although the endosteal blood supply is cut off by this technique, enough blood supply travels longitudinally in the cortex to maintain the nutrition, and there is no doubt that the extra rigidity allows rapid and uneventful healing in most cases. It

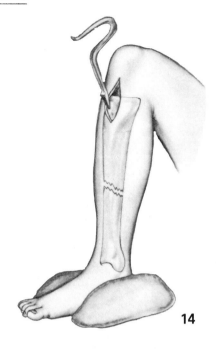

14

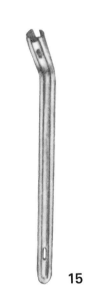

15

must, however, be admitted that much experience is needed to make this procedure safe, and it has no place in segmental fractures nor when there is much comminution. It is quite possible with a segmental fracture for the reamer to spin the middle fragment round, destroying all its soft tissue attachment and therefore killing it.

PLATING OF FRACTURES

With compression

There are now plates that can be used on almost any type of fracture in any long bone in the body.

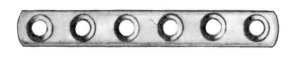

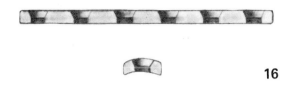

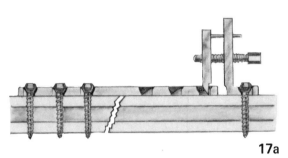

16

16 & 17a, b & c

The design of the plates falls into two main categories; in the first type the plates have circular holes of conical shape into which conical-headed screws are driven, and with these all the screws must be inserted exactly at right angles to the plate. Compression is applied to the bone by using a tension device screwed to the bone beyond one end of the plate, which has first been fixed to the opposite fragment with screws. When the plate has been placed under tension by tightening the compressor, an equivalent amount of positive pressure is applied to the fracture and the screws can then be inserted into the second fragment.

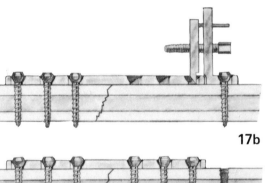

17a

17b

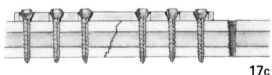

17c

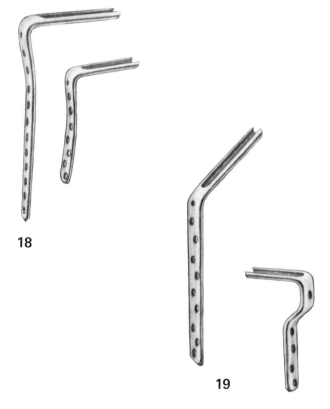

18

19

18 & 19

Different shapes and sizes of plates are available for this technique. There are straight ones of appropriate sizes for use on the diaphysis of femur and tibia, angled condylar plates for use on the lower end of the femur, upper end of the tibia and occasionally the upper end of the femur. There are also angled plates to fix fractures of the neck of the femur and for osteotomy at various sites. Specially shaped plates with clover-leaf outline are made for use on the medial malleolus, and T-plates, particularly for fractures of the neck of the humerus.

20

The A.O. standard plates have the disadvantage that to apply the compression device, extra exposure is needed, which damages muscles and may endanger nerves, especially the radial nerve with high fractures of humerus and radius. It is also possible to insert a screw slightly eccentrically in a screw-hole so that it obtains a purchase at one point only on the plate, leading to an area of high stress which may lead to corrosion.

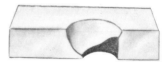

20

21a, b & c

The alternative system is to use a dynamic compression plate (DCP) (Allgöwer, Perren and Matter, 1970). In this the holes in the plate are constructed of two joining cylindrical surfaces and, when the screw is inserted toward the end of the plate-hole away from the fracture, it applies a distracting force to the plate and an equivalent compressing force to the fracture as it is driven home. As the screw head is of spherical shape it is bound to have a semicircular contact with the plate hole, which reduces the chance of corrosion at the point of high stress and gives firmer fixation. A second advantage of this plate geometry is that the screw can be tilted 40° to either side and a similar amount in the axis of the plate without losing its grip on the screw hole. Thus, irregular bone fragments can be captured by the screw, and in porotic bone it is advantageous to insert all the screws at different angles to the plate so that they will get a firmer grip. A third advantage is that the plate can be applied with the central screws inserted eccentrically so that they apply their own compression. There is then no need for the compression device and the increased exposure required for its insertion.

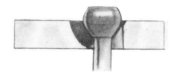

21a

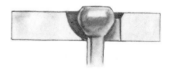

21b

Plates employing this principle are available for the tibia and femur and there is a one-third tubular plate for use on smaller bones as well. The principle of eccentric drilling of holes is also applicable with the special small fragment set designed for the use in hands and feet, clavicles, elbows and fibulae (Heim and Pfeiffer, 1974).

21c

22a, b & c

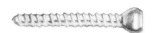

22a

A.O. cortex screws have threads designed for cortical bone, which extend from the neck of the screw to its tip. Cancellous screws have wider threads which only extend for part of the screw length from the tip, the remaining length being smooth. All these screws apply interfragmentary compression. Malleolar screws have a drill point so that they can be driven in without a drill hole after the cortex has been perforated.

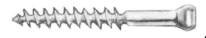

22b

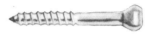

22c

23a & b

Compression plates are often used in combination with independent screws which are not passed through the plate, but pull together independent fragments of bone using the so-called lag principle. The 'lag' screw is inserted so that its tip can obtain a purchase on the cortex of the bone farther from its point of insertion. The threads of the screw nearest to the head must not bite into the bone if compression is to be achieved. Therefore, a hole is drilled in this first cortex wider than the outside diameter of the screw threads. The drill bit is changed to one which matches the core diameter of the screw and this is used to make the hole in the far cortex. This hole is then tapped with the appropriate tap. When the screw is inserted, the threads furthest from the screw head will engage the far cortex and as the screw is tightened, compression will be achieved. This is particularly true with 'butterfly' fragments of the tibia and with comminuted fractures of the upper and lower end of the femur.

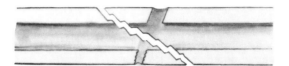

23a

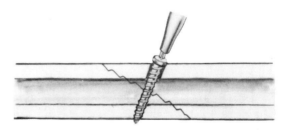

23b

With a single long spiral fracture of the lowest third of the tibia especially, screws may be used by themselves without the addition of a plate. The screws are then inserted to give compression and as the fracture is spiral they will lie in a spiral pattern themselves. With a butterfly fragment, however, a combination of independent screws and a plate with its own screws is necessary.

In a typical case the operation proceeds as follows.

An incision is made longitudinally just lateral to the crest of the tibia so that the suture line does not lie over the plate. It is important to make a long enough incision to avoid the need for vigorous retraction, and a long straight incision is better than a curved or S-shaped incision. The fracture is exposed, and taking care not to disturb soft tissue attachments, the broken surfaces are cleaned of haematoma and any interposed soft tissue. It is determined to which main fragment the butterfly fragment has its major contact and this part of the fracture is then set and fixed with one or more compressing screws. Only one fracture line now remains and this fracture is set and held with bone clamps or a single temporary cerclage wire while the screws are inserted, again to provide compression. It is now important to add a plate to prevent disruptive stresses from falling on the screws themselves. The plate may be one with conical holes, but it is better to use the dynamic compression plate. This plate is applied under slight tension, which gives more rigidity, although the transverse screws are already applying interfragmentary compression. A plate under tension is stronger than an unstressed plate.

24, 25 & 26

Another good indication for fixation by plate and screws is a segmental fracture of a long bone. After exposure and setting of the fracture and temporary fixation with clamps and a loose plate, the definitive plate is applied to the middle segment first and screwed in place. Compression can then be applied at each end to bring both the upper and lower fragments into rigid contact with the intervening fragment. When there is an oblique fracture it is important finally to apply a screw near the middle of the plate to pass obliquely from one fragment to the other. This screw should also be applied so as to exert compression though all the other screws are inserted in the ordinary way, with threads biting in both cortices.

In the femur especially, a segmental fracture may have the two fracture lines so far apart that a single plate cannot span them both. It is then better to apply two plates, the upper one joining the uppermost fragment to the middle fragment, and the lower plate the middle to the distal fragment. Note that as the distances between all the screw holes in the A.O. plates are equal, it is possible to arrange that the screws interdigitate and do not abut against each other when using two plates that overlap.

Positions of plates and contouring

In the case of the tibia, a plate applied to the proximal third or distal third will need to be bent to produce the correct alignment and, because the subcutaneous surface of the tibia, which is where plates are most often applied, has a twist at both ends, the plates used there must be appropriately contoured. A straight plate applied to the lower part of the femur will have to be contoured, but it is often better to apply a

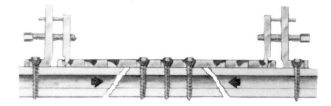

24

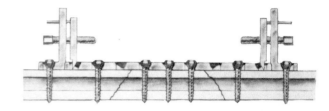

25

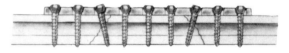

26

condylar plate, of which the 95° angle between blade and plate usually fits well without further bending. It is important to contour plates accurately with a powerfull plate-bender, so that the bend can be placed between screw holes, and not, as is usual with the ordinary manual plate-benders, through the screw holes themselves. This is not so important with the dynamic compression plate because the spherical geometry of the screw/plate interface allows some alteration without disturbing the purchase obtainable by the screw head.

27-30

It must always be determined on which surface the plate will have its main effect and, when applying a plate under tension, it is necessary to discover which is the tension surface of the bone. This may be altered by the fracture shape, but in general the tension surface is on the anterior surface of the tibia and on the lateral surface of the femur. In the case of the tibia a compromise solution is to apply a plate on the medial surface, because the crest is unsuitable. A fracture at the middle of the shaft of either of these bones can usually be fixed with a straight plate which does not need contouring to make it fit. However, when it is applied under compression the effect will be to open up the fracture line on the far side of the bone, unless a precautionary step is taken. This involves bending the plate at its mid-point so that it stands 2 – 3 mm proud of the bone at this point when the bone is straight. When the first two compressing screws are applied adjoining the fracture, the bone is drawn towards the plate, which unbends to fit the bone, and a compressive force is then exerted on the cortex on the far side of the bone as well as under the plate itself. This is a most important step because it is very harmful to apply powerful compression on the cortex just deep to the plate while having a gap which may be of 1 or 2 mm in the cortex on the far side.

There are special needs for modifying the ordinary technique of plating a tibia when the bone is abnormally soft or when the plate has to be applied to the upper or lower end of the bone. To get adequate purchase it may then be necessary to use cancellous screws, which have a special thread to obtain a powerful grip on soft cancellous bone. All A.O. plates are provided with threads in the two holes at each end of the plate to take the wide threads of the cancellous screws. With the dynamic compression plate, cancellous screws can be inserted through any of the holes. Should a normal cortex screw fail to get a purchase on the far cortex, it can be replaced by a screw 2 mm longer, and a small special nut applied to its end, so that a good grip can be obtained beyond the far cortex.

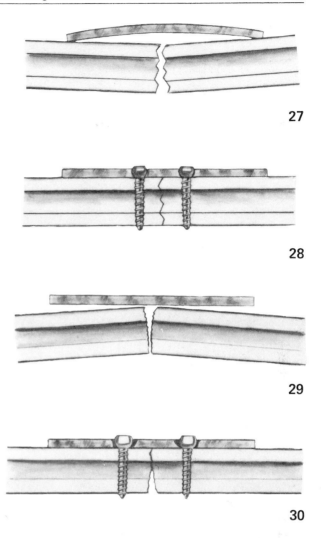

27

28

29

30

Postoperative care

It must be understood that rigid fixation with compression does not allow earlier weight-bearing than any other form of fixation and this must be explained to the patient, preferably both before operation and afterwards.

FRACTURES OF THE UPPER LIMB

These are also amenable to rigid fixation by the application of appropriate compression plates. Tibial plates are adequate for the forearm, and in normal sized adults it is wise to fix any fracture of the shaft of the radius or ulna with a six-hole plate to make sure that there are at least five cortices held on each fragment. It is here that the dynamic compression plate has a special advantage because there is no need for the extra exposure to allow the compression device for an ordinary A.O. plate to be applied. The incision depends on the shape of the fracture but most cases are better exposed using the posterior incision of Henry for the ulna and the anterolateral exposure for the radius. The most important indications for rigid fixation of forearm fractures are the Monteggia fracture for which the ulna must be fixed and the Galeazzi fracture, for which the radius must be fixed.

TIMING OF THE OPERATION

The forearm

Though there is some discussion about the usefulness of delaying internal fixation of many fractures of long bones, it is hard to justify delay with a Galeazzi or Monteggia fracture because of the difficulty of maintaining alignment and length of forearm bones by any other means. A comminuted fracture extending into the wrist joint may need to have a transverse screw applied as well as a dorsal plate.

The humerus

For the shaft of the humerus, when internal fixation is indicated, as with an unstable fracture when there are accompanying major injuries elsewhere, or when an earlier return to work is for some special reason necessary, a compression plate is justified. In an adult it is better to use the femoral DCP for the management of this fracture and it is wise to use the posterior Henry approach for fractures of the shaft of the bone. Fractures of the neck of the humerus are usually managed

without operation, but when there are other fractures in the same limb or multiple injuries, it may be necessary to fix this fracture internally.

31

The special T-plate designed for this particular area is then ideal. It is inserted either via a deltoid-splitting incision or an approach through the deltopectoral groove, depending on the shape and type of the fracture. It is particularly helpful for fracture-dislocation of the humeral head. The upper cancellous screws get a good purchase in the head and the compression is applied distally, using the compressor on the shaft of the bone, because the T-plate for this use has not yet been provided with oval holes.

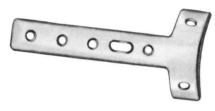

31

It is important to use one drain in the deep layers and one subcutaneously. Closure is in layers, restoring the muscles and nerves to their anatomical positions which may mean, in an upper third fracture, sliding the radial nerve back over the plate when this has been screwed home. There are some situations where the radial nerve is in jeopardy if a plate has to be applied near it, and it is then helpful to transplant the nerve through the fracture line to lie on the opposite surface of the bone so that the plate can be comfortably screwed home.

Postoperative care of upper limb fractures consists of elevating the limb for the first 24 hr and then encouraging active exercises.

APPLICATION OF COMPRESSION TO FRACTURES NEAR TO AND INVOLVING JOINTS

32-35

Lower end of the humerus

With T, Y or other comminuted fractures of the lower end of the humerus, compression techniques play an important part. The patient is first anaesthetized and placed prone on the operating table with the arm supported on an arm board, and the forearm hanging down and securely draped. It is then convenient if there is no fracture in this area to expose the lower end of the humerus by osteotomy of the olecranon, and turning it and the attached triceps upwards. The re-attachment of the olecranon is made easier by first drilling a longitudinal hole through it and into the shaft of the ulna, and tapping this for the cancellous screw that will be inserted finally. The olecranon and triceps now being held proximally with a towel-clip, the whole of the lower end of the humerus can be examined and the ulnar nerve retracted with a tape and watched carefully throughout. The fracture can be repositioned and held temporarily with Kirschner wires while the various components are fixed. With a T-fracture, the first step is to insert a transverse screw to close up the vertical component of the fracture. The re-assembled lower fragment can then be attached to the shaft with a small one-third tubular contoured plate applied to each condylar fragment. When these plates lie on the side of the shaft, compression can be applied by drilling the holes for the screws at the upper end of each hole in the plates, so that when the screws are driven home, compression is applied to the fracture complex. With comminuted fractures, additional screws may be needed at various points but it is usually possible to reconstruct the articular surface of both the capitellum and the trochlea so that the degree of post-traumatic arthrosis is minimal. When the operation on the humerus is completed, the olecranon is replaced and a long cancellous screw is inserted in the hole previously drilled down the shaft. A small transverse hole is drilled in the shaft of the ulna distal to the osteotomy site, and a wire passed through this and upwards as a figure-of-8 round the neck of the screw in the olecranon. This wire is twisted up, the ends buried and the screw driven fully home (*see Illustrations 40* and *41*).

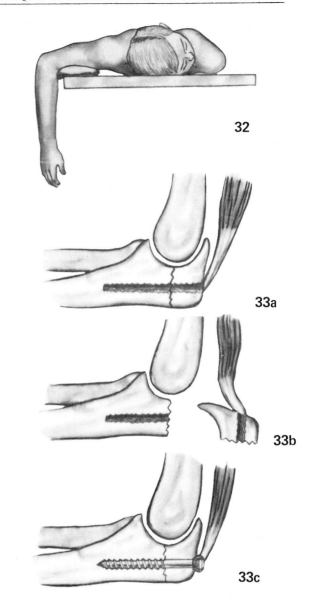

32

33a

33b

33c

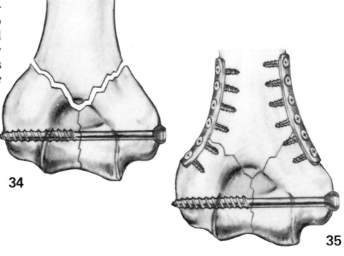

34

35

T-fractures of the knee

Whether these occur in the femur or the tibia, they are well fixed by transverse cancellous screws inserted so as to close snugly the vertical fracture but each fragment may need an additional plate to exert compression axially and thus to stabilize the other parts of these fracture complexes. The special condylar plate has an application both at the lower end of the femur and the upper end of the tibia.

The ankle

Uni-, bi- and tri-malleolar fractures can all be treated by internal fixation, which has the advantage of allowing active movement, as well as making more certain of accurate restoration of the articular surfaces. An especially designed malleolar screw is self-drilling and exerts compression because it is not fully threaded. It can be inserted into the medial malleolus or from the fibula into the tibia in order to close the ankle mortice.

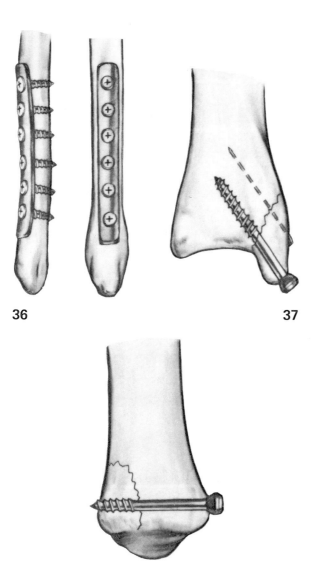

36

37

38

36, 37 & 38

With a comminuted or an oblique fracture causing shortening of the fibula, it is important first to restore the full length of the fibula; this may be done either with one or more small transverse lag screws or by the application of a one-third tubular plate, contoured to fit the outer side of the fibula. The medial malleolus can be satisfactorily fixed by a single malleolar screw, but because the fragment may pivot round this screw, a Kirschner wire should be driven alongside the screw to prevent this. A third posterior tibial fragment can be well fixed by a cancellous screw inserted from the front of the tibia, so that its thread is entirely within the small posterior fragment, and draws it firmly into place.

Suction drains are used after these operations.

39

Plating without compression

Most of the plates that have been used without any attempt at compression are incapable of fixing fractures rigidly. Rigidity can be achieved without compression by using the specially designed and unusually strong plate of Hicks. As with compression plates, however, this needs to be used with both skill and a clear understanding of its proper application. Its strength makes it difficult to alter its shape and its bulk may make it difficult to close skin over it when the plate is subcutaneous.

With these plates it is customary to use self-tapping screws and a drill the size of the core of the screw. Such screws grip well in strong bone, from which they may be impossible to remove later, but they get only a poor grip in soft spongy bone.

Removal of plates

Whether or not plates are used for compression, it is desirable to remove them eventually, partly because of their liability to corrosion (which is not very high in the case of stainless steel plates) and also because

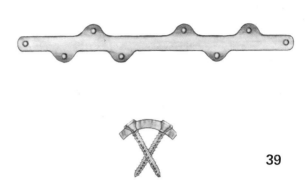

39

a strong plate bears some of the load, which prevents the normal stresses from falling on the bone deep to the plate. These stresses help the bone to remodel and regain its natural strength. It is, therefore, wise to remove plates from the lower limb after 18–24 months, and from the upper limb between 12 and 15 months in most instances. After the removal of a plate the patient must exercise cautiously for some weeks, while the internal architecture of the bone is restored. It has been found that the functional assessment of the limb improves noticeably after the removal of a plate, but in most cases the final functional result depends on the severity of the fracture.

INTERNAL FIXATION USING WIRES

In addition to cerclage wiring, which has an occasional place for fixing a 'butterfly' fragment to the shaft as mentioned above, the main place for wire fixation is in fractures of the olecranon, fractures of the patella and for fixing back comminuted fractures of the greater trochanter of the femur, and of the medial or lateral malleolus. For these fractures the wire is used as a tension wire to resist distraction forces.

Fractures of the olecranon

40

A simple oblique fracture of the olecranon can be conveniently fixed with one compressing screw inserted from the point of the olecranon, directed obliquely downwards and forwards to gain a grip on the coronoid process but with other fractures of the olecranon, especially when there is some comminution or the fracture is transverse, it is better to use two Kirschner wires and a length of flexible wire as described below.

41a & b

A transverse 2 mm hole is drilled through the ulna distal to the site of the fracture. Two Kirschner wires are then driven downwards through the tip of the olecranon parallel with each other but their proximal ends are left projecting an inch or two. A length of wire is then prepared with a small eye at its mid-point and one end is passed through the drill hole and brought up to go round the end of the Kirschner wires. The small eye in the wire is left on one side and the loose ends are twisted together on the other side. The loose ends and the eye in the wire can be tightened simultaneously, thereby applying an equal stress on each side. The ends are buried and the Kirschner wires are each bent to 180°, cut short and hammered flush with the bone from above.

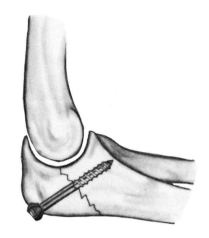

40

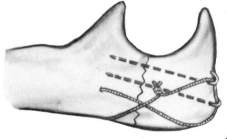

41a

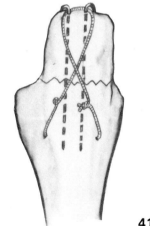

41b

42

Kirschner wires and tension wires can be used in exactly the same manner for awkward fractures of the greater trochanter of the femur, for the medial and lateral malleolus and for the patella.

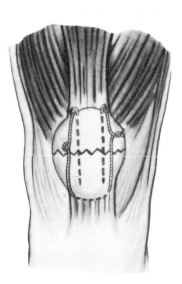

42

Kirschner wires

Kirschner wires may be used for internal fixation of small fragments and especially in phalanges and metacarpals and metatarsals as medullary fixators. It is best to use an open method because it can be difficult to achieve the desired position of the fracture and the wire in any other way. An incision is made over the fractured bone, retracting the extensor tendon, and the wire is then passed through the medullary canal of the distal fragment in a distal direction. When it has emerged through the skin at the appropriate point, it is possible to pass it proximally to its full extent while holding the fracture reduced. Wires may be left buried under the skin or better left bent over or protected with a cork outside the skin over the flexed joint. When the fractures are firm, all the wires are removed and the joints can be exercised.

This method is not very satisfactory with comminuted or oblique fractures and particularly for metacarpals, the plates provided in the A.O. small fragment set give better fixation for irregular fractures and especially those near the joints. For severely smashed hands, it is sometimes helpful to hold some alignment between the metacarpal bones by drilling a Kirschner wire transversely through all the metacarpals; more than one wire may be used in this manner. It may then be possible to institute early activity to keep the metacarpophalangeal joints in action.

Kirschner wires are also useful by themselves for fractures of the epicondyles, condyles or supracondylar region of the lower end of the humerus, especially in childhood. Fractures of the medial or lateral epicondyles in children are safely fixed with temporary Kirschner wires which are left projecting under the skin and removed as soon as stability is obtained. This may be done quite safely without interfering with the growth of the part. In the occasional case of supracondylar fracture for which open reduction is required, it is quite satisfactory to pass a Kirschner wire through each epicondyle in a proximal direction, crossing over each other and obtaining a purchase in the cortex of the metaphysis on each side. These wires may be removed when the fracture is stable.

Cerclage

Loops of wire wrapped round or partly round a bone offer a useful way of holding spiral fragments together, perhaps supplementing a Küntscher nail, or holding in place fragments that for one reason or another cannot be screwed and, temporarily, for assembling comminuted fractures that are to be fixed by other means. Wire loops used definitively in this way should be double and must be applied and remain snugly against bone all the way round; they are dangerous when they are loose, not because they are too tight.

43 a&b

It is important when using cerclage to employ the right thickness of wire, and it is convenient to have spools prepared for use in the theatre marked 'fibula', 'tibia' and 'femur' respectively. Temporary cerclage is of great value when dealing with comminuted fractures, during the application of a plate, or while screwing fragments together: a single loop suffices for this. The most convenient variety for temporary use during an operation is a fairly stout wire with a small eyelet on one end. This is passed round the bone with the help of a tubular wire-passer and the end is then threaded through the eyelet.

A suitable wire-tightener is applied and the wire bent over to hold the bony fragments together. The wire can be left in place while the plate or screws are applied, having just bent it over to hold the wire in a 180° kink. It can be removed before closing the wound but if a plate is applied on top of the wire, it is important to remove the wire before the screws are finally driven home, lest it becomes trapped and cannot be extracted. It is often possible to apply the plate loosely to the bone and then pass the cerclage wire round both the bone and the plate together, holding the fragments up towards it. When the plate has been screwed home and all is secure, it is a simple matter to cut the wire and remove it, together with the wire-twister (Müller, Allgöwer and Willenegger, 1970).

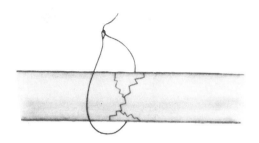

43a

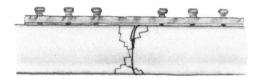

43b

OPEN REDUCTION WITHOUT INTERNAL FIXATION

There are a few occasions when having exposed a fracture it is sufficient to set it in place and close the wound; one such is the overlapped transverse fracture of one or both bones of a child's forearm that has resisted closed manipulation, but even these should be fixed if their shape or a defective hinge makes the fracture unstable in any acceptable position.

EXTERNAL SKELETAL FIXATION

Whenever vessels or nerves are injured and have had to be repaired, it is difficult to hold a fracture by plaster; the soft tissue damage often makes plate or screw fixation impracticable. It is then helpful to have available one or other of the appliances that can give external skeletal fixation. The simplest of these uses two Steinmann pins passed transversely through each of the main fragments of long bones, the ends of the four pins being joined by bars on the medial and lateral sides of the limb. A single pin in each fragment does not prevent movement at the fracture. With a transverse fracture it can be arranged that compression is applied if the lateral bars are provided with thumb screws to push the ends of the Steinmann pins towards each other.

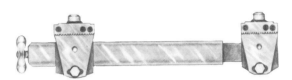

44a

44 a,b & c

The disadvantage of using Steinmann pins is that they may become loose so that pin-track infection is a common complication. This may be avoided by using screws rather than pins and the best apparatus for this purpose is that devised by Wagner; it was originally intended for leg-lengthening operations, but has been found to be just as good for holding a fracture rigidly or for applying compression. This instrument consists of a very strong square-section bar enclosed in a square-section tube, provided with clamps that can be held rigidly at each end by nuts. Screws are driven into the bone, which has been drilled with a 3·6 mm drill. The screws get a very powerful purchase on the bone, penetrating both cortices. Two screws are placed in each main fragment and each pair can be set well apart to allow for dressings and skin grafting procedures or to leave a wound open, if necessary. Each pair of screws is held rigidly by the special clamps to the inside bar and the outside tube of the external fixator. The nuts can be loosened to allow adjustment of the angle of the screws and then tightened to get a very powerful purchase. The fracture is then rigidly stabilized by the outside bar.

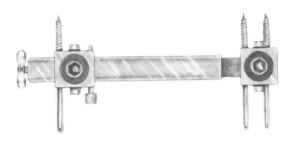

44b

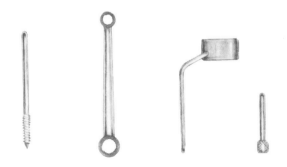

44c

INTERNAL FIXATION IN THE TREATMENT OF NON-UNION

Only the principles are to be dealt with here.

(*1*) Ensure rigid fixation.

(*2*) Do not disturb the fracture except to correct unacceptable deformity.

45

(*3*) Bulging callus may be removed with a chisel for the sake of letting a plate fit snugly, but a plate may be bent to fit offset fragments, which may themselves be trimmed with advantage.

(*4*) Bone grafts should be used to span a gap or a length of dead bone, that is bone that has no callus fixing it.

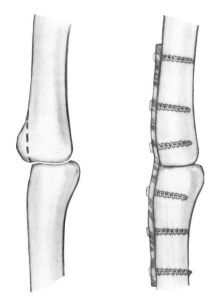

45

ESSENTIAL STEPS FOR SUCCESS IN INTERNAL FIXATION OF OPEN FRACTURES

(*1*) Blood transfusion sufficient to replace blood already lost and that which will be lost, particularly when a tourniquet is not used.

(*2*) Thorough cleansing of the skin around the wound.

(*3*) Gentle but thorough exploration of the wound followed by the painstaking removal of all foreign matter, clot and dead or doomed tissue. In the case of bone, completely separate fragments may have to be retained for the sake of accurate restoration of the fracture.

(*4*) Repeated irrigation of the wound with Ringer's solution helps to remove clot and bacteria.

(*5*) What metal is used must be sufficient for its purpose but should be used in such a way as not further to reduce the ability of the wound to heal.

(*6*) It may be advantageous not to close the wound until 3—5 days after fixation.

Removal of metal

Operations for removal of metal implants may be easy or difficult. The indications for removal of metal depend partly on the type of metal that has been used, what function the implants are performing and whether there have been any complications.

When a fracture that has been internally fixed becomes infected, if the fixation remains firm and is firmly holding a fracture that has become infected, it should be left in position; such operations as are required may proceed and irrigation drainage should be employed. When, however, metal implants are loose in the presence of infection, they are certainly harmful and should be removed, after which treatment can be continued with external splintage, external fixation devices or occasionally the re-application of a better and more rigid implant. It is often helpful in addition even at this stage to insert cancellous bone.

Implants should be removed when there is a danger of corrosion, which may happen with all stainless steel plates and screws in the second or third year, especially if they have been damaged during insertion.

Screws used independently for compression in the medial malleolus, for example, may be left because they do not prevent the transmission of stress in an axial direction and, if not in contact with a plate, they will not corrode. The transverse screw applied in a malleolar fracture from the fibula to the tibia should be removed at 8 weeks in order to restore the normal movement at the inferior tibiofibular joint.

There may be difficulties in the removal of plates and these chiefly concern the shape of the plate, the overgrowth of bone, or the use of self-tapping screws. The plate may be difficult to remove if it is of an irregular shape, or if some of the screw holes have not been filled so that bone has grown into them. If a plate has been inserted under the periosteum it is quite common for bone to grow over the ends of the plate and sometimes over its whole surface so that its removal may require the use of an osteotome. There is finally the difficulty of removing a plate which has been inserted with self-tapping screws, when bone has grown into the flutes at their tips so that it is impossible to turn them. When screws cannot be turned and it is imperative to remove the plate, their heads may be cut off with a diamond wheel and the shafts of the screws removed with the help of a trephine.

Medullary nails are probably better removed in all cases and certainly if they cause discomfort, especially by sticking out too far. It should be remembered, however, that progressive expulsion of a nail is a sign that the fracture is still moving.

The patient should be so placed as to render the proximal end of the nail most easily accessible and this end should then be displayed, which makes it much easier to engage the extractor hook firmly. If it should happen that the nail jams while only partly out, it should be cut short with a hacksaw.

References

Allgöwer, M., Perren, S. M. and Matter, P. (1970). 'A new plate for internal fixation – the dynamic compression plate (DCP).' *Injury* **2**, 40
Heim, U. and Pfeiffer, K. M. (1974). *Small Fragment Set Manual*. Berlin: Springer-Verlag New York: Heidelberg
Lowbury, E. J. L. and Lilley, H. A. (1975). 'Gloved hand as applicator of antiseptic to operation sites.' *The Lancet* **II**, 153
Müller, M. E., Allgöwer, M. and Willenegger, H. (1970). *Manual of Internal Fixation*. Berlin: Springer-Verlag New York: Heidelberg

[*The illustrations for this Chapter on General Techniques of Internal Fixation of Fractures were drawn by Mr. G. Lyth.*]

External Fixation of Fractures

John D. M. Stewart, F.R.C.S.(Eng.)
Consultant Orthopaedic Surgeon, Chichester and Graylingwell,
and Worthing, Southlands and District Groups of Hospitals

INTRODUCTION

The correct management of a fracture entails reduction of the fracture, maintenance of that reduction and exercises, so that union of the fracture occurs in the best functional position as rapidly as possible, the development of joint stiffness is prevented or minimized and as much muscle power as possible is retained. In addition, demineralization of the skeleton is kept to a minimum, and the risk of pneumonia, venous thrombosis and renal calculi occurring is decreased. Traction is often used to achieve these aims.

TRACTION

Traction helps to counteract the deforming forces acting upon a fracture and to control the amount and direction of movement which can occur at a fracture site, thus aiding the healing of bone and soft tissues.

To apply traction a satisfactory hold must be obtained on the affected part of the body. The traction force must be applied, in the case of a limb, through the skin – *skin traction* – or direct to the skeleton – *skeletal traction*.

1&2

When traction is applied, countertraction, acting in the opposite direction, must also be applied to prevent the body from being pulled in the direction of the traction force. When countertraction acts through an appliance which obtains purchase on a part of the body, the arrangement is called *fixed traction*. When the weight of all or part of the body, acting under the influence of gravity, is used to provide countertraction, the arrangement is called *sliding traction*.

Fixed traction can maintain, but not obtain, the reduction of a fracture. Sliding traction can be used for both purposes, but as the initial traction weight required to obtain the reduction of a fracture, in a sliding traction arrangement, is greater than that required to maintain the reduction, great care must be taken to avoid distraction of the fracture.

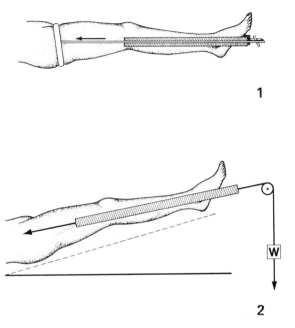

SKIN TRACTION

Skin traction is used in preference to skeletal traction in the treatment of lower limb fractures in children, and in adults when the traction force required is not great.

The traction force is applied over a large area of skin, to spread the load, by using either adhesive or non-adhesive strapping. Skin traction needs frequent re-application.

The maximum traction weight that can be used with skin traction is 15 lb (6·7 kg).

Prepared Elastoplast Skin Traction Kits for use in children or adults are available, or the necessary apparatus can be assembled. For patients who are allergic to adhesive strapping containing zinc oxide, other adhesive preparations can be used.

Contra-indications to skin traction

Contra-indications to skin traction are: abrasions or lacerations of the skin over the area to which the traction is to be applied; impairment of circulation — varicose ulcers, impending gangrene, stasis dermatitis; and marked over-riding of the bony fragments, which indicates that the traction weight required is greater than can be applied through the skin.

Application of non-adhesive (Ventfoam bandage) skin traction

Ventfoam skin traction bandage is applied basically as described above. Shaving is not required. The foam surface lies next to the skin. The traction weight should not exceed 10 lb (4·5 kg).

Complications of skin traction

Complications of skin traction are: allergic reaction to the adhesive; excoriation of the skin from wrinkling or slipping of the adhesive strapping; pressure sores around the malleoli and over the tendo Achillis. Common peroneal nerve palsy may result from pressure on the nerve by the strapping and encircling bandage sliding downwards until they are halted at the head of the fibula, or by the slings, on which the limbs rests, when lateral rotation of the limb is not prevented.

3 a-d

Application of adhesive skin traction

(*a*) The area of skin to which the strapping is to be applied is shaved (shaving is not required with Orthotrac or Skin-Trac).

(*b*) The malleoli are protected with a strip of felt, foam rubber or a few turns of bandage under the strapping.

(*c*) Starting at the ankle but leaving a loop projecting 4–6 inches (10–15 cm) beyond the sole of the foot, the widest possible strapping is applied to both sides of the limb, parallel to a line between the lateral malleolus and the greater trochanter. On the lateral aspect, the strapping must lie slightly behind, and on the medial aspect slightly in front of, this line to encourage medial rotation of the limb. There should be no wrinkles or creases in the strapping, which can be nicked, if necessary, to ensure that it lies flat. The malleoli, tibial crest and patella should be avoided.

(*d*) A crêpe or elasticated bandage is applied over the strapping, again starting at the ankle. A spreader bar or cords are attached to the distal end of the strapping and the required traction weight can then be applied.

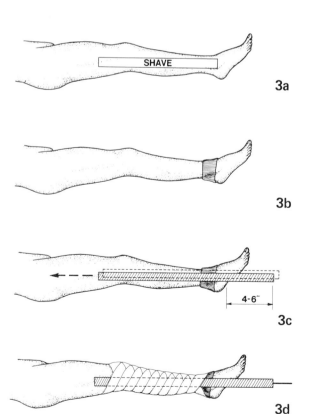

3a

3b

3c

3d

SKELETAL TRACTION

Skeletal traction is used chiefly in adults in the management of dislocations of the hip, certain fractures of the femur and tibia and in fractures and fracture-dislocations of the cervical spine (skull traction). Its use is avoided generally in children and in the management of fractures of the upper limb.

In skeletal traction the traction force is applied directly to the skeleton. For a limb, a metal pin (Steinmann or Denham) or a wire (Kirschner) is driven through the bone. For the cervical spine, a special clamp (Crutchfield tongs) is applied to the skull.

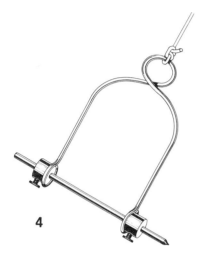

4

Steinmann pin

Steinmann pins are rigid stainless steel pins of varying length, 4–6 mm in diameter. After insertion either a special stirrup (Böhler) or hooks with swivelling connections are attached, to allow the direction of pull to be varied without turning the pin in the bone.

Denham pin

The Denham pin is identical to the Steinmann pin except for a short threaded length, situated towards the end held in the introducer, which engages the bony cortex and thus reduces the risk of the pin sliding in the bone. It is particularly suitable for use in the calcaneus or in osteoporotic bone.

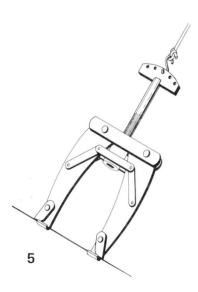

5

Kirschner wire

A Kirschner wire is of small diameter and is insufficiently rigid until pulled taught in a special stirrup (Kirschner). The wire easily cuts out of bone if a heavy traction weight is applied, and rotation of the wire occurs with rotation of the stirrup. It can be used in the lower limb but is used more often in the upper limb.

Common sites for application of skeletal traction

6a

Lower end of femur

Just proximal to the most superior bony protrusion of the lateral femoral condyle. Alternatively, a line is drawn from before backwards at the level of the upper pole of the patella and a second line is drawn from below upwards anterior to the head of the fibula; where these two lines intersect is the point of insertion.

To minimize knee stiffness, the metal pin at the lower end of the femur should be removed after 2–3 weeks and replaced by one through the upper end of the tibia.

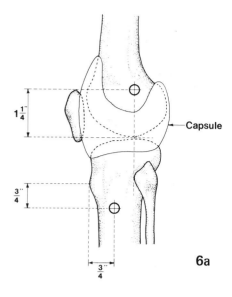

6a

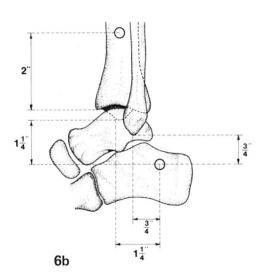

6b

6b

Upper end of tibia

Three-quarters of an inch (2 cm) behind the crest, just below the level of the tubercle of the tibia.

Lower end of tibia

Two inches (5 cm) above the level of the ankle joint, mid-way between the anterior and posterior borders of the tibia.

Calcaneus

Three-quarters of an inch (2 cm) below and behind the lateral malleolus. This corresponds with a point 1 1/4 inches (3 cm) below and behind the medial malleolus.

Insertion of a Steinmann pin

General or local anaesthesia is given. With the latter the skin and periosteum must be infiltrated.

The skin is shaved locally.

Using full aseptic precautions, the skin is painted with iodine and skin towels are draped under and around the limb.

An assistant holds the ankle at right angles, with the toes pointing straight up.

The pin is mounted in the introducer and the site of insertion identified.

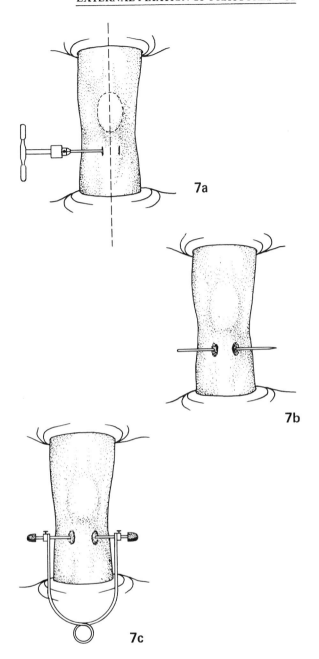

7a

7a

The pin, held horizontally and at right angles to the long axis of the limb, is driven from lateral to medial, through the skin and the bone with a gentle twisting motion of the forearm, while keeping the flexed elbow against the side of the body. The surgeon must take care not to place his other hand over the exit point of the pin. He should also ensure that the skin is not tight around the pin.

7b

7b

A small cotton wool pad, soaked in Benzomastic, is applied around the pin on each side, to seal the wounds. Two separate pads should always be used. A strip of gauze wound back and forth across the shin and around the pin may cause a pressure sore.

7c

The Böhler stirrup is fitted and guards are applied over the ends of the pin.

7c

Complications of skeletal traction

Infection

Unless full aseptic precautions are taken, infection can be introduced into the bone when the metal pin or wire is either inserted or removed. Infection can extend also along the pin tract from the skin wound. This is likely to occur if the skin does not encircle the pin closely or if the pin rotates or moves in and out of the bone.

Delayed union

As a much greater traction force can be applied with skeletal traction, it is possible to distract the fracture, causing delay in union. It is better to allow ½ inch (1·25 cm) of overlap than to risk distraction.

Fracture

The bone may be splintered during insertion of the pin.

Joint stiffness

Stiffness of neighbouring joints can result either from the joint being entered during the incorrect placing of the pin, or by the promotion of fibrosis in the muscles moving the joint.

Pin loosening

Rarely, the pin or wire may cut out of the bone. This is more likely to occur when the bone is porotic or a Kirschner wire is used.

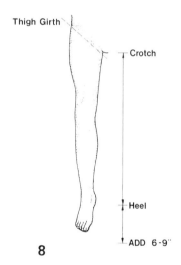

8

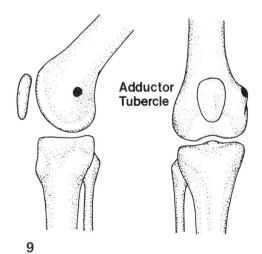

9

SPLINTS

A splint may support a limb only or it may be an integral part of the traction arrangement (fixed traction). The Thomas' splint is used most commonly. The Fisk splint may also be used (*see* page 87).

THOMAS' SPLINT

The Thomas' splint is made in different sizes. It consists of a padded leather covered oval metal ring to which are attached two side-bars. These bars bisect the oval ring, are of unequal length so that the ring is set at an angle of 120° to the inner side-bar, and are joined together distally in the form of a 'W'. The outer side-bar may be angled 2 inches (5 cm) below the ring, to clear a prominent greater trochanter.

8

How to choose a Thomas' splint

To obtain the *internal* circumference of the padded ring, the oblique circumference of the thigh is measured immediately below the gluteal fold and ischial tuberosity, in line with the inclination of the ring of the splint. This measurement must be accurate if fixed traction is intended. Accuracy is not so important with sliding traction. (This measurement can be taken from the uninjured limb to avoid causing pain, but one must remember to allow for swelling of the injured thigh.)

The distance from the crotch to the heel is measured and 6–9 inches (15–23 cm) are added to determine the length of the inner side-bar.

9

Knee-flexion piece

When a knee-flexion piece is used in conjunction with a Thomas' splint, the hinge, to coincide with the axis of movement of the knee joint, must lie level with the adductor tubercle (*see Illustration 11*).

How to prepare a splint

Slings are fashioned between the side-bars.

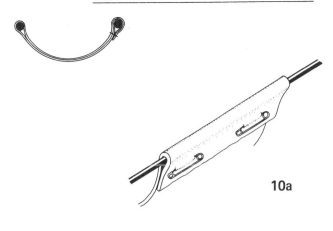

10a

An adequate length of 6 inches (15 cm) wide Domette bandage is cut and passed around the inner side-bar; then the two ends are passed over the outer side-bar and fastened to the sling so formed with two large safety pins. This ensures that later the tension of the sling can be adjusted easily to avoid excessive pressure on the skin or to assist in the management of the fracture.

10a

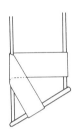
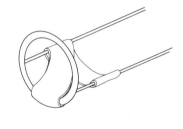

10b

10b

To avoid leaving a triangular area of thigh unsupported proximally, the length of Domette bandage is passed around the ring of the splint and the side-bars.

10c

The distal sling is ended 2$\frac{1}{2}$ inches (6 cm) above the back of the heel to avoid pressure sores developing over the tendo Achillis.

The slings are lined with Gamgee tissue. One large pad 6 by 9 inches (15 by 23 cm) and about 2 inches (5 cm) thick when compressed is fashioned from Gamgee tissue and placed under the lower thigh to maintain the normal anterior bowing of the femoral shaft.

Tubigrip, placed over the end of the splint, instead of individual slings, can be used to support that part of the limb which is not fractured.

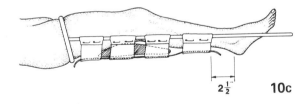

2$\frac{1}{2}$" 10c

Reduction of a femoral shaft fracture and application of fixed traction in a Thomas' splint

Skin traction is used for children, and skeletal traction with an upper tibial Steinmann pin (Denham pin for the elderly) with a Böhler stirrup, for adults.

The prepared splint is passed under the limb.

The dorsalis pedis and posterior tibial pulses are palpated.

The radiographs are studied to determine the type of fracture.

Transverse fractures

An assistant holds the Böhler stirrup and exerts traction in the long axis of the limb, simultaneously forcing the ring of the splint against the ischial tuberosity.

The surgeon stands at the side of the limb, grips the limb above and below the fracture site and manipulates the fracture, reducing the distal fragment to the proximal fragment.

Maintaining traction, he carefully lowers the limb onto the prepared splint, with the large pad under the lower part of the thigh, and then arranges the tension in the other slings to allow 15–20° of flexion at the knee.

Traction cords are attached to each end of the Steinmann pin and tied to the lower end of the splint.

The pull on the Böhler stirrup is released.

Anteroposterior and lateral radiographs are taken to check the reduction of the fracture. If necessary the fracture is remanipulated.

The pulses are palpated and if they are absent the traction force is reduced. If the pulses do not return, the fracture should be very gently remanipulated. If the pulses are still absent, arteriography and open exploration are required. If the pulses are present and the reduction is satisfactory, the Böhler stirrup is removed and the thigh is bandaged into the splint.

The splint is then suspended.

Finally, a 5 lb (2·3 kg) traction weight is attached to the end of the splint to reduce partly the pressure of the padded ring of the splint around the root of the limb.

Oblique, spiral or comminuted fractures

Formal manipulation of these fractures is not required. Traction is applied in the long axis of the limb until the fractured femur is restored to its correct length, and traction is maintained until the traction cords are tied to the lower end of the splint. Placement of the large pad, radiography, palpation of peripheral pulses and suspension of the Thomas' splint are as described above.

*Sliding traction with a Thomas' splint and
Pearson knee-flexion piece*

This method is often used to obtain and then maintain the reduction of a spiral, oblique or comminuted fracture of the shaft of the femur. Knee flexion controls rotation, prevents the development of laxity of the posterior capsule and cruciate ligaments of the knee, and allows variation in the direction of pull when an upper tibial Steinmann pin is used.

11

The correct size of splint is chosen, and the splint and the knee-flexion piece are prepared.

An upper tibial Steinmann pin is inserted.

The prepared splint is passed under the limb, and the limb is rested on the slings. The large pad is placed under the lower part of the thigh.

The hinge of the knee-flexion piece is checked to ensure that it is placed correctly opposite the adductor tubercle.

The distal end of the knee-flexion piece is suspended from the distal end of the splint, by two cords, one on each side, so that the knee is flexed 20–30°.

The splint is then suspended (*see Illustrations 12 and 13*).

The position of the thigh pad and the tension in the sling supporting the pad are adjusted to obtain the normal anterior bowing of the femoral shaft.

The thigh is bandaged into the splint.

A Böhler stirrup and a cord are attached to the Steinmann pin.

The cord is passed over a pulley at the foot of the bed so that the line of the cord is in line with the shaft of the femur.

A weight is attached to the cord.

Finally, the foot of the bed is elevated.

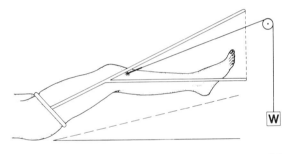

11

The exact traction weight required is determined by trial and observing the behaviour of the fracture, since it depends upon the site of the fracture, the age and weight of the patient, the power of his muscles, the amount of muscle damage, the degree of friction in the traction system and whether the traction weight is being used to reduce the fracture or only to maintain a reduction.

For fractures of the femoral shaft an initial traction weight of 10–20 lb (4·5–9·1 kg) is usually sufficient for an average adult, and 2–10 lb (1·0–4·5 kg) for an average child. The heavier the traction weight used, the higher the foot of the bed must be raised to provide countertraction.

Methods of suspending a Thomas' splint

A Thomas' splint may be suspended from an overhead frame — a Balkan beam — in a number of different ways using cords, pulleys and weights.

12

Method 1

A small loop of cord is formed between the side-bars at each end of the splint.

A suspension cord is tied to the centre of each loop.

The suspension cords are passed up and cranially to two pulleys. From these pulleys the cords are passed over another two pulleys, situated at the head or foot of the bed, and then attached to weights.

Rotation of the splint is controlled by moving the point of attachment of the suspension cords to the proximal and distal loops.

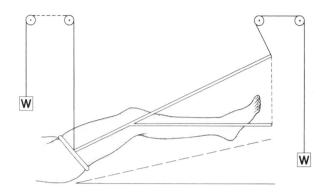

12

13

Method 2

Two lengths of cord are tied, one on each side, to each end of the splint.

Each cord is passed over a pulley.

A suspension weight is attached *firmly* to both cords at a point nearer the pelvis.

Rotation of the splint is controlled by adjusting the length of the cords tied to each end of the splint.

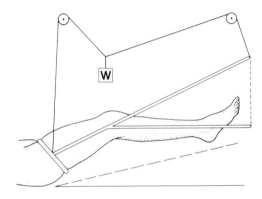

13

FISK SPLINT

14

The groin ring, the front half of which is a padded strap and buckle, is attached by swivel joints to the side-bars, so that the same splint can be used for either limb. The distal ends of the side-bars are connected, just beyond the knee, by a squared-off frame which has two small eyelets at each upper corner. The knee-flexion piece is fixed to the side-bars, just proximal to the squared-off frame, through off-set double-cog hinges. The side-bars of the thigh and the knee-flexion parts of the splint are adjustable telescopically to allow all lengths of lower limb to be accommodated.

Telescopically Adjustable

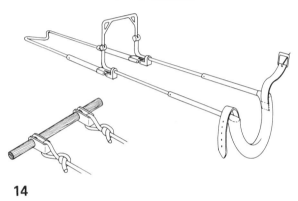

14

Sliding traction with a Fisk splint

The splint is adjusted to fit the limb and then slings are fashioned to support the thigh and calf.

An upper tibial Steinmann pin is inserted.

The prepared splint is passed under the limb.

Traction cords, which must be long enough to clear the foot, are attached to each end of the Steinmann pin and tied to a transverse wooden rod about 6 inches (15 cm) long.

Then the fracture is manipulated.

The position of the thigh pad is adjusted to maintain the normal anterior bowing of the femoral shaft, and the position of the knee hinge is checked.

A single cord is tied to the centre of the wooden rod, passed over a pulley at the foot of the bed and a weight attached. After 6 weeks the initial traction weight is reduced to 6–8 lb (2·6–3·6 kg).

The splint is suspended (*see below*).

Finally, the foot of the bed is elevated.

15

Suspension of a Fisk splint

The ends of a long loop of cord are tied to the eyelets at the corners of the squared-off frame.

The loop is passed upwards and cranially over a pulley situated over the patient's abdomen so that when the hip is flexed to 45°, the cord is at right angles to the long axis of the femur.

A single suspension weight of 4–8 lb (1·8–3·6 kg) is attached to the loop by a slip knot. This loop of cord must be long enough so that the suspension weight hangs within easy reach of the patient.

The distal end of the knee-flexion piece is suspended by a length of cord looped over the overhead frame. The length of this cord is such that when the hip is flexed 45°, the leg is horizontal.

Rotation is controlled by varying the length of the cord attached to the knee-flexion piece and by varying the length of each arm of the loop attached to the squared-off frame.

After suspending the splint, one should check that the *traction* cord is in line with the shaft of the femur when the hip is flexed 45°.

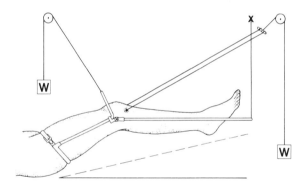

15

In the Fisk splint the patient, as soon as possible, flexes his hip and at the same time flexes his knee and dorsiflexes his ankle, assisting the movement by pulling downwards on the suspension weight. He then actively extends his hip and knee and plantar-flexes his ankle while gradually releasing the pull on the suspension weight. Passive movements are not encouraged.

BUCK'S TRACTION

Buck's traction is used in the temporary management of fractures of the femoral neck in adults and of the femoral shaft in older and larger children. Lateral rotation of the limb is not controlled by this method.

16

Application of Buck's traction

Below-knee skin traction is applied.

The leg is supported on a soft pillow to keep the heel clear of the bed.

The cord is passed from the spreader over a pulley attached to the foot of the bed.

A weight of 5—7 lb (2·3—3·2 kg) is attached to the cord.

The foot of the bed is then elevated.

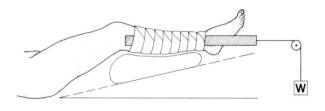

16

HAMILTON RUSSELL TRACTION

Hamilton Russell traction can be used in the management of fractures of the shaft and trochanteric regions of the femur and after arthroplasty operations on the hip.

17

Application of Hamilton Russell traction

Below-knee skin traction is applied.

A pulley is attached to the spreader.

A soft broad canvas sling is placed under the knee.

The limb is supported on two soft pillows, one above and the other below the knee, with the knee slightly flexed and the heel clear of the bed.

A length of cord is tied to the knee sling.

The cord is passed from the knee sling over pulley A, which is placed well distal (*not* proximal) to the knee, around one of the pulleys B, around pulley C and then around the other pulley B before being attached to a weight. The pulleys B must be at the same level as the foot when the leg is lying horizontally on a pillow.

A weight is attached to the cord. Generally, a weight of 8 lb (3·6 kg) is used for adults and 0·5—4 lb (0·28—1·8 kg) for children.

Theoretically the two pulley blocks B double the pull on the limb, but in practice the pull is modified by the friction present in the system. The resultant of the two forces acting along all the cords produces a pull in the line of the femoral shaft. In an alternative arrangement, two cords can be used, each cord passing over pulleys to separate weights.

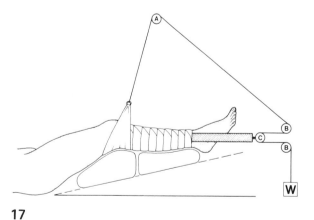

17

TULLOCH BROWN TRACTION

18a

Tulloch Brown, or U-loop tibial pin, traction and suspension with a Nissen foot-plate and stirrup are used in the management of a fracture or fracture-dislocation of the hip, fracture of the shaft of the femur or after an arthroplasty or pseudarthrosis operation on the hip. It is not used in children.

Nissen Stirrup

Footplate

U - Loop

18a

18b

Application of Tulloch Brown traction

A Steinmann or Denham pin is inserted through the upper end of the tibia.

The U-loop is slipped over the ends of the Steinmann pin, ensuring that it lies evenly on each side of the leg.

The leg is supported on slings from the U-loop. The slings which are lined with Gamgee tissue should not be tight; otherwise compression of the tissues of the calf will occur.

The Nissen stirrup is attached to the Steinmann pin.

The detachable Perspex foot-plate is mounted on the U-loop to support the foot.

Two pulleys and cords with weights or the Hamilton Russell system are used for traction and suspension.

The correct rotation of the limb is obtained by varying the attachment of the cord to the Nissen stirrup.

The foot of the bed is elevated.

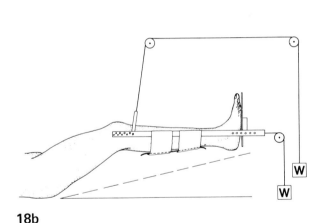

18b

GALLOWS TRACTION

Gallows traction is convenient and reasonably safe for the treatment of fractures of the shaft of the femur in children up to the age of 2 years. Vascular complications may occur in either the injured or the normal limb due to the reduction in blood pressure in the lower limbs which occurs with elevation. These are more likely to occur between the ages of 2 and 4 years, but their occurrence is less likely if posterior gutter splints are applied to keep the knees in slight flexion. *Over the age of 4 years the use of gallows traction is absolutely contra-indicated.*

19

Application of gallows traction

Adhesive skin traction is applied to *both* lower limbs.

The traction cords are tied to an overhead beam.

The cords are tightened sufficiently to raise the child's buttocks just clear of the mattress.

The state of the circulation in the limbs should be checked frequently because of the dangers of vascular complications. (*1*) Observe the colour and temperature of *both feet*. (*2*) Dorsiflex *both ankles* passively. *Dorsiflexion should be full and painless.* If dorsiflexion is limited or painful, muscle ischaemia may be present; therefore the limbs should be lowered and all bandaging and adhesive strapping removed immediately.

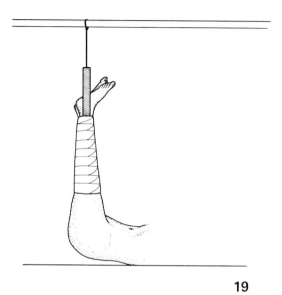

19

SLIDING TRACTION WITH A BÖHLER-BRAUN FRAME

Sliding traction with a Böhler-Braun frame can be used for the management of unstable fractures of the tibia. Skeletal traction is commonly used.

20

Application of sliding traction with a Böhler-Braun frame

Slings are fashioned between the sides of the frame to support the thigh and leg; the slings are covered with Gamgee tissue.

A Steinmann or Denham pin is inserted where necessary. Frequently an above-knee, well-padded plaster cast is applied, incorporating the pin, when a tibial fracture is being treated.

A Böhler stirrup is attached to the pin.

The limb is placed on the slings.

A cord is attached to the stirrup and passed over the required pulley.

A 7–10 lb (3·2–4·5 kg) weight is attached to the cord.

The foot of the bed is elevated.

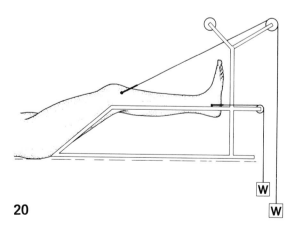

20

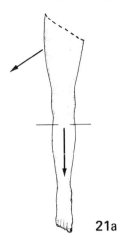

LATERAL TRACTION THROUGH UPPER END OF FEMUR

21a

In central fracture-dislocations of the hip, skeletal traction in the long axis of the femur (Tulloch Brown traction) may be coupled with lateral traction through the upper end of the femur to restore the relationship between the dome of the acetabulum and the weight-bearing portion of the femoral head.

21a

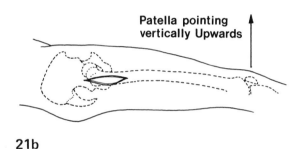

Patella pointing vertically Upwards

21b

Application of lateral traction through upper end of femur

General anaesthesia and full aseptic precautions are used. *Do not place* a sandbag under either buttock.

21b

A small longitudinal incision is made centred just below the most prominent part of the greater trochanter on the affected side and is then deepened down to bone.

21c

The point on the lateral surface of the femur 1 inch (2·5 cm) below the most prominent part of the greater trochanter mid-way between the anterior and posterior surfaces of the femur is identified.

An assistant is asked to rotate medially the lower limb so that the patella points vertically upwards. This eliminates the normal forward angulation (ante-version) of the femoral neck and ensures that the femoral neck is lying horizontally.

A hole is drilled in the lateral cortex of the femur, using the correct size of drill for the coarse-threaded screw or bolt.

A finger is placed on the femoral artery at the groin (this point lies over the head of the femur).

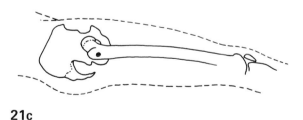

21c

21d & e

The drill is held horizontally and directed cranially and medially towards the finger on the femoral artery. The drill will thus be directed up the neck of the femur.

A hole 1·5—2 inches (3·75—5 cm) deep is then drilled.

The drill is removed and the coarse-threaded screw or bolt inserted. This should be 3—4 inches (7·5—10 cm) long.

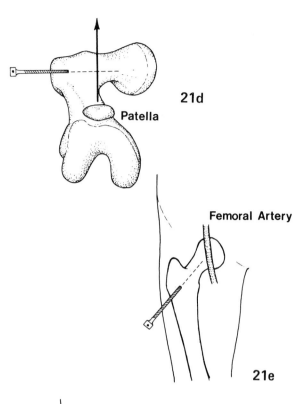

21d

Patella

Femoral Artery

21e

21f

A length of stainless steel wire is attached to the end of the screw or bolt, and brought out through the wound.

The wound is sutured.

A cord is attached to the stainless steel wire and passed over a pulley at the side of the bed to a traction weight of 3—15 lb (3·6—6·7 kg).

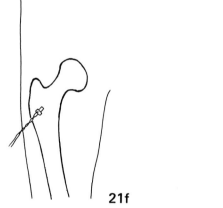

21f

21g

The patient's bed is arranged to tilt in two planes, the foot of the bed being highest on the affected side and the head of the bed lowest on the unaffected side. This is achieved by using three wooden blocks of two different heights.

Active movement of the hip and knee is encouraged.

Lateral traction is continued for 3—4 weeks and Tulloch Brown traction for a total of 8—10 weeks.

As an alternative to a screw or bolt, a Denham pin can be inserted through the greater trochanter in an anteroposterior direction with some lateral inclination. The disadvantages of this method are that pin tract infection is likely to occur, and the posterior end of the Denham pin sticks into the mattress, making it uncomfortable for the patient.

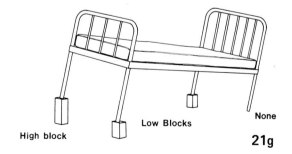

High block

Low Blocks

None

21g

[The illustrations for this Chapter on External Fixation of Fractures were drawn by Mr. J. M. P. Booth.]

Fractures of the Long Bones of the Upper Limb

D. J. Fuller, M.S., F.R.C.S.
Consultant Orthopaedic Surgeon,
Nuffield Orthopaedic Centre and Radcliffe Infirmary, Oxford

INTRODUCTION

The long bones of the upper limb are not as strong as their counterpart in the lower limb and they are, therefore, fractured more easily and frequently. Most fractures of the lower limb require accurate reduction and secure fixation but it is important to appreciate that the majority of the common upper limb fractures are best treated by simple conservative means; surgery must be reserved for special indications. This chapter will cover the principles of the treatment of upper limb fractures and then consider the special indications for surgery. The procedures which have been chosen for illustration combine to give a comprehensive surgical approach to long bones in the arm.

General assessment

Most upper limb fractures result from a fall on to a hand which is thrown out for protection. The impact is thus transferred through the entire length of the limb and it is common to find more than one injury in the same limb. A fracture of the lower radius in a child often occurs together with a supracondylar fracture of the elbow and the commonest of all fractures — a Colles' fracture — is frequently associated with a sprain of the rotator cuff of the shoulder joint and the residual disability usually affects the shoulder rather than the wrist or hand. It is, therefore, recommended that in all cases of upper limb fracture the surgeon should examine the remainder of the limb in detail and the primary x-ray examination must include any suspicious secondary areas.

Most fractures in the upper limb unite readily and the treatment programme need only be designed to achieve good function. Again, this contrasts with fractures of the lower limb where delayed or fibrous union is encountered more frequently. The forces involved in fracturing a lower limb bone are often considerable, whereas the forces generated by a fall on to the hand are less violent and closed indirect injuries usually result in the upper limb. Serious soft tissue damage is, therefore, a less common feature of arm fractures than of broken bones in the leg.

The upper limb bones of the growing child not only unite rapidly after fracture but they also have a capacity for remodelling deformity. Surgery is only required for upper limb long bone fractures in children in specific circumstances and this topic will be expanded in the sections on individual fracture management.

There are three forms of conservative treatment available for fractures of the upper limb — external splintage, longitudinal traction and active joint movement. Each individual fracture must be assessed according to its owner, rather than a plaster timetable in a textbook, and an individual programme of treatment must be designed to give full function as rapidly and safely as possible. *The* complication of upper limb fractures is joint stiffness. The shoulder joint can stiffen permanently if a broken wrist is supported continuously in a sling for too long a period and the fingers can stiffen if a shoulder fracture is treated with a long period of passive dependence of the digits at the other extremity of the limb.

THE HUMERUS

Fractures of the humerus are usually closed injuries caused by indirect force. The vulnerable sites in this bone are the surgical neck and the shaft. A rotating force commonly fractures the neck of the humerus and this injury is frequently seen in the older person with soft bones; the fracture is often highly comminuted. The same force in a younger person is more likely to rupture the capsule of the shoulder joint and result in a dislocation. Surgical reduction of an uncomplicated fracture of the neck of the humerus in an elderly patient should not be contemplated. These fractures unite readily and a combination of longitudinal traction (which is applied very simply by the use of a collar and cuff sling) and early active movement of all the joints of the upper limb leads to restoration of adequate function. Occasionally these fractures combine with a dislocation and it is then necessary to reduce the dislocation element of this combination because a persisting unreduced shoulder dislocation often leads to unacceptable permanent discomfort. If this reduction cannot be accomplished by closed means surgery is required and the anterior approach described in the Chapter on 'Recurrent Dislocation of the Shoulder' (*Orthopaedics Part II*) gives excellent access for both anterior and posterior fracture-dislocations.

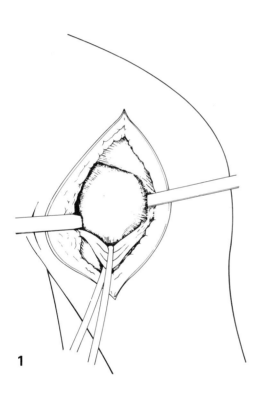

1

Occasionally a young adult will suffer a very violent force to the shoulder area and the neck of the humerus fractures together with the humeral head. Often a large fragment of the humeral head may dislocate and it is impossible to re-align the congruity of the joint without surgery. Operative reduction of the joint is justified in these circumstances and the anterior shoulder joint approach is adequate in most cases. If it is necessary to expose the posterior aspect of the upper humerus a full knowledge of the anatomy of the area is required before surgery. The vulnerable structure during this approach is the axillary nerve and inadvertent damage to this large nerve would lead to a very serious disability resulting from the continuation of post-traumatic shoulder stiffness plus deltoid paralysis. This approach to the posterior aspect of the humerus is only required occasionally in young people and the inexperienced surgeon is advised not to explore this unfamiliar area. The plane between the long head of the triceps muscle medially and the deltoid muscle laterally is readily found through a longitudinal incision centred posteriorly over the upper humerus. The neurovascular bundle containing the circumflex nerve and vessels is identified some 2 inches (5 cm) below the shoulder joint. These are large structures and are shown in the sketch with a protective tape.

Fractures of the surgical neck of the humerus in children are growth plate injuries and the potential for remodelling deformity is extremely high. This remodelling factor combined with the universal nature of the shoulder joint itself ensures a good functional result and these fractures in children should not be treated surgically.

Fractures of the shaft of the humerus are usually closed and uncomplicated. They unite well and, because the humeral shaft is surrounded by good muscle bulk, any minor malunion is well masked by the general contours of the upper arm. A small degree of rotatory malunion is also acceptable because the universal shoulder joint above the fracture ensures the continuing full range of movement of the upper limb. These injuries are usually treated by a combination of plaster splintage and longitudinal traction which is supplied by the weight of the arm when the hand is supported in a collar and cuff sling. This form of treatment has given good results for many years but these fractures may take 2–3 months to unite solidly and the elbow and shoulder stiffness which can result during this period may not resolve quickly.

2

Sarmiento (1977) has demonstrated that humeral shaft fractures can be satisfactorily splinted with a functional brace. Such a brace gives adequate splintage to the fracture and allows free shoulder and elbow joint movements from an early stage. The author recommends that a light, strong, thermoplastic splint (*see Illustration 2*) is moulded and cut to form a supporting cylindrical tube around the humerus. The shoulder joint and elbow joint should have freedom of movement and the splint can be tightened by two Velcro fasteners, as illustrated. During the first 1–2 weeks it is also necessary to wear a collar and cuff support because of the initial discomfort. As soon as possible the patient is encouraged to discard the collar and cuff and actively use the entire upper limb. The splint is worn until consolidated union of the fracture is demonstrated. Many patients using this splint will return to work at an early stage and joint stiffness is reduced to a minimum.

There are few indications for surgical reduction and fixation of fractured shaft of humerus; perhaps the most obvious is the pathological fracture that occurs with metastatic bone cancer (most often breast cancer) where a rapid, strong fixation is required. The simplest and safest approach to the entire shaft of the humerus is the anterior approach.

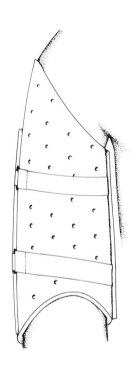

2

ANTERIOR EXPOSURE OF SHAFT OF HUMERUS

A general anaesthetic is recommended and the patient is positioned supine on the operating table. Some form of additional arm rest is required and this procedure is greatly helped if two assistants are readily available. The skin preparation should include the shoulder region and the drapes must be sealed around the root of the limb to give a good exposure of the shoulder area. The hand and forearm need to be draped separately but the elbow joint should be within the prepared sterile area.

3

The incision

The skin incision starts slightly to the lateral side of the anterior aspect of the upper arm and runs vertically down on the lateral side of the biceps muscle towards the elbow joint.

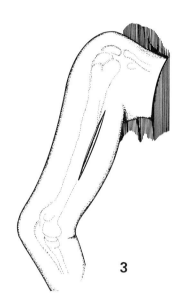

3

4

The exposure

Divide the superficial and deep fascia and locate the cephalic vein in the proximal part of the incision and ligate it. It is necessary now to identify the plane between the biceps muscle medially and the deltoid insertion laterally and this plane is found most easily at the lower level of the deltoid insertion. The biceps muscle is now retracted medially exposing the underlying brachialis muscle and this muscle should be incised in its mid-line longitudinally down to bone. The anterior aspect of the humerus has now been identified and the periosteum can be elevated medially and laterally from this mid-line incision. The radial nerve is well protected by the lateral substance of the brachialis muscle if the exposure is now contained within the humeral periosteum. It is, however, not advisable to use a bone lever on the lateral side of the humerus to aid exposure because this manoeuvre can stretch the radial nerve. If one assistant retracts the musculature with broad soft tissue retractors the second assistant can facilitate the exposure by flexing and extending the elbow as required. Elbow flexion relaxes the anterior structures and simplifies reduction of the fracture.

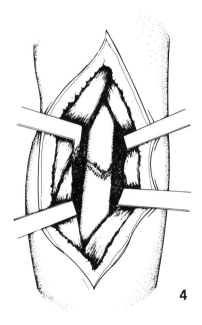

4

Fracture reduction

This approach affords a very wide exposure of the fractured ends of the bone and there should be no difficulty in achieving a ready reduction. A biopsy will often be required if the fracture is a pathological process through a metastasis and this fact should be remembered at this stage.

5

In the operation illustrated it was considered appropriate to internally fix the fracture with an intramedullary Küntscher nail and two cerclage wires. The nail fixation is often required for pathological bone where there is more than one weak area in the shaft. The extent of this exposure makes it an easy matter to apply a six or eight hole plate if necessary.

Closure

This area of the upper limb is highly vascular and it is recommended that a closed suction drain should be inserted before skin closure. The muscles are allowed to regain their normal positions and the author recommends that the deep fascia is not closed and a simple running vertical mattress skin suture is used. This gives a watertight closure and the suction drain prevents haematoma formation.

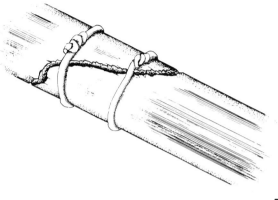

5

THE HEAD OF THE RADIUS

The vast majority of fractures of the head of the radius are comparatively trivial and are best treated conservatively. These injuries are accompanied by haemarthroses in the elbow joint and most patients will appreciate the comfort of a light plaster cast to immobilize the elbow for 1 week. At this stage the pain is diminishing rapidly and it is important to encourage the patient to use the elbow actively. There is usually no difficulty in co-operating with these simple instructions and a ready return of elbow movements can usually be anticipated.

If the fracture is highly comminuted or, if there is serious incongruity of the joint surface, surgery should be considered and the appropriate procedure is to excise the head of the radius. It is recommended that the decision for surgery should be made rapidly and, if operation is required it should be performed as a primary treatment, not after a 2–3 week delay when the elbow joint is beginning to recover from the initial trauma. Before embarking upon this operation the surgeon should have a clear knowledge of the precise anatomy of the posterior interosseous nerve. This nerve (rather like its counterpart, the lateral popliteal nerve in the leg) is particularly vulnerable to rough handling and because the nerve is not visualized during the procedure its exact course must be appreciated. The fragmented head of radius is commonly excised through a lateral approach and this gives good access, but the posterior interosseous nerve is vulnerable at the distal end of this exposure and if the incision has been planned too anteriorly the nerve may well be damaged. The author therefore recommends the posterolateral approach which gives excellent access and carries less risk of damage to this important nerve.

EXCISION OF THE HEAD OF THE RADIUS

The patient lies supine on the operating table and a pneumatic tourniquet is applied. The skin is cleaned and the drapes prepared to give access to the entire elbow joint and the upper half of the forearm. The elbow is flexed and is supported on an arm board and the exposure is assisted by a small sandbag placed beneath the medial aspect of the elbow.

6

The incision

Identify, by palpation, the lateral humeral epicondyle and, just distally, the position of the radial head. The skin incision now runs from the lateral epicondyle across the radial head obliquely towards the posterior surface of the ulna, some 2 inches (5 cm) distal below the tip of the elbow.

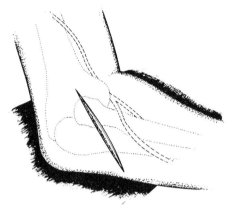

6

7

The exposure

The superficial fascia is divided and elevated and it is now necessary to identify the plane between the anconeus muscle on the ulnar side of the excision and the extensor carpi ulnaris muscle which is arising from the lateral humeral condyle. These two muscles have a confluent proximal tendinous origin and they diverge from each other. It is therefore best to seek the plane between the two muscles in the distal part of the incision. This plane should now be gently opened with dissecting scissors and it may be necessary by sharp dissection to free some of the extensor carpi ulnaris origin. The two muscles are then drawn apart with retractors and the capsule containing the head of the radius lies in the depth of the wound. Open the distal space of the incision to reveal the transverse fibres of the supinator muscles which run across the neck of the radius. These are the deep transverse fibres of the supinator muscle, extending from the posterior upper surface of the ulna to wind around the posterior upper surface of the radius. The posterior interosseous nerve lies superficial to these fibres and well anterior to the exposure. It may be necessary to release these transverse supinator fibres and the proximal inch of this muscle can be divided carefully with scissors. The capsule of the joint is now opened vertically and all of the radial head is well visualized. The fragments are removed and it is recommended that these separate pieces are retained and matched together to ensure that a major fragment is not overlooked. The neck of the radius is inspected, using a

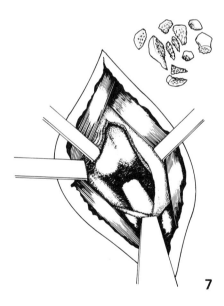

7

soft tissue retractor for the anterior structures (the vulnerable posterior interosseous nerve lies within these structures) and a bone lever only around the *ulnar* side of the neck of the radius. The fractured radial neck should be cleanly severed to leave a 0·75 inch gap between the articular surface of the humerus and the cut surface of the neck.

The capsule is closed with an absorbable suture.

8a & b

Closure

The author's method of closing skin for all medium and small wounds is illustrated. The skin edges are approximated by a subcuticular Dexon suture. The free ends of the Dexon are then pulled tautly and the skin closure is re-inforced with three or four wide Steristrip adhesive paper closures. The ends of the Dexon suture are then severed flush with the skin and they retract leaving a closed wound with no suture material visible. This method gives a satisfactorily cosmetic scar and obviates the need for suture removal. The Steristrips are a necessary adjunct to prevent a tendency for slight wound gaping because the subcuticular suture has no anchorage points.

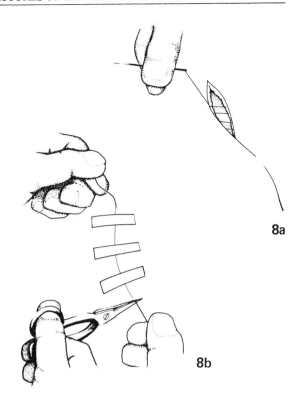

8a

8b

FRACTURES OF SHAFT OF RADIUS AND ULNA

Fractures of the radius and ulna can occur separately, together, with or without dislocations of the superior or inferior radio-ulnar joints in the growing child and in the adult. These many combinations do not make for a complex programme of treatment if certain simple principles are followed.

The shape of the radius and ulna has been designed to allow 180° of rotatory movement of the hand. A minor abnormality of the shape of either bone leads to an abnormal relationship of these two bones during rotatory movement and pronation or supination can be blocked. A loss of pronation or supination is a significant disability and the principle that governs the treatment of fractures of these two bones is that perfect anatomy should be restored. This contrasts with the general principle of the management of upper limb fractures described above. In the mature bones there is no compensatory remodelling process and the author recommends that an early surgical reduction and internal fixation should be performed for these injuries whenever there has been displacement of the original fracture.

Fractures of the radius and ulna in children have a variable capacity to remodel a malunion deformity. This capacity is maximal at the distal end of the radius in infancy. It appears (author's current unpublished research) that the most severe angulation deformities in the lower third of the radius and ulna will remodel satisfactorily up to the age of 12 years. A very young child has considerable capacity to remodel any angulation or even rotational deformity in the mid-shaft of the radius and ulna but this capacity fades rapidly between the ages of 6 and 8 years and a significant malunion of the mid-shaft of radius and/or ulna at the age of 9 years is unlikely to remodel satisfactorily. It is therefore recommended that all forearm fractures in children should be treated by closed reduction and plaster splintage with great care to prevent angular or rotational deformity. If this policy fails, and if the child is aged 9 years or over and the deformity is in the mid-shaft of the radius and the ulna, the fracture should be treated by open reduction and internal fixation.

OPEN REDUCTION OF FRACTURED SHAFTS OF RADIUS AND ULNA

The patient is positioned supine on the operating table and a pneumatic tourniquet is applied. The limb should be rested on an additional arm support and the skin is prepared and the towels are draped to expose the elbow joint and all of the forearm to the wrist joint. The arm is laid on the support with the hand facing downwards.

9

The incision

The radial exposure is performed first. A 6 inch (15 cm) skin incision is centred over the site of the fracture and runs longitudinally down the dorsolateral aspect of the forearm.

10

The exposure

The superficial fascia is opened and the deep fascia which is a strong envelope in the forearm is incised along the line of the bone. It is necessary to open the plane between extensor digitorum communis and extensor carpi radialis brevis and this division is readily found at the junction of the middle and lower thirds of the forearm where the long thumb extensor and abductors emerge from the depths of the forearm to pass between these two muscles. The proximal plane between the two muscles is opened further by separation with dissecting scissors. This manoeuvre reveals the tendon of the pronator teres inserting into the radius and, more proximally, the lower fibres of the supinator muscle which are running from the ulna obliquely into the radius — these fibres are running in the opposite direction to the insertion of the pronator teres. Again, the vulnerable structure is the posterior interosseous nerve and the nerve appears on the superficial surface of the supinator muscle about three fingers' breadth down from the elbow joint.

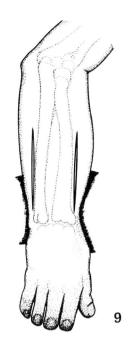

9

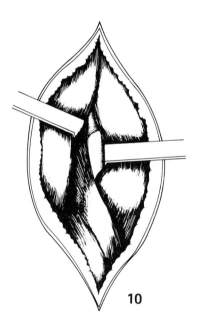

10

11

The radial fracture can now be exposed by subperiosteal dissection and in the distal part of the incision care has to be exercised in the handling of the thumb muscles and tendons which run superficially over the distal fragment. In the proximal part of the wound the incision of radial periosteum should be carried around to the extreme radial side of the bone beyond the insertion of the supinator muscle into the bone. A subperiosteal exposure of the radius now elevates the insertion of the supinator muscle and the posterior interosseous nerve is well protected. It must now be ensured that the fractured radius can be accurately reduced by manipulation. Do not fix the radial fracture at this stage because it may not be possible to reduce the ulnar fracture if the radius is immobilized.

It is now necessary to expose the ulnar fracture.

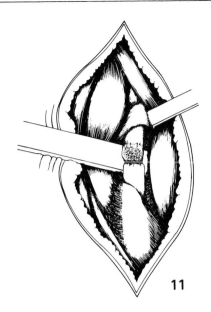

The incision

Palpate the posterior surface of the ulna and identify the subcutaneous border. This lies between the extensor and flexor carpi ulnaris muscles and the skin incision should run vertically along this surface. Again, some 6 inches (15 cm) of skin incision will be re-quired and this should be centred on the fracture. It is a little more difficult to approach the ulna with the arm lying palm down on an arm support and the exposure is facilitated by lifting the arm upwards on sandbags and fully pronating the hand.

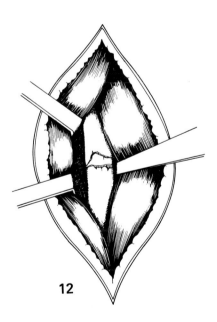

12

The exposure

Open the superficial and deep fascia and carefully define the subcutaneous border some distance away from the fracture site. Make a periosteal incision along this border and reflect the periosteum to give an easy exposure of the ulna and its fracture. Manipulate the broken ends of the ulna to secure an accurate reduction of the fracture and apply a six-hole plate (the A.O. equipment is recommended and a flat dynamic compression plate is ideal for this fracture) and lightly clamp the plate in position.

13

Now return to the radial fracture and again reduce this fracture. If this manoeuvre is prevented by the fixation of the ulna, the ulnar clamps and plate can be temporarily removed. There is usually no difficulty in re-reducing the radius once the ulna is held in its correct alignment. A semitubular six-hole plate is appropriate for the radius and the radial fixation should now be secured. Considerable care should be taken during the drilling of the radius because the anterior interosseous nerve is a relatively immobile structure on the deep surface of the bone. The drill should be protected by a sleeve which prevents over-drilling of the anterior compartment of the arm.

The ulnar plate can now be screwed in position and the wounds closed with suction drainage to each compartment.

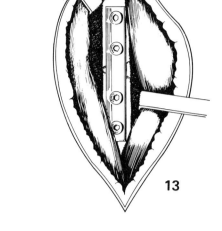

13

SMITH'S FRACTURE

14

A fall on to the dorsum of the hand can fracture the lower radius with anterior displacement of the distal fragment. This injury can present in one of three distinct patterns (Thomas, 1957). The true Smith fracture is a transverse fracture about 1 inch (2·5 cm) proximal to the wrist joint and it differs from a Colles fracture in the direction of the displacement. Closed reduction and plaster splintage is excellent treatment for this injury. The commonest of the three patterns is the highly comminuted fracture of the distal 1 inch (2·5 cm) of the lower radius and the many fragments displace anteriorly with no loss of overall congruity of the wrist joint. The author advises surgery (*see* below) whenever there is difficulty in maintaining a reduction by closed means or if a significant period of plaster immobilization is unacceptable. The third pattern of injury – Thomas' Type 2 fracture – is illustrated in the line drawing of a radiograph of such a fracture. The plane of the fracture is oblique and disrupts the anterior distal fragment of the lower end of the radius. The wrist joint capsule is not ruptured and the carpus is therefore carried anteriorly with the small fragment and there is a consequent subluxation

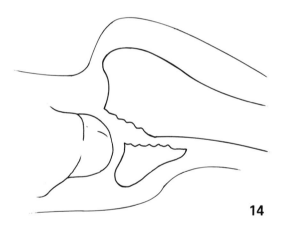

14

of the wrist joint. This fracture occurs characteristically in young adults and a perfect reduction is required to restore the congruity of the articular surface of the wrist joint. It is difficult to obtain and hold such a reduction by closed means and the author (Fuller, 1973) recommends that this injury should be treated electively by surgical reduction and internal fixation with an Ellis plate.

THE ELLIS PLATE OPERATION FOR SMITH'S FRACTURE

The patient lies supine on the operating table and a pneumatic tourniquet is employed. The skin of the hand and forearm are prepared for surgery and the drapes are secured to expose these areas. The hand is supinated and supported on an arm board attachment and a folded sterile towel positioned at the level of the wrist assists the hyperextension manoeuvre which is usually required later in the procedure when the fracture is reduced.

15

The incision

Incise the skin longitudinally on the ventral surface of the forearm over the front of the shaft of the lower radius. The incision should be 3 inches (7·5 cm) long and extends down to, but not across, the joint crease.

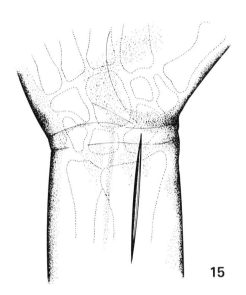

15

16a & b

Exposure

The superficial and deep fascia are divided and the tendon of flexor carpi radialis and the muscle of flexor pollicis longus which is inserted into its tendon at this level are identified. The plane between these two structures is opened and the thumb flexor retracted radially (this protects the radial artery) and the flexor carpi radialis to the ulnar side — the median nerve is retracted with the tendon. The pronator quadratus is seen at the base of the wound and in a recent fracture this muscle will be bulging with dark red haematoma from the underlying fracture. There is no structure between the pronator quadratus and the radius and the muscle is divided longitudinally on to bone in the same line as the skin incision. The fracture is now exposed and a subperiosteal clearance of the pronator quadratus muscle gives a full exposure of the lower anterior aspect of the radius and the fracture. The wrist joint capsule should be clearly identified at the distal end of the radius.

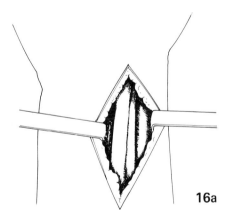

16a

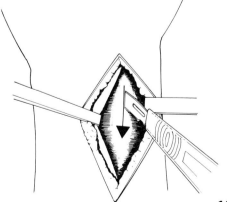

16b

17a & b

Reduction and fixation

The fracture is opened by hyperextension of the wrist and the fragments can usually be readily reduced. Two small bone levers, one around each side of the lower radius just proximal to the fracture, give excellent exposure during this procedure and an Ellis plate is chosen and contoured to fit on to the anterior surface of the radius with its buttress extending across the level of the fracture towards the wrist joint. This small buttress supports the distal fragment but the distal transverse edge of the plate should not extend beyond the wrist joint. The plate is held in position by an assistant (it is not possible to clamp the plate to the radius at this stage) and the two screw holes are drilled. As the screws are tightened the Ellis plate is fixed securely against the shaft of the radius and the fracture reduction is held very securely by the buttress. Suction drainage is not routinely required and the author recommends simple skin closure without deep sutures. No external fixation is needed to supplement the Ellis plate and early wrist movements are encouraged.

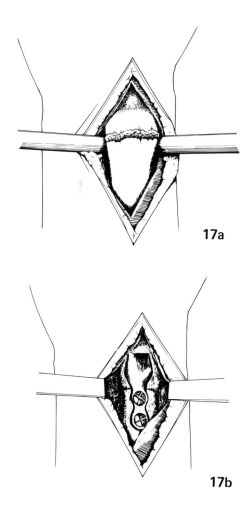

17a

17b

References

Fuller, D. J. (1973). 'The Ellis plate operation for Smith's fracture.' *J. Bone Jt Surg.* **55B,** 173

Sarmiento, A. *et al.* (1977). 'Functional bracing of fractures of the shaft of the humerus.' *J. Bone Jt Surg.* **59A,** 596

Thomas, F. B. (1957). 'Reduction of Smith's fracture.' *J. Bone Jt Surg.* **39B,** 463

[*The illustrations for this Chapter on Fractures of the Long Bones of the Upper Limb were drawn by Mr. G. Bartlett.*]

Operative Management of Fractures of the Lower Limb

Christopher E. Ackroyd, M.A., F.R.C.S.
Clinical Reader, Nuffield Department of Orthopaedic Surgery,
University of Oxford

INTRODUCTION

Fractures of the lower limb produce particular problems for every patient owing to the need to restrict the considerable forces occurring in the limb on weight-bearing during the healing period. The treatment of fractures of the lower limb should be modified for the future needs of the patient and the method of treatment chosen may vary depending on the type of injury sustained and the general condition of the patient. It has long been recognized that prolonged immobilization and restriction of weight-bearing lead to the complication of fracture dystrophy. This has been described as the pathological changes that result from a fracture, and consists of joint stiffness, muscle atrophy, oedema and osteoporosis. These changes may persist after union of the fracture and be irreversible. It is well recognized that irregularity of joint surfaces following intra-articular fractures, and mal-union leading to unequal distribution of forces across a joint, strongly predispose to future osteo-arthrosis. The philosophy of fracture treatment from both the operative and non-operative schools emphasizes the importance of early functional treatment of joints and muscles, with the additional stimulus of weight-bearing to reduce the incidence of these complications (Dehne *et al.*, 1961; Sarmiento, 1967; Müller, Allgöwer and Willenegger, 1970; Mooney *et al.*, 1970). Conservatism has no place in the management of fractures. Perkins (1953) has drawn attention to the early inflammatory phase following injury which requires immobilization and cessation of function, and the late repair phase when activity and resumption of function should occur. London (1967) has pointed out that the objective in the management of injuries is the restoration of function to the part in the shortest time.

Many surgeons agree with the principle of introducing early function; however, there is radical disagreement on how this should be achieved. Aggressive non-operative treatment, with functional activity, usually involves a period of skeletal traction and bed-rest. The development of functional braces for both the femur and the tibia has, however, dramatically reduced the time required in traction and produced excellent results when these methods are applied to certain fractures (Sarmiento, 1967; Connolly, Dehne and Lafolette, 1973). Properly performed, rigid internal fixation provides the best opportunity for early functional treatment. Immobilization of the part is only necessary for a short time in order to allow soft tissue healing; weight-bearing may also be introduced at an early stage if there is a stable and satisfactory fixation (Rüedi, Webb and Allgöwer, 1976).

For some fractures in the lower limbs, most surgeons would agree that the advantages of internal fixation far outweigh the disadvantages. There is another group of fractures for which most surgeons agree that internal fixation should not be employed. However, there is a large area of middle ground where specific surgical philosophies are the determining factor, rather than clear-cut scientific evidence, of the benefit to be obtained. It is clear therefore that dogmatic rules cannot be employed and it is necessary to develop general guiding principles. London (1967) has emphasized that internal fixation is a potentially dangerous method of treatment and in each case definite identifiable gains should be pursued. Few properly controlled studies of treatment methods have yet been carried out, although it is evident from the literature that properly conducted treatment, with careful attention to detail, will lead to good short-term results after widely diverse forms of management.

In the pages that follow, the general principles underlying the indications for operative treatment will be discussed. Detailed consideration of the main injuries to the lower limb will be covered in the sections on each topographical area.

BONE HEALING AND UNION

The process of fracture healing of an unsplinted long bone has been described for many years. However, a full understanding of the mechanisms initiating and controlling the healing process has yet to be achieved. McKibbin (1978) has recently reviewed the subject with particular reference to the clinical implications. He has emphasized that there are four main biological processes which may be evoked in the healing of a fracture and these have different characteristics and can be modified by the physical environment. Primary callus response and external bridging callus can occur in the presence of movement of the fracture ends although under some conditions the external bridging fails and delayed or non-union of the fracture may occur. Danis (1949) observed that, under conditions of rigid internal fixation, fracture healing took place with minimal callus formation. Schenk and Willenegger (1967) demonstrated that this was due to cortical

Haversian remodelling and in areas of bone contact, primary bone union could occur. In areas of gap between the fracture ends, the space is filled by woven bone probably derived from the medullary callus, the fourth type of healing. This then undergoes remodelling by new Haversian systems. The effectiveness of this form of union depends on the vascularity of the bone ends and if there is a considerable length of necrotic bone, the remodelling process may take many months, or even years, to reach completion. In the presence of minor degrees of movement, external and medullary callus will form and these will produce a major contribution to fracture healing. Under these circumstances, fatigue failure of the metallic implant may occur prior to union and cause disruption of the fracture. For this reason, the appearance of external callus is a warning sign that the implant is being overstressed and the forces acting across the fracture should be reduced.

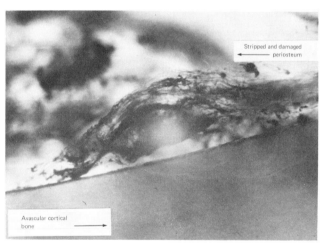

Stripped and damaged periosteum

Avascular cortical bone

1

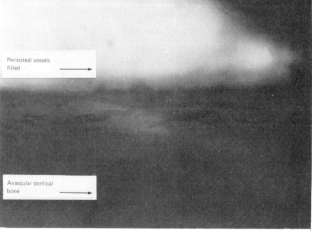

Periosteal vessels filled

Avascular cortical bone

2

1 & 2

It thus becomes clear that the primary damage occurring to bone and soft tissue at the time of injury is of vital importance in determining the subsequent behaviour of the fracture. *Illustration 1* shows a fracture of a long bone after a high-velocity missile injury. The periosteum and the endosteum are stripped from the bone surface and this micro-angiogram shows no perfusion of the cortex over a distance of 1·5 cm. There has also been damage to the blood supply to the periosteum itself. *Illustration 2* shows a bone fragment with intact soft tissue attachments, with filling of periosteal vessels. However, the endosteal surface has been completely stripped and there is little evidence of cortical vessel filling. Rhinelander (1968) in his microvascular studies of the response of the diaphyseal cortex to fracture has shown that when the medullary circulation is disrupted, there is rapid ingrowth of new vessels to the periosteum which takes up a dominant role in the early period of fracture healing. When the medullary circulation has been reestablished, it once more becomes predominant, sending vessels through the cortex and even supplies the periosteal callus itself. It is also evident from Rhinelander's work that intact periosteum is necessary to preserve the normal centrifugal flow of blood from the medullary to the periosteal circulation. Support for these findings comes from Kolodny (1923) and Holden (1972).

It would thus seem wise to avoid stripping the periosteum from cortical bone in the early period after fracture, as this may increase the amount of cortical bone without a blood supply. However, interference with the blood supply of the periosteum itself should also be avoided as the muscle-periosteal anastomoses are important in the early period of fracture healing, when primary callus and external bridging callus are the predominant form of healing (Zucman, 1960; Whiteside and Lesker, 1978). It is clear that there is a dilemma between the plane of dissection which will tend to damage the cortical bone and one which will tend to damage the periosteum. In carrying out internal fixation, attention must therefore be paid to the type of healing to be expected and the anatomical conditions of the area so that the plane of dissection chosen will be that which produces the least possible damage.

Evidence is accumulating to suggest that the conditions for bone healing are more favourable when internal fixation for shaft fractures is delayed 1–2 weeks (Charnley and Guindy, 1961; Lam, 1964; Smith, 1964; Emery and Murakami, 1967; Piekarski, Wiley and Bartels, 1969; Ellasser et al., 1974). However, in all these studies, internal fixation was not rigid and healing was by external bridging callus. Hicks (1961) and Rüedi, Webb and Allgöwer (1976) have shown that after primary rigid fixation excellent bone healing is obtained. When delayed operation is carried out, the periosteum is thickened and firmly attached to the surrounding soft tissues. There has been a general increase in the blood supply to the area and the layer of dissection must at this stage be between bone and periosteum.

If bone healing is delayed, application of rigid internal fixation, together with bone grafting when necessary, provides an excellent method of achieving union with high success rates (Weber and Cech, 1976; Watson-Jones, 1976).

FRACTURES AT DIFFERENT AGES

Immobilization of fractures in childhood by plaster-of-Paris fixation seldom produces long-term consequences provided satisfactory reduction has been obtained. With increasing age immobilization of joints can lead to more serious consequences. This is particularly so when there is severe soft tissue injury and the institution of early functional treatment is desirable. In elderly patients, ambulation with crutches and non-weight-bearing is seldom a practical proposition. Prolonged bed-rest may produce the well-known complications of thrombo-embolism, chest infections, pressure sores, urinary tract infection and confusional states. In this group of patients particularly, there is much to be gained from effective stabilization of the fracture which will allow immediate ambulant treatment. It must, however, be borne in mind that the strict criteria for a satisfactory reduction which may apply in the younger age groups may not be quite so important in patients with a limited life expectancy.

ADEQUATE REDUCTION OF THE FRACTURE

Reduction of most fractures can be achieved satisfactorily by closed means when the mechanism of injury is understood (Charnley, 1970). There are, however, some circumstances where interposition of muscle, tendon, periosteum or other soft tissue structures, makes it impossible to achieve adequate bony contact. In other circumstances gross displacement of bony fragments, often with rotation, may make it impossible to reduce the fracture by closed means. This is particularly true with intra-articular fractures. In some circumstances imbalanced muscle activity may prevent an adequate reduction or make maintenance of the position difficult. When there has been a significant delay in treatment, reduction becomes increasingly difficult and closed methods may not be successful after the first week, particularly in children, when healing can occur very rapidly. All these factors may lead to a decision to carry out an open reduction with internal fixation (Watson-Jones, 1976).

When closed reduction has been carried out satisfactorily, maintenance of the position may be difficult. This is particularly true for intra-articular fractures where the criteria for adequacy of reduction are much more exact. This also occurs with juxta-articular fractures, where maintenance of an adequate reduction may be difficult. In general, length can be maintained satisfactorily with skeletal traction for most shaft fractures, although if there is a segmental fracture, difficulties in maintaining length and alignment may occur.

The criteria for an acceptable reduction vary considerably with each anatomical area and with the age of the patient. In childhood, fractures near the growing epiphysis may undergo significant remodelling if there is adequate growth potential. However, a rotational mal-alignment is seldom significantly altered. In adults, suggested guidelines are available, but there is little clear-cut evidence to relate degrees of mal-union with the amount of disability or incidence of post-traumatic arthrosis. Clearly in borderline cases it will depend on the judgement of the surgeon and the needs and wishes of the patient as to whether the position is no longer acceptable. This Swiss A.O. school has popularized the idea of achieving an anatomical reduction. This is an essential requirement when internal fixation is being carried out, for an adequate rigid fixation relies on an anatomical reconstruction of the bone fragments to produce a mechanically stable unit. However, there is little evidence to support this concept when non-operative treatment is being carried out, provided the defined limits of reduction are achieved and early functional treatment is instituted.

INTRA-ARTICULAR FRACTURES

It is never possible to predict accurately the degree of damage that has been inflicted on a joint until the articular surfaces have been inspected. Much information is available about the ankle joint with evidence to suggest that only minor degrees of incongruity may be important. An anatomical reduction of the fractured fragments, rigidly fixed to allow early functional treatment, produces good results and reduces the risks of post-traumatic arthrosis (Klossner, 1962; Burwell and Charnley, 1965; Joy, Patzakis and Harvey, 1974). There is however little information available for the knee joint and the exact criteria of reduction have not yet been clearly defined. While restoration of the normal anatomy would seem desirable, there is no indication that minor degrees of articular incongruity lead on in the short term to painful arthrosis, particularly when early functional treatment has been instituted, allowing moulding of the articular surfaces to encourage the maturation of fibrocartilage in the fracture gaps (Apley, 1956; Courvoisier, 1973). Malunion of the fracture leading to axis deviation at the knee joint should be avoided as this will lead to increased loading of one or other compartment of the knee joint, with subsequent degenerative changes.

Reconstruction of the main weight-bearing areas of the hip joint seems to be important in obtaining satisfactory long-term results after fracture-dislocation (Judet, Judet and Letournel, 1964; Epstein, 1974). However, it has not been conclusively shown that accurate anatomical reconstruction of the entire articular surface is essential for good long-term results.

Clearly there are different considerations for the three main weight-bearing joints of the lower limb, partly due to their different anatomical shapes, the different forces that cross them and the salvage procedures that are available should degenerative changes ensue.

OPEN FRACTURES

Open fractures can conveniently be classified into three main groups, depending on the degree of damage and contamination to skin, muscle and other soft tissues (Matter and Rittman, 1978; Clancey and Hansen, 1978). The care of an open fracture is basically in two parts: firstly, wound care and secondly, immobilization of the bone fragments. The principles of care of the wound have been delineated for many centuries and this involves debridement or opening of the skin to reveal the full extent of the deeper tissue damage and contamination. This is followed by excision of dead, damaged and contaminated tissue which is of no further use for reconstruction of the tissues and may predispose to infection. The decision to carry out primary repair of the structures involved is one which depends to some extent on the tissues involved and the experience of the surgeon. Even primary closure of the skin is a decision which should not be taken lightly. Suture of the skin under tension may result in skin necrosis with the inevitable dangers of infection. After adequate surgical excision, clean vascularized wounds can safely be left open, although if possible, vascularized tissue should cover exposed bone or implants. In most cases, delayed primary closure of the skin can be carried out in 7–10 days, either by direct suture or with the use of skin grafting. In rare circumstances, when the recipient surface is unsuitable for split-thickness skin grafting, full-thickness flap cover may be carried out. Great advances have been made in this field in recent years and the use of free vascularized skin flaps, possibly incorporating vascularized bone graft, can be considered (Watson and Taylor, 1978).

The second phase in the treatment of an open fracture is immobilization of the bony fragments. Rigid fixation of the fragments without plaster or traction allows easy access to the wounds and joint function may be commenced at an early stage. Gustilo and Anderson (1976), in a study of over 1000 open fractures, have laid down clear treatment guidelines. The use of rigid external skeletal fixation devices provides ideal immobilization of the skeleton for severe Grade III fractures, where the wounds should be left open. In Grade I and II fractures, primary skin closure may be considered and external skeletal fixation may be used to advantage (Connes, 1977). There is considerable controversy over the use of internal fixation in shaft fractures with a Grade I or II open wound. Good results have been reported after primary internal fixation (Varma and Rao, 1974; Rüedi, Webb and Allgöwer, 1976). Other authors have suggested that delayed primary internal fixation should be carried out when primary skin suture has resulted in a satisfactorily healed wound (Smith, 1964; Gustilo and Anderson, 1976).

The management of open intra-articular fractures may present great problems to the surgeon. Primary internal fixation has been widely accepted in Grade I and II open fractures, where primary stabilization of the skeleton will allow earlier joint function and delayed internal fixation is often difficult. In Grade III fractures, the more versatile external skeletal fixation devices can be used to immobilize the fracture in the correct anatomical position (Connes, 1977).

MULTIPLE INJURIES

Patients with multiple injuries pose particular problems for management. It is often the case that the optimum nursing position for one injury may produce adverse effects on another. Management of patients with injuries to the trunk may be considerably more difficult with the limbs in skeletal traction. In view of these factors, careful assessment of the individual needs of each case is necessary in order to arrive at a rational plan of treatment which will produce positive gains and a correct order of priorities. In general, most peripheral limb injuries can be managed by non-operative treatment until the full extent of the patient's injuries have been evaluated and the respiratory and cardiovascular systems satisfactorily stabilized. Primary internal fixation may be indicated in some instances especially when it fits into the general programme of management (Border, La Duca and Seebel, 1975). Some authors have suggested that primary internal fixation of the main shaft fractures reduces the risk of adult respiratory distress syndrome (shock lung syndrome) (Riska *et al.*, 1976; Rüedi, 1977). In many instances delayed internal fixation is advisable when the general condition of the patient is satisfactory and the local conditions at the fracture site are favourable.

BIOMECHANICS OF INTERNAL FIXATION

Before embarking on the operative treatment of fractures it is essential that the surgeon has a thorough understanding of both the biomechanical and biological conditions in the fracture area as well as their limitations. The biomechanical principles underlying internal fixation are well described by Frankel and

Table 1

The Properties of Fixation Techniques in Resisting the Deforming Forces Acting upon a Fracture

Fixation technique	Tension	Compression	Bending	Torsion
Intramedullary nail	–	+ + +	+ + +	+
Interfragmentary screws	+	+	+ +	+ +
Tension band-plate	+ + +	+ +	+ +	+
Cantilever blade-plate	–	+	+ +	+ +

Burstein (1971), there being four types of loading to which a fracture may be exposed — tension, compression, torsion and bending.

There are essentially four different types of fixation devices which can be used to resist these deforming forces acting on the fracture. These are the intramedullary nail, interfragmentary screws, the tension band-plate and a cantilever blade-plate. The mechanical properties of these devices are shown in *Table 1* and each one is good at resisting forces in some directions and less good at resisting forces in other directions. In order to provide a satisfactory rigid internal fixation, it may therefore be necessary to utilize two differing techniques in combination in order to get adequate stability. Precise definition of the forces that may act on any particular fracture depends entirely on the characteristics of that fracture, whether it be transverse, short oblique, long oblique or comminuted. In order to assemble the fragments into a mechanically stable unit, it is necessary to insist on an accurate anatomical reconstruction.

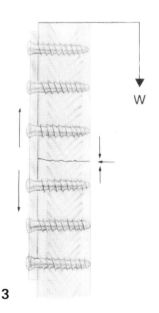

3

3

Wherever possible interfragmentary compression should be applied between the separate fracture fragments. If a nail or plate is merely used to connect two main fracture fragments, it may be subject to considerable bending strains which may ultimately lead to fatigue failure. A complementary point is the necessity of having accurate cortical contact in all areas of the fracture so that there is no gap at one point, producing a weakened area. It is particularly important when using the tension band principle to have cortical contact on the side opposite the plate.

Many bones of the body have a tension and compression surface under the normal loads applied during functional activity. The tension surface can usually be identified as the convex surface and greater muscle forces acting along the bow-string of the curved concave surface produce the compression surface. In biomechanical terms, a stronger fixation is obtained if the plate, which is designed to resist tension rather than compression, is applied on the tension surface. This means that when the normal muscle forces are acting on the limb, the amount of tension in the plate will increase and this will correspondingly produce compression across the fracture site. Here it is of vital importance that there is continuity of the bone on the compression side; otherwise this will merely result in bending of the plate. Thus, if it is not possible during a fracture fixation to get accurate cortical contact on the concave compression side, either due to difficulty in reduction, or because of comminution or absence of bone fragments, special precautions must be taken to prevent the generation of excessive bending strains in the plate. At the time of operation a cancellous bone graft should be applied to such an area of cortical defect or comminution and it is advisable to restrict the forces going through the limb during the postoperative period until sufficient new bone has formed in this area to support the compressive loads (Müller, Allgöwer and Willenegger, 1970).

In some instances, it may not be possible to produce a rigid internal fixation either due to extreme comminution of bone or osteoporotic bone with poor screw fixation. In these instances, it is always advisable to apply additional external splintage for a period, together with restriction of weight-bearing. With the advent of the functional braces for both the knee and the ankle, the application of external splintage need not mean the abolition of joint movement. In general, if a moderate range of joint movement is developed in the early postoperative period, the application of an immobilizing plaster will not lead to any significant or prolonged joint stiffness after its removal.

The implant itself should be sufficiently rigid to provide adequate fixation and sufficiently flexible to allow the normal bone structure to bear a percentage of the load. When very rigid implants are used, the underlying bone undergoes porotic changes with canalization by large medullary spaces. This means that, when the plate is removed, the bone may be significantly weaker and it may take several months for the remodelling process to restore it to normal compact cortical bone under the influence of the increased stresses passing through the bone. This factor is particularly important when double plating is carried out and it is recommended that the plates are removed separately, even with the addition of cancellous bone at the time of the first plate removal.

4

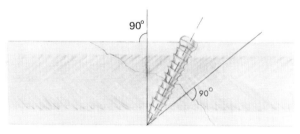

4

The placement of interfragmentary screws may involve some compromises, for to resist torsion and bending forces the screws should be placed at right-angles to the fracture line and to resist compression forces they should be placed at right-angles to the long axis of the bone. It is therefore often better to place the screw in a compromise angle, halfway between these two positions (Danis, 1949).

The neck of the femur is an area where great forces may be exerted on the bone due to the lever arm effect of the neck and the large pelvitrochanteric muscles acting in this area to control the body stability during walking. Special precautions are necessary here as not only is it essential to use an implant of sufficient strength, but it may also be necessary to alter the bony anatomy to increase the inherent stability of the fracture and so reduce the bending forces acting at the area. This is discussed in more detail in the Chapter on 'Subcapital Fractures of the Neck of the Femur', pages 113–119.

OPERATIVE TECHNIQUE AND EQUIPMENT

The Swiss A.O. equipment offers the surgeon a comprehensive mechanical kit designed to deal with every eventuality and capable of producing rigid fixation in almost any fracture. While the basic equipment is very straightforward the surgeon and theatre staff should be thoroughly familiar with the various instruments. They should have a thorough understanding of the principles underlying their application in order to fulfill the ideals of the A.O. group, of putting the mechanical fixation of bone onto a sound biomechanical basis. Use of the basic equipment is well described by Müller, Allgöwer and Willenegger (1970), and use of the small fragment set is similarly well covered by Heim and Pfeiffer (1974). There is a profusion of other implants available to the surgeon for use in the lower limb, most of which have specific application to one particular area. However, it is often the practice of the surgeon which will dictate their use rather than any particular qualities of their effectiveness.

Open operation on a fracture should be regarded as no different from any other orthopaedic procedure and attended by the same attention to detail and precautions against infection. The operation should be carefully planned and carried out in proper facilities under optimum conditions. There is little to recommend the rush to theatre in the middle of the night with theatre and medical staff working under pressure, unless there is an adequate team properly trained and organized to provide a 24 hr service.

The skin should be in good condition before operation is carried out and it is inadvisable to operate through contused or abraded areas. Adequate preparation of the skin should be carried out with suitable antiseptic, and shaving of the skin surface should be kept to a minimum and carried out just prior to operation. The use of the tourniquet is of great advantage for operations on the distal part of the lower limb and its practice and use are well reviewed by Klenerman (1962). Many surgeons now recommend the use of prophylactic chemotherapy given with the premedication, peroperatively and for 48 hr postoperatively. Murray (1944) described the detailed operative techniques for the fixation of fractures of the long bones and these principles are as applicable today as they were 35 years ago. Anderson (1971) has brought these recommendations and details up to date with a comprehensive description of operative practice. These authors emphasize the great importance of care of the soft tissues, the avoidance of excessive retraction and the use of tissue planes rather than a direct approach through muscle. Similarly, the bone and periosteum should be treated with respect; wherever possible the bone should be manipulated with small bone hooks rather than large bone clamps which unnecessarily destroy the soft tissue attachments. The question of whether to preserve the periosteal attachment to bone remains controversial. This has been discussed earlier. It is recommended that the plane of dissection chosen should be that which produces the least damage to periosteum and bone, having taken account of the anatomy of the vascular anastomoses in the particular area under consideration. Copious irrigation of the wound site should be carried out during operation, preferably with an antibiotic solution such as Ringer's Polybactrin. As well as having a cooling effect, this helps to clear the operative debris during the drilling of the bone. The use of sealed suction drains is of importance in the prevention of haematomas and great care should be taken in the closing of the soft tissues particularly with the avoidance of tension on the skin edges utilizing fine nylon sutures. Hilton stated in 1863 that wounds heal better if subjected to a short period of rest; immobilization in a plaster splint for 5–7 days is often advantageous, particularly in areas where skin healing may be delayed. The object of the internal fixation is therefore the insertion of the minimum amount of metal which will result in the maximum amount of stability in order to allow function of the limb against gravity. With careful attention to operative detail and proper supervision of the postoperative programme, excellent results can be obtained with no additional risk to the patient and full function can be restored to the part.

References

Apley, A. G. (1956). 'Fractures of the lateral tibial condyle treated by skeletal traction and early mobilization.' *J. Bone Jt Surg.* **38B**, 699

Anderson, L. D. (1971). 'Fractures.' In *Campbell's Operative Orthopaedics,* Vol. 1, 5th Edition. Edited by A. H. Crenshaw. St. Louis: Mosby

Border, J. R., La Duca, J. and Seebel, R. (1975). 'Priorities in management with polytrauma.' *Prog. Surg.* **14**, 84

Burwell, H. N. and Charnley, A. D. (1965). 'The treatment of displaced fractures at the ankle by rigid internal fixation and early joint movement.' *J. Bone Jt Surg.* **47B**, 634

Charnley, J. (1970). *Closed Treatment of Common Fractures.* 3rd Edition. Edinburgh and London: Livingstone

Charnley, J. and Guindy, A. (1961). 'Delayed operation in the open reduction of fractures of long bones.' *J. Bone Jt Surg.* **43B**, 664

Clancey, G. J. and Hansen, S. T. (1978). 'Open fractures of the tibia: A review of one-hundred-and-two cases.' *J. Bone Jt Surg.* **60A**, 118

Connes, H. (1977). *The Hoffmann's External Fixation. Techniques, Indications and Results.* Paris: Editions Gead

Connolly, J. F., Dehne, E. and La Folette, B. (1973). 'Closed reduction and early cast-brace ambulation in the treatment of femoral fractures.' *J. Bone Jt Surg.* **55A,** 1581

Courvoisier, E. (1973). *Fractures of the Tibial Tables.* AO Bulletin. Swiss Association for the Study of Internal Fixation

Danis, Robert (1949). *Theorie et Pratique de l'Osteosynthèse.* Paris: Masson

Dehne, E., Metz, E. W., Deffer, P. A. and Hall, R. M. (1961). 'Non-operative treatment of the fractured tibia by immediate weight-bearing.' *J. Trauma* **1,** 514

Ellsasser, J. C., Moyer, C. F., Lesker, P. A. and Simmons, D. J. (1974). 'Improved healing of experimental long bone fractures in rabbits by delayed internal fixation.' *J. Trauma* **15,** 869

Emery, M. A. and Murakami, H. (1967). 'The features of fracture healing in cats after immediate and delayed open reduction.' *J. Bone Jt Surg.* **49B,** 575

Epstein, H. C. (1974). 'Posterior fracture-dislocation of the hip.' *J. Bone Jt Surg.* **56A,** 1103

Frankel, V. H. and Burstein, A. H. (1971). 'Design.' In *Orthopaedic Biomechanics.* Philadelphia: Lea & Febiger

Grantham, S. A. (1974). 'Discussion.' *J. Trauma* **14,** 835

Gustilo, R. B. and Anderson, J. T. (1976). 'Prevention of infection in the treatment of one thousand and twenty-five open fractures of long bones.' *J. Bone Jt Surg.* **58A,** 453

Heim, U. and Pfeiffer, F. (1974). *Small Fragment Set Manual.* Berlin, Heidelberg, New York: Springer-Verlag

Hicks, J. H. (1961). 'Fractures of the forearm treated by rigid fixation.' *J. Bone Jt Surg.* **43B,** 680

Hilton, J. (1863). *Rest and Pain.* London: Bell

Holden, C. E. A. (1972). 'The role of blood supply to soft tissues in the healing of diaphyseal fractures.' *J. Bone Jt Surg.* **54A,** 493

Joy, G., Patzakis, M. J. and Harvey, J. P. (1974). 'Precise evaluation of the reduction of severe ankle fractures.' *J. Bone Jt Surg.* **56A,** 979

Judet, R., Judet, L. and Letournel, E. (1964). 'Fracture of the acetabulum: Classification and surgical approaches for open reduction.' *J. Bone Jt Surg.* **46A,** 1615, 1675

Klenerman, L. (1962). 'The tourniquet in surgery.' *J. Bone Jt Surg.* **44B,** 939

Klossner, O. (1962). 'Late results of operative and non-operative treatment of severe ankle fractures.' *Acta chir. scand.,* Suppl. 293

Kolodny, A. (1923). 'The periosteal blood supply and healing of fractures. An experimental study.' *J. Bone Jt Surg.* **5,** 698

Lam, S. H. (1964). 'The place of delayed internal fixation in the treatment of fractures of the long bones.' *J. Bone Jt Surg.* **46B,** 393

London, P. S. (1967). *A Practical Guide to the Care of the Injured.* Edinburgh and London: Livingstone

Matter, P. and Rittman, W. W. (1978). *The Open Fracture.* Bern, Stuttgart, Vienna: Huber

McKibbin, B. (1978). 'The biology of fracture healing in long bones.' *J. Bone Jt Surg.* **60B,** 150

Mooney, V., Nickel, V. L., Harvey, J. P. and Snelson, R. (1970). 'Cast-brace treatment for fractures of the distal part of the femur.' *J. Bone Jt Surg.* **52A,** 1563

Müller, M. E., Allgöwer, M. and Willenegger, H. (1970). *Manual of Internal Fixation.* Berlin, Heidelberg, New York: Springer-Verlag

Murray, C. R. (1944). 'The detailed operative technique for open reduction and internal fixation of fractures of the long bones.' *J. Bone Jt Surg.* **26,** 307

Perkins, G. (1953). 'Rest and movement.' *J. Bone Jt Surg.* **35B,** 521

Piekarski, K., Wiley, A. M. and Bartels, J. E. (1960). 'The effect of delayed internal fixation on fracture healing: An experimental study.' *Acta orthop. scand.* **40,** 543

Rhinelander, F. W. (1968). 'The normal microcirculation of diaphyseal cortex and its response to fracture.' *J. Bone Jt Surg.* **50A,** 784

Riska, E. B., Bonsdorff, H. von, Hakkinen, S., Jaroma, H. and Kiviluoto, O. (1976). 'Prevention of fat embolism by early internal fixation of fractures in patients with multiple injuries.' *Injury* **8,** 110

Rüedi, T. (1977). *Multiple Injuries,* 24th AO Course, Davos

Rüedi, T., Webb, J. K. and Allgöwer, M. (1976). 'Experience with the dynamic compression plate (DCP) in 418 recent fractures of the tibial shaft.' *Injury* **7,** 252

Sarmiento, A. (1967). 'A functional below-the-knee cast for tibial fractures.' *J. Bone Jt Surg.* **49A,** 855

Schenk, R. and Willenegger, H. (1967). 'Morphological findings in primary fracture healing.' *Symposia Biologica Hungarica* **8,** 75

Smith, J. E. M. (1964). 'The results of early and delayed internal fixation of fractures of the shaft of the femur.' *J. Bone Jt Surg.* **46B,** 28

Varma, B. P. and Rao, Y. P. C. (1974). 'An evaluation of the results of primary internal fixation in the treatment of open fractures.' *Injury* **6,** 22

Watson, N and Taylor, G. T. (1978). 'Microvascular free flaps and free bone transfer.' *J. Bone Jt Surg.* **60B,** 141

Watson-Jones, R. (1976). In *Fractures and Joint Injuries.* 5th Edition. Edited by J. N. Wilson. Edinburgh, London, New York: Churchill Livingstone

Weber, B. G. and Cech, O. (1976). *Pseudarthrosis.* Bern, Stuttgart, Vienna: Hans Huber

Whiteside, L. A. and Lesker, P. A. (1978). 'The effects of extraperiosteal and subperiosteal dissection, I: On blood flow in muscle.' *J. Bone Jt Surg.* **60A,** 23

Whiteside, L. A. and Lesker, P. A. (1978). 'The effects of extraperiosteal and subperiosteal dissection, II: On fracture healing.' *J. Bone Jt Surg.* **60A,** 26

Zueman, J. (1960). 'Studies on the vascular connections between periosteum bone and muscle.' *Br. J. Surg.* **48,** 324

[The illustrations for this Chapter on Operative Management of Fractures of the Lower Limb were drawn by Miss S. Baker.]

Subcapital Fractures of the Neck of the Femur

Christopher E. Ackroyd, M.A., F.R.C.S.
Clinical Reader, Nuffield Department of Orthopaedic Surgery,
University of Oxford

INTRODUCTION

Fracture of the neck of the femur is one of the commonest and most disabling injuries sustained by the elderly. It is estimated that there are 30,000 new cases per year and of these approximately half are of the subcapital type (Office for Population Censuses and Surveys, 1976). These fractures have been classified in several different ways. Garden's stages are probably the most useful and widely used (*see Illustrations a–d*)(Garden, 1961). Pauwels' classification of the obliquity of the frature should still be considered (Pauwels, 1934). When the fracture line runs horizontally, the forces of weight-bearing produce compression which tends to increase the stability. When the fracture line is more vertically orientated, shear forces are generated which tend to cause instability and fracture displacement. Bingold (1977) has recently drawn attention to these fractures and has divided them into six groups: those with horizontal fracture lines and those with vertical fracture lines, and within these groups are displaced, undisplaced and impacted fractures. He distinguishes the different mechanical characteristics of each group which therefore require different methods of treatment.

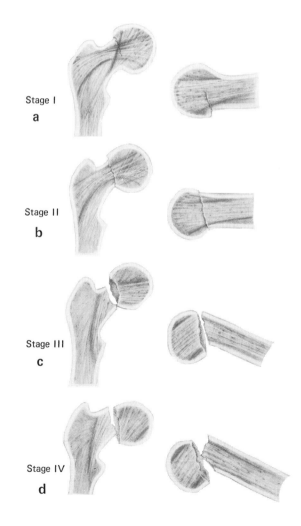

Stage I

a

Stage II

b

Stage III

c

Stage IV

d

PRE-OPERATIVE

Indications

The benefits of operative treatment in this elderly group of patients are considerable. Pressure sores, chest infections, thrombo-embolic complications, and confusional states are a constant hazard for the bedridden elderly patient. There is much discussion in the literature of whether primary prosthetic replacement, or reduction and internal fixation, produces the best results. There is, however, general agreement that for the frail and elderly patient, with a life expectancy of 5 – 10 years or less, and a displaced Stage III or IV fracture, primary prosthetic replacement carefully performed produces most gratifying results. Reduction and internal fixation can be reserved for the younger patient in whom total joint replacement can be performed as a secondary procedure if non-union or avascular necrosis occurs. Certainly a united fracture with an intact femoral head produces a better long-term result than a primary hemi-arthroplasty.

Femoral neck fractures in children and adolescents are uncommon injuries. When the fracture is displaced, it is probably best treated by some form of screw or pin fixation (Ratcliffe, 1962; Lam, 1971). In younger patients a failed internal fixation can be salvaged by a valgus subtrochanteric osteotomy, designed to render the fracture line more or less horizontal so that healing can occur in compression (Pauwels, 1935).

Internal fixation should not be carried out in patients with severe osteoporosis because the bone is not strong enough to hold the metallic implants. It is also wise to avoid internal fixation in patients with neurological disorders. Pathological fractures due to secondary deposits should be treated by a long-stemmed prosthesis cemented into the femoral shaft.

1

2

1&2

Fixation devices

Numerous internal fixation devices have been designed to stabilize this difficult fracture since Smith-Petersen revolutionized the treatment with his Trifin nail in 1931. In order to choose an appropriate method of fixation it is necessary to take into account the direction of the fracture line and the degree of displacement. Impacted horizontal fractures may rarely be treated by early weight-bearing. Bingold (1977) recommends cancellous screw fixation for undisplaced horizontal (*see Illustration 1*) and impacted vertical fractures, both of which have some intrinsic stability. Displaced fractures and those with a vertical fracture line are unstable and require extensive internal fixation, provided the femoral head possesses the necessary mechanical strength. Considerable success has been reported with the use of a telescoping nail (Fielding, Wilson and Ratzan, 1974). However, the multicentre Medical Research Council review (Barnes *et al.*, 1976) could find no difference between this and other methods of rigid internal fixation with crossed compression screws. It is undesirable to hammer any type of nail into the femoral head as this may produce fissuring of the articular surface. Compression at the fracture line decreases the shear forces and this has led to the design of a compression screw which allows impaction of the fracture (*see Illustration 2*). A device of this type was designed by Charnley, Blockey and Purser (1957) and more recently, other similar implants have been recommended although the long-term results have yet to be fully evaluated (Muckle, 1977).

Pre-operative preparation

Reduction should be carried out as soon as possible in order to safeguard the blood supply to the head of the femur. However, in this elderly group of patients, special attention must be given to their general medical condition. Screening for intercurrent infection, particularly that of the urinary tract, should be carried out and general medical conditions, such as cardiac failure and bronchopneumonia, should be effectively treated before operation. It is often advisable to cover the operative period with prophylactic antibiotics. When operation is delayed for more than a few hours skin traction should be applied with up to 6 lb (3 kg) of weight in order to relieve pain and perhaps improve the position of the fracture.

Anaesthesia

Modern anaesthesia has greatly improved the safety of operating on these elderly patients. A general anaesthetic is preferable although satisfactory reduction can be obtained with the use of local anaesthesia (Ackroyd, 1973).

THE OPERATION

3

Technique of closed reduction

It is most convenient to use an orthopaedic table which holds the legs in the required position and allows access for an image intensifier or x-ray machine. The patient is placed on the operating table and the intact limb secured in the usual way, with the patella slightly internally rotated in order to control the pelvis. Several methods of reduction have been described, most recently by Flynn (1974). Reduction should be a gentle manoeuvre and its success relies entirely on absolute muscle relaxation. The surgeon should stand beside the injured limb, just below the knee. The upper hand is placed over the front of the thigh to grip the medial side, the lower hand grips the limb at the level of the knee with the calf supported against the body. The thigh is flexed some $20°-30°$ in the neutral plane and gradually increasing traction is exerted along the line of the femoral neck. When it is felt that complete muscle relaxation has occurred, the thigh is then gradually internally rotated and extended so that the knee describes a gentle arc. The thigh is now internally rotated some $15°$ and abducted to $20°$ and the foot secured. Tension in the limb is adjusted so that it is just possible to spring the knee. The uninjured limb is now abducted further to allow access for the radiographic equipment, and check radiographs are taken in the anterior and lateral planes.

The experienced surgeon will usually be able to feel whether the reduction is satisfactory and if an image intensifier is available, screening of the hip while gently rotating the limb will aid visualization of the fracture. Care should be taken to ensure correct interpretation of the radiographs and a metal marker may help orientation. The skin is now prepared with three applications of suitable antiseptic and the patient draped with sterile towelling to allow access for radiography.

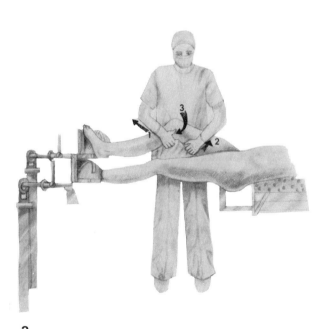

3

4

The incision

A mid-lateral incision should run from the tip of the greater trochanter 10 — 20 cm along the line of the shaft of the femur. After division of the deep fascia, the greater trochanter and vastus lateralis and its ridge of origin are clearly seen. When exposure of the neck is required, the upper part of the incision may be curved forwards towards the anterior superior iliac spine (Watson-Jones incision).

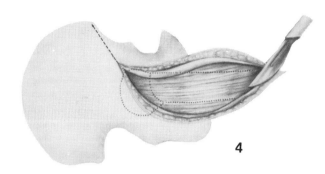

4

5

Exposure of the femur

A muscle-splitting incision may be used for placement of pins or screws; however, when a plate is being inserted on the lateral side of the femur it is preferable to lift the entire flap of vastus lateralis from its origin at the vastus lateralis ridge and along the linea aspera. This ensures that a well-vascularized muscle flap covers the entire length of the plate. A transverse incision is made in vastus lateralis just below the trochanteric ridge, extending from the anterior to the posterior surface of the femur. The incision then curves posteriorly to run along the linea aspera, retaining a small cuff of fascia for re-attachment. It is necessary to divide the transverse branches of the lateral circumflex femoral artery and, as vastus lateralis is elevated from the lateral surface of the femur, the first of the perforating branches of the profunda femoris is encountered. A Hohmann retractor is now inserted round the medial side of the shaft so that the femur is satisfactorily exposed.

If reduction of the fracture is satisfactory, the first guide wire may now be inserted. However, if reduction is poor, a choice must be made between an open reduction or proceeding to prosthetic replacement of the femoral head.

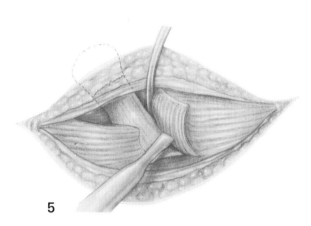

5

6

Exposure of the neck of the femur

To approach the neck of the femur the skin incision is extended from its upper end towards the anterior superior iliac spine. The deep fascia is split in line with the incision and the anterior margin of the gluteus medius muscle is identified and retracted upwards. The space between the gluteal muscles and tensor fascia latae is developed and the ascending branch of the lateral circumflex femoral artery is identified and ligated. The extracapsular fat is cleared to expose the capsule of the hip joint. This is now incised in line with the axis of the femoral neck and carefully retracted to expose the fracture. Insertion of bone levers inside the capsule greatly improves the exposure; however, this interferes with the already tenuous blood supply to the femoral head and is best avoided. If access is difficult the capsular incision may be extended to a T or L at its proximal end, running near the edge of the acetabulum.

Reduction of the fracture can now be carried out under direct vision and temporary fixation with Kirschner wires is advisable while preparations are being made for insertion of the main fixation device. It has been suggested that aspiration of the haemarthrosis is beneficial in all cases. This reduces the intra-articular pressure which may cause obstruction to the veins draining the femoral head.

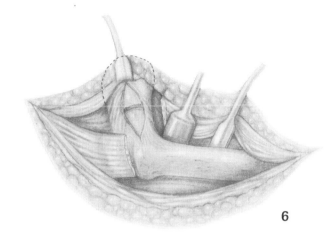

6

7

Insertion of the guide wire

The first guide or Kirschner wire is inserted along the anterior surface of the femoral neck and driven a short distance into the head. This determines the amount of anteversion of the femoral neck and the second guide wire is inserted parallel to the first in the lateral plane. Penetration of the lateral cortex should be some 2 cm below the vastus lateralis ridge, level with the lesser trochanter and situated mid-way between the anterior and posterior surfaces of the femur. A preliminary 3·2 mm drill hole will allow for fine adjustments in angulation. When a 130° fixed angle appliance is being used, a 50° drill guide will allow correct insertion in the anteroposterior plane. The guide wire may be introduced by hand or using a power drill and should slide easily along the soft trabecular bone in the inferior part of the femoral neck. It is often advisable to penetrate across the joint space in order to avoid movement of the fracture whilst the implant is being introduced along the femoral neck. A rough guide of the alignment may be obtained by aiming the guide wire towards the opposite anterior superior iliac spine. If resistance is encountered as the guide wire is inserted, it is likely that contact has been made with the calcar femoralis or posterior cortex. If this occurs, the guide wire should be re-inserted and the alignment rechecked.

The position of the guide wire may now be confirmed radiographically and with a little experience it will soon be found possible to insert this correctly on the first occasion. When several cancellous screws have been inserted, it is important that they should be spread out to grip different parts of the femoral head rather than converging on a single point.

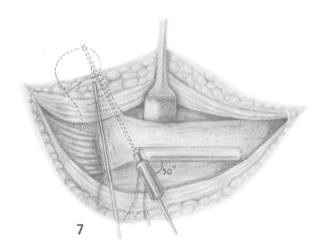

7

8

Insertion of the nail or screw

When the guide wire has been placed in a satisfactory position along the inferior aspect of the femoral neck, the lateral cortex of the femur is prepared to allow insertion of the fixation device. Appropriate reamers are slid over the guide wire and a channel prepared. The correct length of nail, or screw, is determined so that the tip of the device lies 1 cm from the sub-chondral bone of the femoral head. A tap may be used to prepare the threads when inserting a screw, although when the bone is soft this is not necessary and better grip is obtained without previous tapping. The screw is then inserted over the guide wire and tightened to get a good grip of the femoral head. It is often advisable to place a Kirschner wire high in the neck to maintain the reduction which can be lost when inserting the screw or nail. If a nail is used, heavy blows should be avoided as these can produce fragmentation of the articular surface.

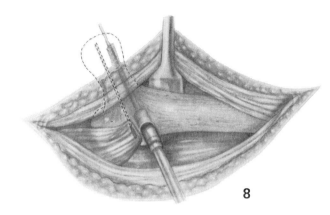

8

9

Fixation of the plate to the lateral cortex

The guide wires are now removed and the plate is applied to the lateral surface of the femoral shaft and secured with screws. Impaction of the fracture may be carried out with a few blows on the impactor punch sited on the lateral surface of the femur. When a compression screw and plate are being used, tightening of the screw in the plate will produce compression at the fracture site. In cases with a large femoral neck, a further cancellous screw can be inserted above the nail for additional stability.

The wound is now closed and vastus lateralis is folded over the plate and resutured to its site of origin. One or two suction drains are inserted to prevent deep haematoma formation. The deep fascia and subcutaneous tissues are closed with absorbable Dexon sutures and the skin closed with nylon sutures.

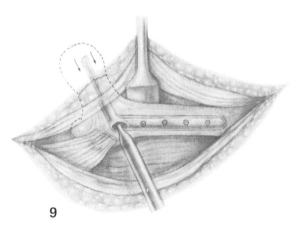

9

POSTOPERATIVE CARE

The patient is nursed in bed and movement of the hip and knee are encouraged from the start. The suction drains should be removed by 48 hr and a check radiograph will have confirmed the position of fixation. The patient should be got out of bed as soon as possible and when the drains have been removed walking can commence. In elderly patients, in whom a satisfactory fixation has been achieved, partial or non-weight-bearing is seldom possible and the patient should be encouraged to bear as much weight on the limb as is comfortable. In younger patients, or in cases where the stability of the fracture is poor, partial weight-bearing is advised for up to 6 weeks. There is little evidence that restriction of weight-bearing improves fracture healing and it is probable that it merely protects the fixation from excessive load. Routine anticoagulation of patients with femoral neck fractures has been shown to reduce the incidence of thrombo-embolic complications (Sevitt and Gallagher, 1959). However, the surgeon should balance the advantages and disadvantages of such a policy in each individual case.

References

Ackroyd, C. E. (1973). 'Treatment of subcapital femoral fractures fixed with Moore's pins: a study of 34 cases followed for up to 3 years.' *Injury,* **5,** 100

Barnes, R., Brown, J. T., Garden, R. S. and Nicoll, E. A. (1976). 'Subcapital fractures of the femur. A prospective review.' *J. Bone Jt Surg.* **58B,** 2

Bingold, A. C. (1977). 'The science of pinning of the neck of the femur.' *Ann. R. Coll. Surg. Engl.* **59,** 463

Charnley, J., Blockey, N. J. and Purser, D. W. (1957). 'The treatment of displaced fractures of the neck of the femur by compression.' *J. Bone Jt Surg.* **39B,** 45

Fielding, J. W., Wilson, S. A. and Ratzan (1974). 'A continuing end-result study of displaced intracapsular fracture of the neck of the femur treated with the Pugh nail.' *J. Bone Jt Surg.* **56A,** 1464

Flynn, M. (1974). 'A new method of reduction of fractures of the neck of the femur, based on anatomical studies of the hip joint.' *Injury* **5,** 309

Garden, R. S. (1961). 'Low-angle fixation in fracture of the femoral neck.' *J. Bone Jt Surg.* **43B,** 647

Lam, S. F. (1971). 'Fractures of the neck of the femur in children.' *J. Bone Jt Surg.* **53A,** 1165

Muckle, D. S. (1977). *Femoral Neck Fractures and Hip Joint Injuries.* Chapter 2. London: Chapman & Hall

Pauwels, F. (1934). 'Grundlagen des Heilungsvorganges bie Schenkelhalsbrüchen.' *Verh. dt. orthop. Ges.* **29,** 54

Pauwels, F. (1935). *Der Schenkelhalsbrüch. Ein Mechanisches Problem.* Stuttgart: Ferdinand Enke Verlag

Ratcliffe, A. H. C. (1962). 'Fractures of the neck of the femur in children.' *J. Bone Jt Surg.* **44B,** 528

Report on Hospital in-Patient Enquiry for the Year 1973 (1976). Department of Health & Social Security and Office for Population Censuses and Surveys. H. M. S. O.

Sevitt, S. and Gallagher, N. G. (1959). 'Prevention of venous thrombosis and pulmonary embolism in injured patients. A trial of anticoagulant prophylaxis with phenindione in midde-aged and elderly patients with fractured neck of femur.' *Lancet* **2,** 981

Smith-Peterson, M. N., Cave, E. F. and van Gorder, G. W. (1931). 'Intracapsular fractures of the neck of the femur: treated by internal fixation. *Archs Surg.* **23,** 715

Watson-Jones, R. (1976). In *Fractures and Joint Injuries,* 5th Edition. Edited by J. N. Wilson. Edinburgh: Churchill Livingstone

[The illustrations for this Chapter on Subcapital Fractures of the Neck of the Femur were drawn by Miss S. Barker and Mrs. P. Dewhurst.]

Pertrochanteric Fractures of the Femur

Christopher E. Ackroyd, M.A., F.R.C.S.
Clinical Reader, Nuffield Department of Orthopaedic Surgery,
University of Oxford

PRE-OPERATIVE

1a & b

Introduction

Fractures of the base of the neck of the femur and of the pertrochanteric region make up approximately half the fractures of the femoral neck in the elderly. They are of two different types. The first type is a relatively stable fracture, often with minimal displacement which when reduced has good apposition of the medial cortex in the region of the calcar femoralis. The second is an unstable fracture with comminution and three or four main fragments often with considerable displacement which, after reduction, does not have an intact medial cortex and calcar femoralis. The obliquity of the fracture is also important in determining the stability, the more vertical the fracture line the greater shear force that is exerted on weight-bearing.

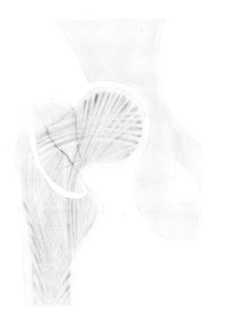

1a

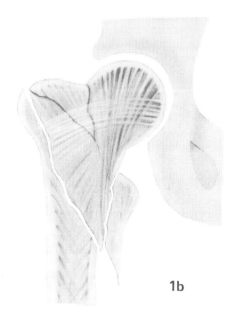

1b

Indications

Pertrochanteric fractures carry a high mortality rate and it is a great advantage in the general care of the patient to carry out an internal fixation that will produce sufficient stability to allow early weight-bearing (Clawson and Melcher, 1975). In cases where the general condition or wishes of the patient militate against operative treatment, traction can be applied and the fracture will usually unite satisfactorily in 8–12 weeks. There is seldom difficulty in maintaining satisfactory alignment of the fragments and the main indication for internal fixation is to allow early mobilization in order to prevent the numerous complications of bed-rest and to ease the difficulties of nursing these patients.

Techniques of fixation

Frankel (1963) has pointed out that the forces acting on the head of the femur during walking and standing are considerable. Although the use of a walking aid will reduce these forces, the loads will still be high

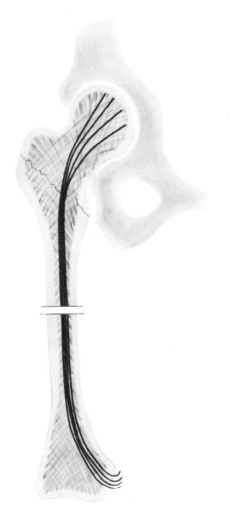

2

because of the pelvitrochanteric muscle forces. Even during recumbency, the forces acting on this region may be great and of sufficient magnitude to cause implant failure. Stable pertrochanteric fractures produce few real problems in treatment and 130° fixed angle nail-plates, such as the Jewett or the A.O. blade-plate, produce very satisfactory fixation allowing early ambulation and carrying little risk of implant failure. The technique of insertion is exactly the same as that described for the treatment of subcapital fractures, with the sliding compression screw-plate.

The unstable four-part fractures pose a much greater problem in providing sufficient stability to allow immediate weight-bearing while fracture union occurs. Many authors have sought to overcome this problem by increasing the strength and the size of the metallic plate (Holt, 1963; Sarmiento, 1963). Others have sought to alter the biomechanical forces exerted on the fracture by carrying out a valgus or displacement osteotomy (Dimon and Hughston, 1967; Sarmiento and Williams, 1970; Müller, Allgöwer and Willenegger, 1970). Kaufer, Matthews and Sonstegard (1974) carried out studies on simulated unstable pertrochanteric fractures and concluded that the main factor in maintaining stability of fixation was the strength of the implant and a nail of sufficient strength should be chosen when treating unstable fractures. While these methods seem to produce an improvement in the stability of fracture fixation, it is as yet uncertain whether they produce any functional improvement in this frail and elderly group of patients (Hubbard et al., 1978).

2

More recently several intramedullary devices have been designed which seem to give satisfactory stability in the upper part of the femur. The flexible Ender's nails are inserted by a closed technique through the medial femoral condyle and this is reported to give good results (Ender, 1970; Jones et al., 1977) although a large properly controlled trial is awaited before this method can be generally adopted.

Müller, Allgöwer and Willenegger (1970) have suggested the use of the 95° condylar blade-plate for fixation of the stable pertrochanteric fracture with an intact calcar femoralis. While in their hands excellent results are produced, considerable experience with this technique is required. It relies on an accurate anatomical reconstitution of the calcar. The blade should be placed in 5°–10° of valgus, allowing impaction of the fracture, and at least two screws should firmly grip the calcar to produce interfragmentary compression at the oblique fracture line.

Pre-operative preparation

As in treatment of the subcapital fracture, operation should be carried out as soon as the patient is fit for a general anaesthetic. Temporary skin traction may be applied to make the patient more comfortable. Careful screening should be carried out for general medical conditions, such as cardiac failure and bronchopneumonia, which should be effectively treated before operation. The use of short-term prophylactic antibiotics can reduce the infection rate in operations on these fractures to less than 2 per cent (Tengue and Kjellander, 1978). General anaesthesia is usually essential for this operation.

The patient is placed on an orthopaedic table and the intact limb secured. Closed reduction of the stable fractures is carried out in a similar way to the reduction of the subcapital fracture. In comminuted unstable fractures there is little connection between the head and the neck of the femur and the shaft. It is therefore seldom possible to carry out a closed reduction and the affected leg should be secured in 20° of abduction and 10° of internal rotation. Moderate traction is applied to the limb and the opposite limb is adjusted to allow access for the radiographic apparatus.

THE OPERATION

VALGUS OSTEOTOMY TECHNIQUE

3

Exposure of the fracture

Exposure of the lateral side of the shaft of the femur is exactly as described in the section on subcapital fractures. A longitudinal incision is made from the tip of the greater trochanter, running along the line of the shaft of the femur. The deep fascia is divided to expose the greater trochanter, vastus lateralis ridge and the muscle. Vastus lateralis is divided from its origin transversely below the trochanteric ridge and the incision is curved downwards to skirt alongside the linea aspera. The muscle is reflected forwards and medially to expose the upper part of the shaft of the femur and the intertrochanteric region. If the lateral cortex is intact, this is divided with a 20° oblique osteotomy at the level of the fracture of the medial cortex. The divided proximal fragment of bone is lifted upwards with a bone hook to give good access to the neck of the femur and enable reconstruction of the medial buttress. If the lateral cortex is fractured with the main part of the greater trochanter separated, a similar 20° oblique osteotomy is carried out at the level of the fracture of the medial cortex and the loose wedge of bone is removed giving access to the neck of the femur.

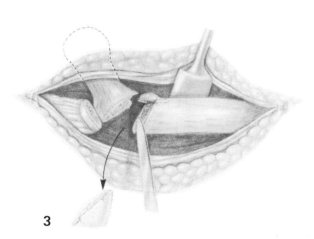

3

4

Reconstruction of the medial cortex

The next stage should be assessment of the integrity of the medial cortex. The lesser trochanter is often fractured taking with it a fragment of the postero-medial area of the shaft. The anteromedial aspect of the shaft can be clearly visualized. Reduction of a large piece of lesser trochanter may be carried out at this stage and it should be reduced and fixed with a cortical or malleolar interfragmentary screw to the main part of the shaft of the femur. In some cases, the fracture of the lesser trochanter has removed little of the medial femoral cortex and fixation is not necessary, or can be deferred until later in the operation. In any event it is now important to ensure that the proximal fragment of the neck rests firmly on the medial surface of the shaft with adequate bony contact and no tendency to displacement. If necessary any bony spikes can be trimmed off to ensure smooth edge-to-edge apposition.

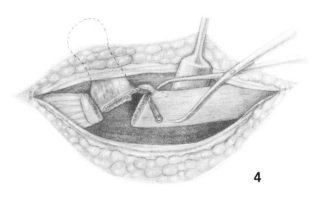

4

5

Preparation of the femoral neck

The remaining proximal fragment of the lateral femoral cortex and the greater trochanter is now lifted up with a bone hook to expose the medullary cavity of the neck of the femur. A guide wire is slid along the anterior aspect of the femoral neck and impacted into the inferior quadrant of the head in order to determine the plane of anteversion. The second guide wire is now inserted high into the neck in the same plane as the first approximately at right angles to the long axis of the femur. The position of this guide wire may now be checked with a radiograph and the AO seating chisel is then inserted into the neck of the femur directly beneath this guide wire and parallel to it in both planes. The chisel should enter the neck through the fracture as far superiorly as possible and should be aimed at the postero-inferior quadrant of the femoral head. With experience, insertion of the seating chisel can be carried out without the use of the second guide wire and without radiographic control. The chisel now has a firm grip of the head and neck fragment which can now be brought into the valgus position, allowing contact of the fracture surfaces, particularly ensuring that there is accurate reduction of the medial buttress. Radiographs are helpful at this stage to ensure that the seating chisel is correctly placed in the head and neck of the femur and the reduction is satisfactory. It should be noted that the upper fragment often lies in external rotation and it is necessary to rotate it internally, so that the neck lies horizontally, in order to re-establish the correct relationship between the neck and shaft of the femur.

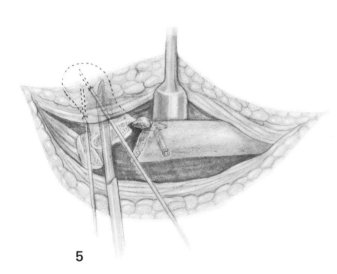

5

6

Insertion of the 130° blade-plate

Measurement of the length of the blade should now be carried out and this should be at least 1 cm short of the subchondral bone of the femoral head in order to allow for possible impaction. A four- or six-hole 130° angled blade-plate is inserted along the channel prepared by the seating chisel.

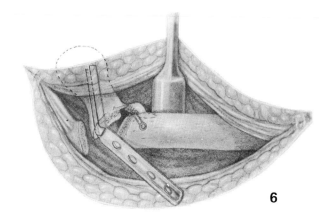

6

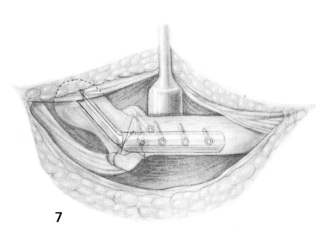

7

7

Reduction and fixation of the plate

The plate is brought to lie against the femoral shaft and secured in this position, care being taken to ensure that there is a correct rotational relationship between the femoral neck and shaft. The proximal fragment should lie in a valgus position and the shaft itself should be displaced a little inwards. Now that the fracture line has been rendered more or less horizontal, provided there is good medial contact, satisfactory stability should result. If there is considerable comminution of the medial buttress, then it is advisable to pack cancellous bone chips, taken from the region of the greater trochanter, in this area prior to wound closure.

The displaced fragments of the greater trochanter are now brought down to the correct position and may be fixed with a figure-of-eight tension band wire or cancellous screws. In some cases the greater trochanter may have sufficient soft tissue attachment not to require separate fixation. The flap of vastus lateralis is now returned to its correct position covering the plate and sutured to the periosteum of the greater trochanter and along the linea aspera. A deep suction drain is inserted and the deep fascia is closed. The superficial tissues are now closed and a sterile occlusive dressing is applied to the wound.

8

Alternative techniques of fixation

There are a number of nail-plate devices which can be used in this area with differing neck shaft angles. Those with greater angles allow the valgus configuration of the neck to be achieved while placing the blade in the usual line along the inferior part of the neck of the femur; for example, with this 150° Jewett nail plate. The essential requirement in this operation is to get adequate stability so that immediate weight-bearing can take place. There are a variety of different fracture patterns in this area and several additional techniques may be required. Dimon and Hughston (1967) describe a medial displacement osteotomy where the calcar of the femoral neck is impacted into the medullary cavity of the shaft and fixed with a 130° blade-plate. This may be necessary if sufficient contact between the fragments on the medial side cannot be obtained. In severely osteoporotic bone where the blade and screws do not hold sufficiently, it may be necessary to pack the medullary cavity with bone cement in order to aid fixation; alternatively, a high-density polyethylene plate may be applied on the medial side in order to aid a screw fixation.

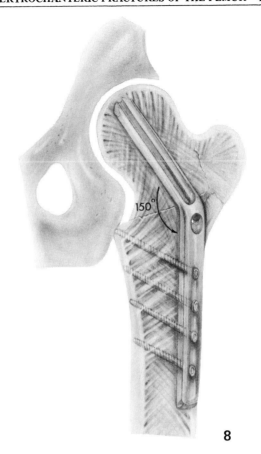

8

POSTOPERATIVE CARE

The patient is nursed in bed with an air-ring under the sacrum and pillows to support the leg maintaining some flexion of the hip and knee joint. Early mobilization is of extreme importance in these elderly patients and can usually be commenced within 48 hr. The suction drain is removed on the second day and a check radiograph should be carried out to confirm adequate stability of the fracture. The patient may get up and start walking with crutches or a frame and the elderly patient may put as much weight as is comfortable on the affected limb. In younger patients it is advisable to restrict weight-bearing for 4—6 weeks until there is some evidence of healing. When an osteotomy has been carried out, this inevitably leads to some shortening of the femur. However,

this is compensated for by the valgus position of the femoral neck and results in little overall shortening. Prophylactic anticoagulation may be carried out in suitable cases to prevent thrombo-embolic complications.

Failure of the fixation and development of a varus deformity may delay union. However, this usually impacts into a stable position and produces little functional disability. Rarely non-union may occur after failure of the plate and this will necessitate re-operation. It is seldom necessary to remove the implant which can be safely left in position unless there is discomfort over the lateral aspect of the thigh, or intrusion of the nail into the hip joint.

References

Clawson, D. K. and Melcher, P. J. (1975). 'Fractures and dislocations of the hip.' In *Fractures*. Edited by C. A. Rockwood and D. P. Green. Philadelphia, Toronto: Lippincott

Dimon, J. H., III and Hughston, J. C. (1967). 'Unstable intertrochanteric fracture of the hip.' *J. Bone Jt Surg.* **49A**, 440

Ender, J. (1970). 'Probleme beim frischen per-und aubtrochanterem Oberschenkelbruch.' *Hefte Unfallheilkd.* **106**, 2

Frankel, V. H. (1963). 'Mechanical fixation of unstable fractures about the proximal end of the femur.' *Bull. Hosp. Jt Dis.* **24**, 75

Holt, E. P. (1963). 'Hip fractures in the trochanteric region: treated with a strong nail and early weight-bearing.' *J. Bone Jt Surg.* **45A**, 687

Hubbard, M. J. S., Burke, F. D., Bracey, D. J. and Houghton, G. R. (1978). 'A prospective controlled trial of valgus osteotomy in the fixation of unstable pertrochanteric fractures of the femur.' *J. Bone Jt Surg.* **60B**, 144

Jones, C. Wynn, Morris, J., Hirschowitz, D., Hart, G. M., Shea, J. and Arden, G. P. (1977). 'A comparison of the treatment of trochanteric fractures of the femur by internal fixation with a nail plate and the Ender technique.' *Injury* **9**, 35

Kaufer, H., Matthews, L. S. and Sonstegard, D. (1974). 'Stable fixation or intertrochanteric fractures.' *J. Bone Jt Surg.* **56A**, 899

Müller, M. E., Allgöwer, M. and Willenegger, H. (1970). *Manual of Internal Fixation*. Berlin, Heidelberg, New York: Springer-Verlag

Sarmiento, A. (1963). 'Intertrochanteric fractures of the femur.' *J. Bone Jt Surg.* **45A**, 706

Sarmiento, A. and Williams, E. M. (1970). 'The unstable intertrochanteric fracture: treated with a valgus osteotomy and I-beam nail plate.' *J. Bone Jt Surg.* **52A**, 1309

Tengue, B. and Kjellander, J. (1978). 'Anti-biotic prophylaxis in operations on trochanteric femoral fractures.' *J. Bone Jt Surg.* **60A**, 97

[*The illustrations for this Chapter on Pertrochanteric Fractures of the Femur were drawn by Miss S. Barker and Mrs. P. Dewhurst.*]

Fractures of the Femoral Shaft

Christopher E. Ackroyd, M.A., F.R.C.S.
Clinical Reader, Nuffield Department of Orthopaedic Surgery,
University of Oxford

PRE - OPERATIVE

Indications

Fractures of the middle and lower thirds of the femur are relatively easy to control by closed means and are eminently suitable for early ambulant treatment in a functional brace (Mooney *et al.*, 1970, Connolly, Dehne and LaFollette, 1973). While transverse and short oblique fractures of the mid-shaft of the femur are suitable for operative treatment with an intramedullary nail, ease of operation alone should not constitute a valid reason for operative treatment. Dencker (1965) in his large review of femoral shaft fractures, could show little difference between the results of operative and non-operative treatment. He recommended that operation should be carried out if reduction was unsatisfactory, or when fracture healing was slow. The age of the patient may influence the decision to carry out internal fixation, particularly in the elderly who may not be suitable for a functional brace and are more prone to develop complications after prolonged bed-rest. The presence of multiple injuries, particularly in the same limb, often constitutes a good indication for primary or delayed primary internal fixation, which will greatly simplify medical and nursing treatment. Internal fixation may also be indicated when there is arterial damage, for a pathological fracture, or in the treatment of non-union.

Methods of fixation

Most transverse and short oblique fractures of the middle two quarters of the femoral shaft are best fixed with an intramedullary nail. Fractures in the lower third of the shaft may be treated with a nail. However, difficulty in controlling rotation often occurs and a small antirotation plate may be added. In these fractures it is often more satisfactory to use tension band-plate fixation, if possible incorporating interfragmentary screws across the fracture (Müller, Allgöwer and Willenegger, 1970). Comminuted fractures pose great problems for fixation and are best treated non-operatively. If internal fixation is considered necessary, several interfragmentary screws will be required in combination with a neutralization plate. The results of plate fixation in the femur suggest that this method should be used with extreme care and reserved only for fractures which cannot be fixed in any other way (Gant, Shaftan and Herbsman, 1970; Solheim and Vaage, 1972; Jensen, Johansen and Mørch, 1977).

1&2

Fractures in the subtrochanteric region may be difficult to control by non-operative methods and internal fixation may be carried out more regularly. Müller, Allgöwer and Willenegger (1970), report the use of the A.O. 95° condylar blade-plate, which is designed specifically for use in the upper or lower parts of the femur. The blade produces a good fixation of the proximal fragment and allows axial compression to be obtained, although interfragmentary screws should also be incorporated into the fixation if at all possible. In any plate applied as a tension band, an intact medial cortex is essential and if there is a gap or comminution in this area, supplementary cancellous bone graft must be added. Zickel (1976) has introduced an intramedullary nail, which controls rotation of the proximal fragment, which is a useful alternative to plating and provides an implant which is less likely to suffer fatigue failure.

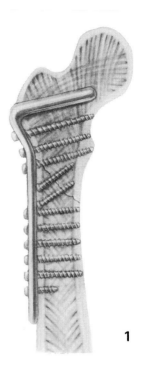

1

Pre-operative preparation and anaesthesia

In most cases operation should be carried out as a delayed procedure after an interval of 2–3 weeks. Temporary skeletal traction is therefore instituted with a tibial pin and the leg placed on a Thomas splint in order to immobilize the fracture and maintain leg length. The general condition of the patient should be assessed prior to operation so that this can be carried out as a planned procedure under optimum conditions. Blood loss from the fracture should be replaced. If shaving of the area of the incision is necessary, this should be carried out on the day of operation and a suitable antiseptic applied.

The operation should be carried out under general anaesthesia and blood should be cross-matched and ready for transfusion.

Position of patient

Plating of the femur

The patient should be placed supine on the operating table with a sandbag under the ipsilateral buttock. The operation site is prepared with three applications of an appropriate antiseptic and the leg draped with sterile towelling so that it is free for manipulation. It is often helpful to leave the skeletal traction and stirrup *in situ* until the end of the operation so that traction can be applied with greater ease. The skin over the operative site is covered with adhesive plastic.

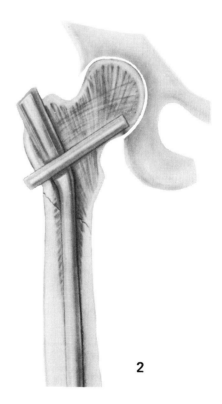

2

THE OPERATION

PLATING OF THE FEMUR

3a&b

The incision

The plate should always be applied to the lateral tension surface of the femur and this is best approached through a lateral incision. Reflection of vastus lateralis allows the plate to be covered with a well vascularized muscle flap and this approach involves minimal interference with the quadriceps mechanism. A mid-lateral incision, some 15–20 cm in length, is made at the level of the fracture. This is deepened and the deep fascia is split along the same line. Cutaneous bleeding points are controlled with diathermy.

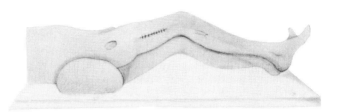

3a

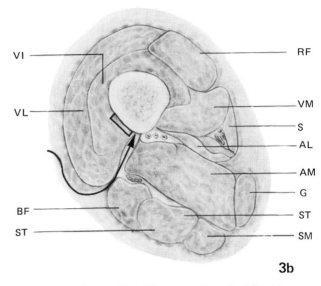

3b

VI = vastus intermedius; VL = vastus lateralis; BF = biceps femoris; ST = semitendinosus; RF = rectus femoris; VM = vastus medialis; S = sartorius; AL = adductor longus; AM = adductor magnus; G = gracilis, SM = Semimembranosus

4

Exposure of the fracture

The deep fascia is elevated from the muscle along the posterior border of the incision as far as the lateral intermuscular septum. Vastus lateralis is then reflected forwards and separated from the lateral intermuscular septum towards the linea aspera. The muscle is now detached from the linea aspera and any perforating vessels that may be encountered are ligated. Vastus intermedius is now encountered and together with vastus lateralis they are reflected forward and separated from their attachment to bone. Bone levers may now be placed round the femur to produce good exposure of the lateral surface of the shaft and the fracture site. In fresh fractures the periosteum should be left undisturbed as far as possible, although when delayed internal fixation is carried out, it is usually better to elevate the periosteum over a short distance to expose the fracture rather than attempting to fashion a plane of dissection between the periosteum and muscle.

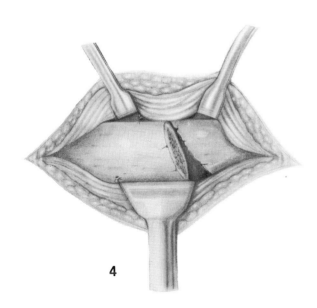

4

5

Fixation of the fracture

The fracture ends are separated using a small bone hook and the surfaces cleaned with a curette. Reduction is carried out using two bone hooks and traction on the limb. It may be necessary to increase the angulation of the fracture in order to oppose the fracture surfaces. When using bone hooks, care must be taken to ensure that there are no secondary fractures which may be separated.

The reduction is held with a reduction clamp or temporary cerclage wire. Whenever possible an interfragmentary screw should be placed across the fracture producing interfragmentary compression which greatly enhances the stability. A 4·5 mm cortical screw is used and therefore the proximal cortex is drilled out to 4·5 mm, while the distal cortex is drilled to 3·2 mm, prior to tapping. If necessary this screw may be incorporated into the plate which is now applied to the lateral surface of the femur. A large dynamic compression plate is chosen which will allow at least four screw holes above and below the fracture and this is fixed by a single screw placed 1 cm away from one side of the fracture. Some tension should always be applied to the plate, even when it acts as a neutralization plate, supplementing interfragmentary screws. The eccentric yellow drill guide is, therefore, used for the second screw on the opposite side of the fracture so that when the screw is tightened tension is generated in the plate. When carrying out plating of a long bone, it is important that there is an intact cortex on the opposite side of the plate. Comminution of the medial cortex, or bone loss, may lead to instability and result in fatigue failure of the plate. If there is insufficient contact at this point, the defect should be filled with a cancellous bone graft at the time of operation. Cancellous bone may easily be obtained from the greater trochanter or the femoral condyles.

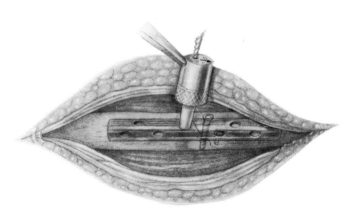

5

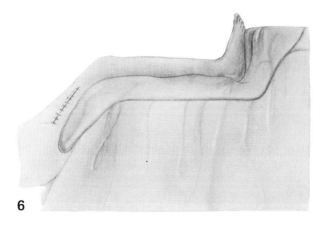

6

6

Wound closure

The wound is thoroughly irrigated with Ringer's Polybactrin solution and the vastus lateralis muscle flap is closed over the plate. A deep suction drain is inserted into the wound and the remaining layers are closed using absorbable polyglycolic acid (Dexon) sutures. The skin is closed with a nylon suture and a sterile dressing applied to the wound. The limb is elevated on a foam frame with the hip and knee joints at 90°.

POSTOPERATIVE CARE

The suction drain is removed at 48 hr and quadriceps exercises are commenced as soon as possible. The limb is maintained in a 90/90 splint for the first week. However, the knee should be extended at least twice daily for a period of static quadriceps exercises. When satisfactory quadriceps control has been achieved, the patient may mobilize with crutches non-weight-bearing. Care must be taken to avoid excessive force through the femur, particularly in comminuted fractures and weight-bearing may need to be restricted for at least 6–10 weeks. In suitable cases where there is little comminution the use of a cast brace to protect the internal fixation will allow earlier weight-bearing with function at the knee. If any of the signs of loosening of the implant occur, weight-bearing should be restricted or additional external splintage applied.

Considerable stress protection osteoporosis occurs in the bone underlying the large femoral plates. These should be removed at approximately 2 years after injury. Some care is necessary after removal of the plate as the bone will be weaker. Restriction of activities is recommended for several months.

References

Connolly, J. F., Dehne, E. and LaFollette, B. (1973). 'Closed reduction and early cast-brace ambulation in the treatment of femoral fractures.' *J. Bone Jt Surg.* **55A**, 1581
Dencker, H. (1965). 'Shaft fractures of the femur.' *Acta chir. scand.* **130**, 173
Gant, G. C., Shaftan, G. W. and Herbsman, H. (1970). 'Experience with the ASIF compression plate in the management of femoral shaft fractures.' *J. Trauma* **10**, 458
Jensen, J. S., Johansen, J. and Mørch, A. (1977). 'Middle third femoral fractures treated with medullary nailing or AO compression plates.' *Injury* **8**, 174
Mooney, V., Nickel, V. C., Harvey, J. P. and Snelson, R. (1970). 'Cast-brace treatment for fracture of the distal part of the femur.' *J. Bone Jt Surg.* **52A**, 1563
Müller, M. E., Allgöwer, M. and Willenegger, H. (1970). *Manual of Internal Fixation.* Berlin, Heidelberg, New York: Springer-Verlag
Solheim, K. and Vaage, S. (1972). 'Operative treatment of femoral fractures with the A.O. method.' *Injury* **4**, 54
Zickel, R. E. (1976). 'An intramedullary fixation device for the proximal part of the femur.' *J. Bone Jt Surg.* **58A**, 866

[*The illustrations for this Chapter on Fractures of the Femoral Shaft were drawn by Miss S. Barker and Mrs. P. Dewhurst.*]

Küntscher's Closed Intramedullary Nailing Technique for the Treatment of Femoral Shaft Fractures

Kevin F. King, F.R.C.S., F.R.A.C.S.
Senior Orthopaedic Surgeon, Western General Hospital, Melbourne;
Orthopaedic Surgeon, St. Vincent's Hospital, Melbourne

INTRODUCTION

Küntscher first described his closed femoral nailing operation in 1940 and over the next 30 years he gradually improved the technique, particularly by the introduction of flexible intramedullary reaming over guide wires and by the use of the image intensifier x-ray unit in the late 1950s. Using this technique, a femoral shaft fracture can be fixed rigidly through a single small incision over the lateral aspect of the buttock. The procedure can be carried out with minimal trauma, with little interference to the fracture haematoma and without further disruption to the periosteal blood supply of the femoral shaft.

PRE-OPERATIVE

Indications

The prime indication for the closed nailing operation is a traumatic fracture of the mid-shaft of the femur. It is also suitable for use in some subtrochanteric fractures in the proximal one-third, and with modifications (e.g. cross-bolts) it can be used to fix internally fractures of the lower third of the shaft. It is also readily applicable to the treatment of pathological fractures, particularly those due to secondary neoplastic deposits where the patients are often frail and minimal operative trauma is even more desirable than usual.

Technical requirements

The following items of equipment are required.

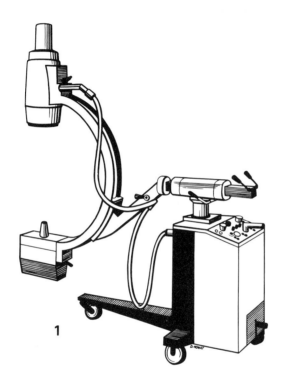

1

A mobile image intensifier x-ray unit and a television screen

With this sophisticated x-ray equipment it is possible to reduce the fracture, pass guide wires and to perform intramedullary reaming under direct x-ray screening. A very desirable extra piece of equipment is a video storage unit which allows x-ray images to be recorded, stored and recalled at will. This attachment not only makes the operative technique easier, but it also greatly diminishes the radiation to the patient and the theatre staff.

An orthopaedic operating table

This must be of a modern design with low slung horizontal leg extension pieces which allow access for the image intensifier unit to be swung around the thigh through an arc of at least 110° from vertical to horizontal screening positions. It must have various types of perineal support bars, both of the horizontal and vertical variety, allowing the patient to be positioned either on the side or supine.

A complete set of Küntscher's instruments

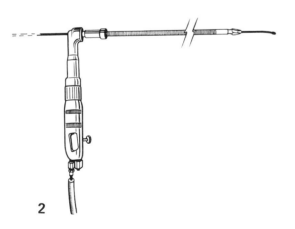

2

A slow speed (up to 400 rev/min) right-angled air-powered drill with a cannulated chuck allowing the reaming bit to operate along a guide wire.

A full set of flexible cannulated intramedullary reamers increasing in size from 9 mm to 18 mm by 0·5 mm increments.

A ball-tipped guide wire (3 mm diameter, length 950 mm) over which the cannulated flexible intramedullary reamers are threaded. In the event of reamer breakage, the ball tip allows for easy removal of the broken bits by withdrawal of the guide wire with the attached fragments.

3

A medullary tube. This is a plastic tube used for changing from reaming rod to inserting rod.

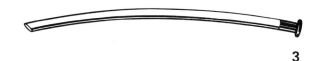

3

4

Inserting rod (4 mm diameter, length 950 mm) over which the Küntscher's nail is inserted.

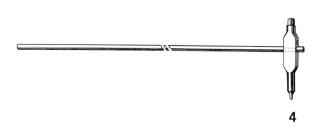

4

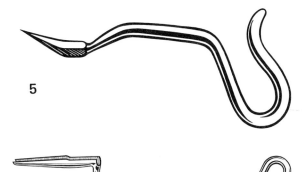

5

6

5 & 6

Awls. A pointed awl is used for perforating the tip of the greater trochanter. The cannulated enlarging awl is used to enlarge and to straighten the initial hole in the greater trochanter and also gives some control over the proximal fragment of femur.

7

A soft tissue guard to protect the skin of the thigh at the upper margin of the incision.

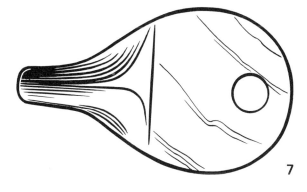

7

8

A cannulated punch and split hammer for the insertion of the nail over the guide wire.

A full set of Küntscher's nails. The minimum requirements are a set of nails varying in diameter from 10 to 15 mm and in length from 36 to 46 cm.

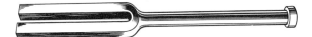

8

9

Supracondylar skeletal traction

A Steinmann's pin should be inserted through the femoral condyles at the beginning of the operation. By means of a long stirrup connected to the footpiece of the orthopaedic table, routine traction forces of 50–150 lb (24–74 kg) can be applied to the lower femoral fragment, all traction through the knee itself being avoided. It is essential to the success of this operation that distraction of the bone ends should be achieved to permit reduction at the fracture site.

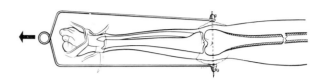

9

External correcting devices

These are designed to apply two-point pressure to the proximal and distal fragments, in a line at right angles to the line of the shaft and are designed to be applied once the fracture site has been distracted by supracondylar traction.

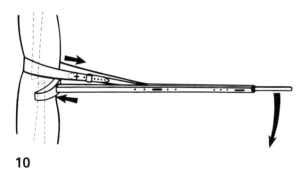

10

10

Küntscher used a crutch and strap technique which was effective but can be clumsy to use.

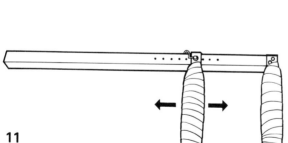

11

11

An alternative apparatus preferred by the author is made of square section aluminium tubing which is radiotranslucent. It has padded jaws, the distance between which can be adjusted to fit varying thicknesses of thigh. With this instrument it is possible to apply corrective pressure and, possessing a long handle, it keeps the manipulator clear of the x-ray beam.

Protective lead-impregnated wrap-around aprons

These should be worn by all members of the surgical team working in the operating theatre.

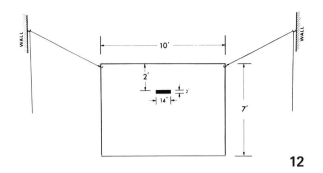

12

12, 13 & 14

Special draping

A large vertically-hung sheet with an operating slit
14 inches × 2 inches (36 cm × 5 cm) fitting over the
lateral part of the buttock and upper thigh allows the
surgeon access to the trochanteric region. It also leaves
free access to the patient for radiographer and anaesthetist. It is suspended by its upper corners from
opposite walls of the theatre and the upper free margin
of the sheet lies over the mid-line of the patient. The
surface of the sheet thus flows downwards and towards the surgeon over the curve of the buttock,
allowing room for the use of reaming drills and other
instruments. The long skirt of this sheet allows the
image intensifier to swing up to the horizontal position
without disturbing the sterile field. The margins of
the operating sheet are sutured to the lateral aspect of
the upper thigh and buttock and further secured with
a Steridrape to seal off the margins.

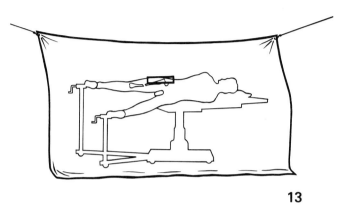

13

A Küntscher's nail extractor

This should always be available in case of need.

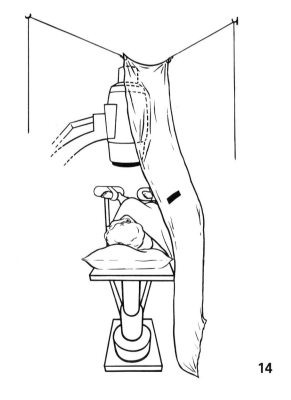

14

THE OPERATION

Positioning of patient

The patient is anaesthetized on the anaesthetic trolley. The subsequent transfer to the orthopaedic table requires the co-operation of at least four people directed by the surgeon. The anaesthetist controls the head and shoulders, two assistants on opposite sides of the trolley and table lift the trunk, using a narrow lifting sheet under the buttocks and a third assistant holds the feet and legs. The first stage is to transfer the patient onto the top of the orthopaedic table in a supine position, the perineal support having first been removed. At this stage the third assistant is supporting the weight of both legs. The next co-ordinated step is to switch the patient from a supine to a lateral position with the injured leg uppermost and the buttocks facing where the surgeon will stand.

15

The L-shaped perineal support is then attached to the orthopaedic table and its padded horizontal component is positioned in the perineum, separating the thighs. Both feet are now strapped to the footplates, the lower limb fully extended at knee and hip, the top limb fully extended at the knee but flexed 30° at the hip. This flexion of the injured limb at the hip allows radiological screening in vertical and horizontal planes. The mobile image intensifier unit is now positioned with the plane on the C-arm at right-angles to the line of the upper thigh. The beam is first centred in the vertical screening position and once a satisfactory image has been obtained on the television screen, the C-arm is swung to the horizontal position and height adjusted until a satisfactory x-ray image is obtained in this plane as well.

16

If the fracture is of the upper third of the femur, purely vertical screening may result in supra-imposition of the two thighs with a poor image. Therefore, in upper third fractures, the C-arm is swung 30° beyond the vertical to clear the lower thigh.

17

The above positioning is the optimal one for standard closed nailing. Another position is with the patient supine, the uninjured leg widely abducted and the image intensifier positioned between the legs. This arrangement is used when closed nailing of the femoral shaft is combined with fixation of a fracture of the neck of the femur in the same limb using Knowles pins. An alternative lateral position is with the upper injured limb flexed 30° at the hip as described above, but the lower limb flexed as far as possible at both hip and knee with the subcutaneous surface of the tibia resting on a padded gutter support. This is an awkward position if there are other injuries affecting the opposite limb or if the patient has any stiffness at all of the knee and hip in the opposite limb.

18

Insertion of supracondylar Steinmann's pin and application of external correcting force

The outline of the femoral condyles is marked on the skin with a felt pen, the skin is prepared with iodine and a threaded Steinmann's pin is drilled through the posterior halves of the lateral and medial femoral condyles, the placement avoiding the risk of the Küntscher's nail impacting on the Steinmann's pin later in the operation. The long Steinmann's pin stirrup is then attached and hooked around the footplate; through it, longitudinal traction may be applied without any strain being placed on the knee joint. Heavy traction forces of between 50 and 150 lb (24–74 kg) (as can be measured on a spring balance) are then applied and distraction of the bone ends is demonstrated on the x-ray screen. Once distraction is achieved, the external correcting device is applied and the bone ends are reduced under x-ray screening. *The operation does not proceed unless preliminary reduction can be demonstrated on the image intensifier television screen.* When reduction is achieved, the traction is partly released and the area of the greater trochanter is prepared and draped.

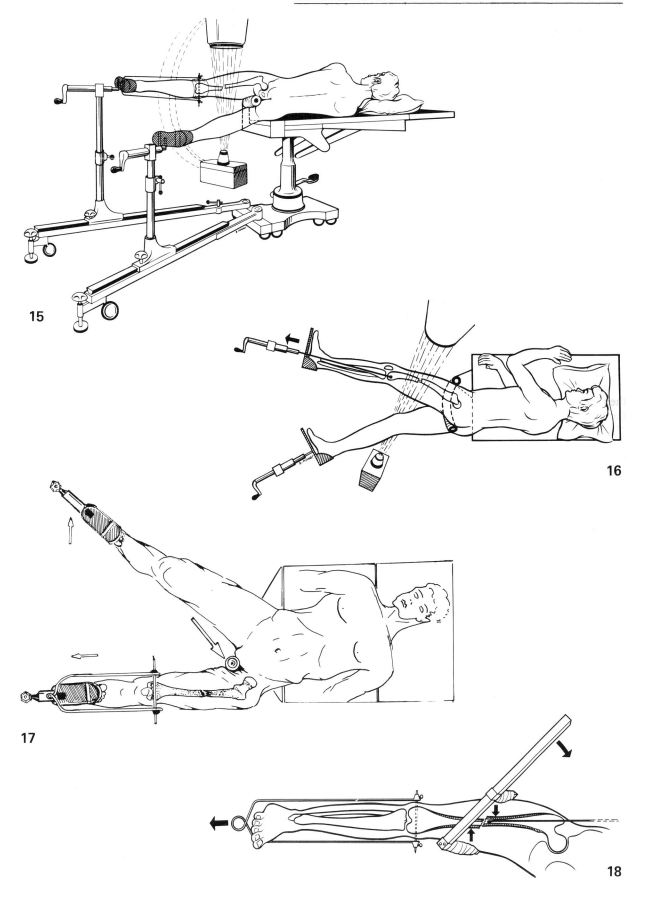

15

16

17

18

19 & 20

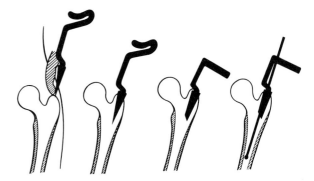

19

The incision

A small 2-inch (5 cm) incision is made proximally from the tip of the greater trochanter in the line of the femoral shaft. The tip of the trochanter is palpated with a double-gloved finger, the conjoined fibres of the gluteus maximus and tensor fascia lata are split in the line of their fibres, as also are the distal fibres of gluteus medius. The upper border of the greater trochanter can then be palpated and seen and it is perforated with an awl mid-way between the anterior and posterior margins and as far medially as is possible without actually passing over into the piriform fossa and on to the top of the femoral neck. Before making this awl hole it is essential to check once more the alignment of the proximal fragment of femur by placing a guide wire over the outer aspect of the thigh and screening both vertically and horizontally. If the awl hole is not made in the line of the medullary canal, a false passage may result and great difficulty can then be experienced in passing the guide wire down the femoral shaft. This initial awl hole is then enlarged with the enlarging awl, which also gives the operator some control over the proximal fragment. Through it, the ball-tipped guide wire is passed into the proximal shaft of the femur and heavy skeletal traction is re-applied. The external correcting device is used to reduce the bone ends and under x-ray screening the guide wire is passed into the distal fragment and advanced until it reaches the level of the femoral condyles. *If the distal 1 inch (2·5 cm) of the guide wire is curved slightly this greatly assists its manipulation into the medullary canal of the distal fragment.*

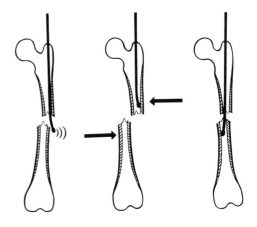

20

21

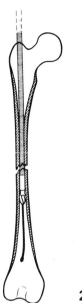

21

Flexible intramedullary reaming

Using the flexible intramedullary reamers over the ball-ended guide wire and starting at a diameter of 9 mm, the proximal and distal medullary canals are reamed in 5 mm increments. In the average-sized adult, routine reaming up to 14 or 15 mm diameter is used, the general principle being that the size of the reamer is increased until it can be felt to bite solidly on both proximal and distal medullary canals. When this occurs it is then advisable to ream at least several sizes above this. The larger the diameter of nail used the stronger and more rigid is the fixation.

Insertion of the nail

The length of the nail is gauged either by preliminary measurement of the opposite femur from tip of trochanter to upper border of patella (plus 1 cm) or, alternatively, by means of the intramedullary guide wire. *The diameter of the nail must be 1 mm less than that of the largest reamer used to avoid any possibility of jamming.* An inserting rod without a ball tip is then substituted for the reaming guide wire, this manoeuvre being facilitated by the use of a plastic medullary tube which is temporarily passed down through the medullary canal while the exchange is being made. Over the inserting rod the appropriate Küntscher's nail is then slowly tapped into the femur using the cannulated punch and split hammer.

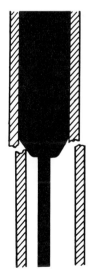
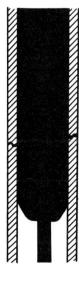

22

22

As the tapered tip of the nail crosses the fracture site it corrects the last few millimetres of lateral displacement and this stage must be closely observed under x-ray screening to make sure the tip of the nail does not impact onto the distal fragment.

Traction is then released, and the rest of the nail is hammered into place, leaving 1 cm of nail exposed proximally above the tip of the greater trochanter to facilitate later removal.

Wound closure

The wound over the trochanter is now sutured and the Steinmann's pin removed from the supracondylar region of the femur.

COMPLICATIONS AND THEIR MANAGEMENT

Failure to reduce the bone ends pre-operatively

If reduction cannot be demonstrated with supra-condylar traction and external correcting force, the closed procedure should be abandoned.

23

Failure to pass the guide wire into the proximal medullary canal of the femur

This occurs if the awl hole in the tip of the trochanter is not made in the right direction at the correct point of entry. The direction in which the awl is inserted must be carefully checked by x-ray screening in two planes before the hole is made. If the guide wire does not glide easily into the medullary canal of the proxmal fragment, the initial track is best made with a 9 mm diameter solid hand reamer.

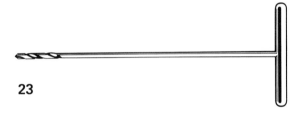

23

Jamming and breaking of reamers

If the full set of graduated reamers is used with a proper reaming drill and matching guide wires, this complication is rare. If, however, breakage or jamming does occur, then the remnants of the remaining drill can be removed by pulling out the guide wire. The ball on the end of the guide wire usually ensures that no fragments are left behind. Small broken metallic fragments lying loose in the medullary canal can be removed with sigmoidoscopy biopsy forceps, using the image intensifier for x-ray control.

Impaction of the drill or nail on the edge of the distal cortex at the fracture site

This is avoided by reaming and inserting the nail under x-ray control in two planes and by screening continuously as the tip of the nail passes the fracture site.

A stuck nail

This should not happen if the femoral shaft in normal bones has been adequately reamed and if the diameter of the nail is 1 mm less than that of the largest reamer. In the case of Paget's disease affecting the femoral shaft, jamming may occur readily if the nail is not prebent to the shape of the bowed shaft.

SPECIAL INDICATIONS
24

Fractures of the lower third of the femoral shaft are unsuitable for closed femoral nailing alone, as the nail will not grip on the distal fragment and thus will not control rotation or, in the case of comminution, shortening. This problem can be overcome by inserting a threaded cross-bolt through the lower eye of the Küntscher's nail under x-ray control, making a small stab incision over the lateral aspect of the lateral femoral condyle at the level of the lower eye of Küntscher's nail. If more stability is required, a second bolt can be passed through the upper eye of the nail. This is a reasonably straightforward procedure but requires practice.

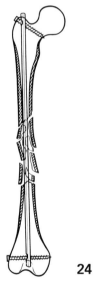

24

POSTOPERATIVE CARE

The limb is suspended in a sling or Thomas' splint for 7 days, but quadriceps exercises and knee bending are started within 24 hr. In the average patient with an uncomplicated middle-third fracture of the femoral shaft, where a firm grip is obtained on both proximal and distal fragments, full weight-bearing can be commenced within 7–10 days and discharge from hospital within 14–21 days is usual.

APPENDIX

AVAILABILITY OF EQUIPMENT

The most complete and technically the most satisfactory set of instruments is that designed by the A.O. group and manufactured by Synthes. They have copied and improved Küntscher's original instruments, the only item missing being the enlarging trochanteric awl.

Zimmer (U.K.) produce a basic set of instruments including the trochanteric enlarging awl and a right-angled air drill designed for reaming. This is neither as complete nor as technically satisfactory as the A.O. set but is significantly cheaper.

Howmedica supply a good set of flexible cannulated reamers produced by Ortopedia, a German subsidiary, but supporting instruments are limited.

In his last years Küntscher himself had his instruments and implants supplied by an American Company, the Orthopaedic Equipment Co. The author has had no experience of this particular set.

The long traction stirrups for supracondylar traction can be inexpensively made to order by any surgical supply firm or hospital splint shop.

The aluminium external correcting device was designed and made in his own workshop by Mr. E. Talkish, a radiographer at Western General Hospital. The design is simple and the instrument can be easily reproduced by any hospital engineer or splintmaker.

There are various designs of mobile image intensifier units available. The C-arm must rotate through an arc of at least 110°. Video storage units are expensive and are not essential. However, they are valuable, not only because they reduce radiation, but also because they make the operation technically easier.

References

Decoulx, J., Kempf, I., Jenny, G., Schvingt, E., Petit, P. and Vives, P. (1975). 'Enclouage à foyer fermé avec Alésage du femur selon Küntscher'. *Revue Chir. orthop.* **61**, 465
Kootstra, G. (1973). *Femoral Shaft Fractures in Adults*. Assen, The Netherlands: Van Gorcum & Coy
Küntscher, G. (1967). *Practice of Intramedullary Nailing*. Springfield: Charles C. Thomas

[*The illustrations for this Chapter on Küntscher's Closed Intramedullary Nailing Technique for the Treatment of Femoral Shaft Fractures were drawn by Mr. D. Howat and Mr. T. King. Illustrations 10, 19, 20 and 22 were redrawn after Küntscher.*]

Supracondylar Fractures of the Femur

Christopher E. Ackroyd, M.A., F.R.C.S.
Clinical Reader, Nuffield Department of Orthopaedic Surgery,
University of Oxford

PRE-OPERATIVE

1, 2 & 3

General considerations

Fractures of the supracondylar and intercondylar region of the femur are difficult to treat satisfactorily and require careful management to obtain good cosmetic and functional results. The main difficulty is obtaining and maintaining an adequate reduction while allowing function of the knee to start at an early stage. Neer, Grantham and Shelton (1967) have designed a classification based on anatomical deformity. Supracondylar fractures (*Illustration 1*), may be undisplaced, impacted, displaced or comminuted. However, it is the intercondylar fractures, with their extension into the knee joint, which are more serious in nature. Neer, Grantham and Shelton describe three types of fracture. First, undisplaced, secondly, displaced fractures (*Illustration 2*) with medial or lateral displacement of the distal fragment and, finally, comminuted fractures (*Illustration 3*), where there is considerable displacement and rotation of the condyles, together with comminution of the shaft. Closed methods have traditionally been used for these injuries, utilizing tibial traction or occasionally using the two-pin skeletal traction technique described by Modlin (1945). Watson-Jones (1976) recommended the use of tibial traction for most fractures provided a satisfactory reduction could be obtained. However, if there is severe displacement and particularly rotation of the condyles, closed reduction may not be possible, and he recommended open reduction.

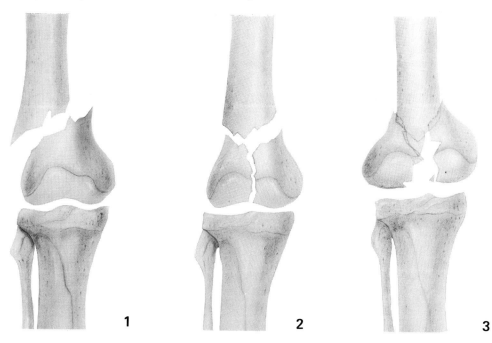

1   2   3

Stewart, Sisk and Wallace (1966) reviewed 442 fractures at the Campbell Clinic and found that the best results tended to occur with non-operative treatment. They therefore concluded that simple non-operative treatment produced good results in the majority of these fractures. Neer, Grantham and Shelton (1967) emphasized the problem of closed treatment, suggesting careful attention to detail. More recently, Mooney *et al.* (1970) and Connolly, Dehne and LaFolette (1973) have reported the use of the cast brace to allow early ambulant treatment of these fractures. Treatment time has been considerably shortened with good results.

Methods of internal fixation of these fractures have generally been unsatisfactory and given poor results. More recently, effective implants have been designed which allow rigid fixation of cancellous bone fragments in this area, together with sufficient stability to allow immediate functional treatment. Several preliminary reports have recorded good results (Müller, Allgöwer and Willenegger, 1970; Olerud, 1972; Shelton *et al.*, 1974). Hohl (1975) has detailed the various techniques of treatment and emphasized that open operation can be extremely difficult and require considerable experience to achieve a satisfactory fixation. Though closed reduction also requires considerable attention to detail, the risks of failure would appear to be less.

Indications

In the absence of any long-term comparative trials, most fractures should be treated by the technique of skeletal traction with early active joint movement followed by the use of a functional brace when swelling has subsided. When adequate reduction cannot be obtained by closed means, particularly in younger patients, open reduction and internal fixation should be carried out as a planned procedure under optimum conditions. The precise criteria of an adequate reduction have yet to be clearly defined, although excessive varus or valgus displacement, separation of the condyles of more than 3—4 mm, or malrotation of the condyles with joint incongruity, will suggest a surgical approach. Specific indications for open reduction and internal fixation may occur in patients with neuromuscular disorders, where active control of the limb in traction may not be possible.

Single fractures of a condyle, if displaced by more than 2—3 mm, may be fixed by interfragmentary compression using one or two cancellous screws. Fractures with a supracondylar component require the use of the 95° condylar blade-plate as described by the AO group.

Pre-operative preparation

If a satisfactory closed reduction has not been obtained, intra-articular fractures are best treated within the first 12 hr before significant swelling and soft tissue oedema have developed. If the operation cannot be performed within this time, then it should be delayed for at least 5—7 days until the swelling has decreased. After 2 weeks have elapsed, operation becomes much more difficult and if mal-union occurs this will require corrective osteotomy as a secondary procedure.

Operation is carried out under general anaesthesia and the use of a tourniquet is helpful. The limb is exsanguinated with an Esmarch bandage and a pneumatic tourniquet applied to the upper part of the thigh, with the knee in the flexed position over a layer of wool, and inflated to 400 mmHg for a maximum time of 2 hr. A diathermy pad is inserted under the buttock.

The patient should be positioned with a sandbag under the ipsilateral buttock and the skin at the operative site prepared with three applications of a suitable antiseptic. It is often helpful to be able to break the operating table at the level of the knee joint. The limb is draped in sterile towelling so that it is free for manipulation. It is often necessary to take additional cancellous bone graft, and the area of skin overlying the greater trochanter or the iliac crest should be prepared for this procedure.

THE OPERATION

4

The incision

The approach to the supracondylar region of the femur should be from the lateral side and the skin is incised in the mid-lateral position just in front of the iliotibial tract. The incision starts 10–15 cm above the lateral joint line and its lower end curves forward medially towards the tibial tubercle. The deep fascia is divided along the line of the incision to expose the vastus lateralis and the quadriceps expansion. An alternative approach has been described by Olerud (1972) where a U-shaped incision is made on both medial and lateral sides of the knee, the tibial tubercle is osteotomized and the patella reflected upwards to expose the whole of the anterior aspect of the knee joint. This approach may be necessary when there is extensive comminution of bone and displacement of the medial femoral condyle.

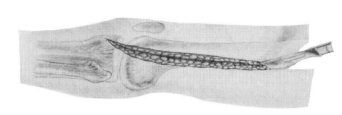

4

5

Exposure of the fracture

Vastus lateralis is lifted forward from the lateral intermuscular septum and separated from its attachment to the linea aspera. As in the approach to the femoral shaft, the perforating branches of the profunda femoris artery are divided and ligated. This line of dissection is continued downwards, and the quadriceps expansion and capsule of the knee joint are divided to expose the synovium which is opened to gain wide exposure to the anterolateral aspect of the knee joint. Exposure of the joint is only necessary when there is an intercondylar fracture, so that reduction of the joint surfaces can be carried out under direct vision. Vastus lateralis is further reflected forwards and detached from its origin on the femur with a periosteal elevator so that the anterolateral surface of the femur is exposed. The patella is reflected medially and the fracture surfaces now come into view.

The fractured fragments are gently separated using a small bone hook and the fracture edges carefully cleaned, care being taken to maintain soft tissue attachments. Careful inspection of the fracture should be carried out at this stage in order to define precisely the number of fragments present and the orientation of the fracture lines. Copious irrigation should be carried out with Ringer's Polybactrin solution to remove blood clot and small detached bony fragments.

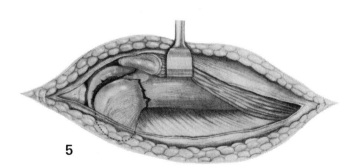

5

6

Reduction of the intercondylar fracture

Reduction of the intercondylar fracture is now carried out and held with temporary Kirschner wires. Two 3·2 mm drill holes are made in the lateral femoral condyle, crossing into the medial condyle. Two cancellous screws are inserted after preliminary tapping of the proximal cortex. These screws should be placed in the anterior part of the condyles, one sited more proximally than the other. Care should be taken to ensure that they do not interfere with placement of the blade-plate. As the screws are tightened, interfragmentary compression is applied to the intercondylar fracture, which is now satisfactorily stabilized.

The Kirschner wires are removed and it is necessary to determine precisely the alignment for the blade of the condylar plate. Three Kirschner wires are used. The first is inserted under the patella so that it lies on the anterior surface of the femoral condyles. The second is inserted transversely through the knee joint, parallel to the surfaces of the femoral condyles and in the same plane as the first wire. The third wire is passed through the middle of the femoral condyle 1 cm above the articular surface, parallel to both the first and second wires, and this serves as the guide for the blade of the condylar plate.

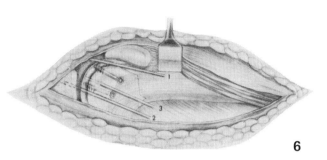

6

7

Alignment of the plate

The condylar template should now be applied to the lateral surface of the femur, preliminary reduction of the supracondylar component of the fracture having been carried out and held with provisional Kirschner wires. It is now possible to check that the plate will lie satisfactorily against the side of the femur. The site of insertion of the blade is marked with an osteotome. In some cases, reduction of the main fracture may not be possible until control of the distal fragment is obtained with the blade and the site of its insertion should lie in the centre of the anterior half of the femoral condyles.

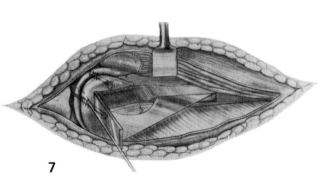

7

8

Preparation of the femoral condyles

A slot is now made in the lateral cortex of the femoral condyle, 16 × 10 mm in size, in line with the femoral shaft. This can be made by utilizing the 4·5 mm triple drill guide followed by the router, or by using an appropriately sized osteotome. The special seating chisel should now be inserted in line with the third Kirschner wire at approximately 81° to the long axis of the femur. The chisel guide ensures that alignment with the shaft of the femur is maintained. The chisel should be inserted with sharp blows of the hammer, firm pressure being applied to the medial side of the knee to resist the disruptive forces acting on the inter-condylar fracture. It is important to maintain the chisel parallel to the articular surface of the knee joint, heading very slightly down towards the medial femoral condyle. This will ensure that when the supracondylar fracture is reduced and compression applied, the cortex furthest from the plate is compressed first, followed by the cortex nearest the plate.

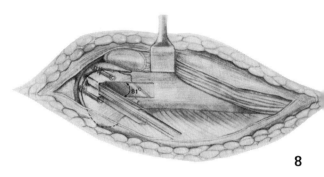

8

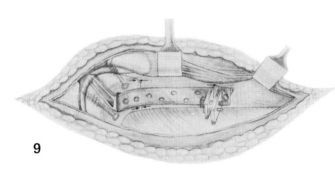

9

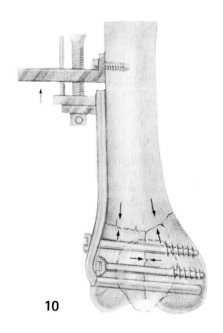

10

9 & 10

Insertion of the condylar blade-plate

The seating chisel is removed and a suitably-sized 95° blade-plate is inserted along the groove prepared in the femoral condyles. The blade is impacted into the condyles and secured with one or two cancellous screws which may allow additional interfragmentary fixation of the intercondylar fracture. If reduction of the supracondylar fracture has not yet been carried out, the plate will allow better control of the distal fragment and once anatomical reduction has been obtained a bone clamp is applied to maintain the position. Axial compression can now be exerted at the fracture site, utilizing the tension device. This necessitates drilling a single cortex hole proximal to the plate to secure the tension device. *Illustration 10* shows the appearance in diagrammatic form. When the fracture has been adequately compressed the remaining 4·5 mm cortical screws are inserted into the shaft. If an accurate reduction has been obtained and a dynamic compression plate is being utilized, it is not necessary to use the tension device.

Impaction of cancellous bone usually occurs in these fractures leaving a defect at the fracture site. This should be filled with cancellous bone graft, and if necessary a small window should be made in the supracondylar region so that it can be packed with cancellous bone to support the articular surfaces. After irrigation with Ringer's Polybactrin solution wound closure is carried out in layers using a poly-glycolic acid (Dexon) suture. Suction drainage helps to prevent haematoma formation. Vastus lateralis is resutured to the linea aspera, so providing good soft tissue cover of the plate. The skin is sutured with interrupted 3/0 nylon sutures and a wool and crêpe bandage dressing applied.

POSTOPERATIVE CARE

In the postoperative period the limb should be nursed with the hip and knee flexed to 90° as for femoral shaft fractures. A Robert Jones bandage should be applied to the flexed knee and the limb should then be supported on a foam splint. Provided that there is satisfactory stability of the fracture, assisted active movements may be commenced within the first few days. The suction drain is removed at 48 hr and the Robert Jones bandage removed and the knee extended at least twice daily for a period of static quadriceps exercises. As the patient develops quadriceps control, he may sit with his legs over the edge of the bed and begin active flexion and extension movements. The 90/90 splint is discarded by the end of the first week, by which time a good range of flexion has been established. During the second week the patient should concentrate on developing full control of extension. The sutures are removed at the fourteenth day and if wound healing is satisfactory the patient may be allowed out of bed to commence walking with crutches non-weight-bearing. The programme of active exercises should be continued under supervision of the physiotherapist, together with the use of hydrotherapy if this is available.

Partial weight-bearing may be introduced at between 4 and 6 weeks after operation, depending on the stability of the fixation and the co-operation of the patient. If the fixation is poor, or the signs of loosening of the implant develop, additional external splintage can be applied with the use of a cast brace which will allow weight-bearing and knee function.

Large implants such as the condylar blade-plate should be removed in most patients approximately 18 months after injury. Stress protection osteoporosis occurs in the bone underlying the plates and care should be taken in the first few months to avoid excessive activity which can produce the risk of a refracture.

References

Connolly, J. P., Dehne, E. and LaFolette, B. (1973). 'Closed reduction and early brace ambulation in the treatment of femoral fractures. Part II. Results in 143 fractures.' *J. Bone Jt Surg.* **55A**, 1581

Hohl, M. (1975). 'Fractures about the knee.' In *Fractures,* Edited by C. A. Rockwood and D. P. Green. Philadelphia, Toronto: Lippincott

Modlin, J. (1945). 'Double skeletal traction in battle fractures of the lower femur.' *Bull. U.S. Army Med. Dept.* **4**, 119

Mooney, V., Nickel, V. L., Harvey, J. P. and Snelson, R. (1970). 'Cast-brace treatment for fractures of the distal part of the femur. A prospective controlled study of 150 patients.' *J. Bone Jt Surg.* **52A**, 1563

Müller, M. E., Allgöwer, M. and Willenegger, H. (1970). *Manual of Internal Fixation.* Berlin, Heidelberg, New York: Springer-Verlag

Neer, C. S., Grantham, S. A. and Shelton, M. L. (1967). 'Supracondylar fractures of the adult femur. A study of one hundred and ten cases.' *J. Bone Jt Surg.* **49A**, 591

Olerud, S. (1972). 'Operative treatment of supracondylar–condylar fractures of the femur.' *J. Bone Jt Surg.* **54A**, 1015

Shelton, M. C., Grantham, S. A., Neer, II, C. S. and Singh, R. (1974). 'Fixation device for supracondylar and low femoral shaft fractures.' *J. Trauma* **14**, 821

Stewart, M. J., Sisk, T. D. and Wallace, S. L. (1966). 'Fracture of the distal third of the femur. A comparison of methods of treatment.' *J. Bone Jt Surg.* **48A**, 784

Watson-Jones, R. (1976). *Fractures and Joint Injuries.* Chapter 27, 5th Edition. Edited by J. N. Wilson. Edinburgh, London, New York: Churchill Livingstone

[*The illustrations for this Chapter on Supracondylar Fractures of the Femur were drawn by Miss S. Barker.*]

Fractures of the Patella

Christopher E. Ackroyd, M.A., F.R.C.S.
Clinical Reader, Nuffield Department of Orthopaedic Surgery,
University of Oxford

PRE - OPERATIVE

Indications

Fractures of the patella are caused by direct or indirect violence. This results in varying degrees of displacement of the fragments and interrupts the quadriceps mechanism. Accurate reconstruction of the articular surface is important in safeguarding the long-term health of the joint. Loss of active extension of the knee, with fragment separation of more than 2 – 3 mm, and a step in the articular surface of more than 2–3 mm are indications for operation (Boström, 1972). In older patients a more conservative approach can be adopted if there is gross continuity of the quadriceps mechanism. In children small avulsion fractures, of either pole, may be difficult to see on the radiographs and consist of a considerable portion of the articular surface. If displacement is more than 2 – 3 mm, operation should be carried out.

Restoration of normal anatomy is recommended for transverse fractures and for comminuted fractures when the articular surface is not severely damaged and can easily be reduced. Where there is a small upper or lower pole fragment bone reconstruction to restore the quadriceps mechanism is preferable to fragment excision and re-insertion of the tendon. In severely comminuted fractures reconstruction of the bone may be impossible and excision of the patella should be carried out with repair of the quadriceps expansion (Hohl, 1975). The decision whether or not to attempt reconstruction depends upon the integrity of the articular surface of the patella and may thus only be carried out at the time of operation. Significant fissuring or fibrillation of the articular cartilage, except in the young patient, or evidence of osteo-arthrosis, will favour patellectomy. The patella should be preserved, if at all possible, as excision may result in considerable residual disability (Scott, 1949) although Sanderson (1974) suggested that good results could be obtained from total excision and this was better done as a primary procedure.

Pre-operative preparation

Operation should be performed as soon as possible after injury unless there is local skin infection, extensive abrasions, or other more serious injuries that demand priority. The skin in the operative area is lightly shaved and a suitable antiseptic applied. While awaiting operation, the patient's leg should be rested in a foam gutter splint.

Anaesthesia

The operation should be carried out under general anaesthesia. The limb should be exsanguinated with an Esmarch bandage and a pneumatic tourniquet applied high up on the thigh over a layer of wool. The tourniquet should be inflated to 400 mmHg and may be left in position for up to 2 hr.

Position of patient

The patient is placed supine with the knees straight. The operative area is prepared with at least three applications of antiseptic and the whole limb draped in sterile towelling. The skin around the site of the incision may be protected by adhesive plastic.

THE OPERATION

1

The incision

A slightly curved transverse incision, 10 cm long, is made on the anterior aspect of the knee. The incision should be centred over the lower half of the patella with the knee extended. During flexion and extension of the knee, the skin on the anterior aspect slides in relation to the aponeurosis with the intervening pre-patellar bursa. Scar adherence between these layers may lead to long-term discomfort. The loose areolar tissue is usually infiltrated with haematoma and identification of the layers of the deep fascia may be difficult.

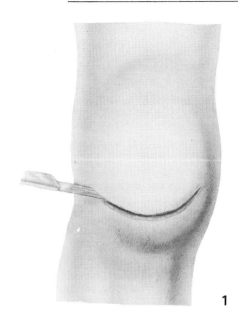

1

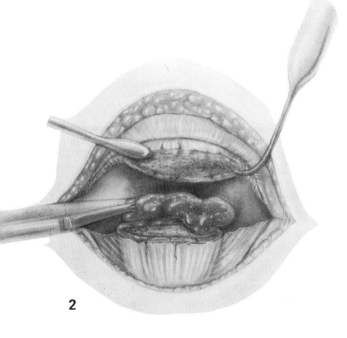

2

2

Exposure of the fracture

The deep fascia is divided and the skin flaps are elevated and retracted using sharp dissection. The fractured patella and torn patellar retinacula are now exposed. The blood clot is removed from both the fractured surfaces using a dissector or small curette. A small bone hook is used to elevate proximal and distal fragments so that the articular surface of the patella can be inspected and the knee joint cleaned and irrigated with Ringer's Polybactrin solution. The periosteum and retinacular fibres are scraped back from the edge of the fracture some 2 — 3 mm, using a small periosteal elevator so that reduction is not obstructed.

3

Reduction of the fracture

The bone fragments are now reduced. It is important that there should be perfect apposition, particularly of the articular surface. Difficulty with reduction may be due to small bone fragments or soft tissue which have not been removed from the fracture surface. The reduction is maintained with reduction clamps or a temporary Kirschner wire, which is inserted with the power drill. It may be necessary to enlarge the tear of the medial retinaculum and make a small medial arthrotomy incision in order to inspect the articular surface, to ensure its accurate reconstitution. Alternatively, a check radiograph can be obtained at this time.

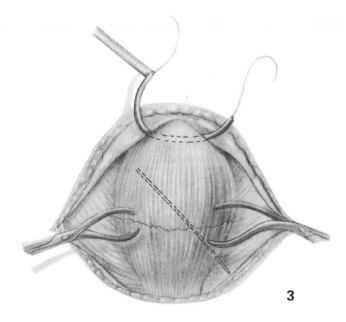

3

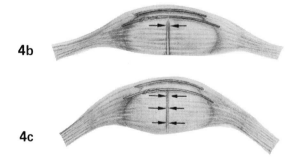

4a

4b

4c

4a,b&c

Rigid internal fixation

In transverse fractures the double tension band wiring technique provides excellent fixation. The first wire is passed deep to the quadriceps tendon and patellar tendon. The second wire lies more superficially and passes through the Sharpey's fibres of the two tendons. The wires are tightened on opposite sides to ensure equal distribution of tension. The wire ends are turned in so as not to cause pressure areas and the patellar retinacula are repaired over the wire with interrupted sutures. When the wires are tightened, slight over-correction at the fracture occurs. On flexing the knee, or contraction of the quadriceps, the over-correction vanishes and the fracture surfaces are squeezed together under compression. In T-fractures or other more comminuted types, Kirschner wires, or interfragmentary screws may be used to create two main fragments suitable then for the tension band wiring technique.

A suction drain is inserted and the deep fascia is closed with Dexon sutures, ensuring good soft tissue cover of the wires. The skin is closed with interrupted 3/0 nylon sutures.

POSTOPERATIVE CARE

A sterile dressing is placed on the wound and a generous layer of plaster wool applied to the entire limb. The limb is then immobilized in a plaster-of-Paris cylinder. The tourniquet is removed and the surgeon awaits return of the circulation to the foot. The limb should be elevated on pillows or a frame at 45° for 5 days and quadriceps activity encouraged within the plaster cylinder. Mobilization with crutches and weight-bearing is commenced when the general condition of the patient is satisfactory and the leg is comfortable. The patient may be discharged when he is walking satisfactorily.

The plaster cylinder is bivalved and the sutures are removed at between 10 and 14 days and provided wound healing is satisfactory, knee flexion may be commenced together with static quadriceps exercises. A removable plaster-of-Paris back splint may be used with advantage during weight-bearing for a further 2 weeks and is essential if there is inadequate control of the quadriceps muscle.

Experimental studies have confirmed that with secure tension band wire fixation, early active movement and weight-bearing may safely be allowed without loss of reduction. If there is any doubt about the fixation, the plaster cylinder may be maintained for 4 – 6 weeks (Müller, Allgöwer and Willenegger, 1970).

The institution of early active movement, seldom results in postoperative stiffness and a full range of movement should be achieved within 8 – 10 weeks. However, manipulation, if it becomes necessary, should not be carried out until at least 3 months or when radiological union has been demonstrated. Removal of the metal is often necessary as it may cause some discomfort under the skin. This should be carried out after 6 – 9 months when clear radiological union of the fracture has taken place.

References

Boström, A. (1972). 'Fractures of the patella.' *Acta orthop. scand.,* Suppl. 143
Hohl, M. (1975). 'Fractures of the patella.' In *Fractures,* Edited by C. A. Rockwood and D. P. Green. Philadelphia, Toronto: Lippincott
Müller, M. E., Allgöwer, M. and Willenegger, H. (1970). *Manual of Internal Fixation.* Berlin, Heidelberg, New York: Springer-Verlag
Sanderson, M. C. (1974). 'The fractured patella.' *J. Bone Jt Surg.* **56B,** 391
Scott, J. C. (1949). 'Fractures of the patella.' *J. Bone Jt Surg.* **31B,** 76

[*The illustrations for this Chapter on Fractures of the Patella were drawn by Miss S. Barker.*]

Fractures of the Tibial Condyles

Christopher E. Ackroyd, M.A., F.R.C.S.
Clinical Reader, Nuffield Department of Orthopaedic Surgery,
University of Oxford

INTRODUCTION

Fractures of the tibial condyles occur in a variety of different patterns. However, the most common injury is the so-called bumper (syn. fender) fracture of the lateral condyle. The mechanisms of injury are probably complex and there is invariably a combination of bony and soft tissue damage. Road traffic accidents account for about half of these injuries (Barr, 1940; Hohl, 1975). However, with the adoption of a higher bumper on domestic vehicles there may be a change in the patterns of injury. Many systems of classification have been designed, but none is completely satisfactory. Palmer (1951) evolved a classification of three types. However, the more comprehensive system described by Hohl (1967) of six types has been widely accepted. Courvoisier (1973) has devised a similar classification in which the medial or lateral condylar injury may be of three main types.

1–4

First (*Illustration 1*), a cleavage or separation fracture with essentially no compression of the cancellous bone; second (*Illustration 2*), an impacted fracture where the articular surface is compressed with crushing of the cancellous bone; and third (*Illustration 3*), a mixed fracture where there is both crushing of the cancellous bone and a large fragment separated from the peripheral part of the condyle. *Illustration 4* shows a fourth variety — the well recognized comminuted fracture of the T- or Y-type, affecting both condyles. Further groups include marginal fractures and tibial spine avulsions. All authors emphasize the importance of accurate diagnosis of the precise area of fracture and this relies on additional oblique radiographs and, in some instances, tomography to reveal a depressed segment. Damage to the menisci and the ligaments may accompany a fracture of the tibial plateau and an examination under anaesthesia with stress radiography may be necessary to diagnose ligamentous disruption, which, if present, should in general be repaired.

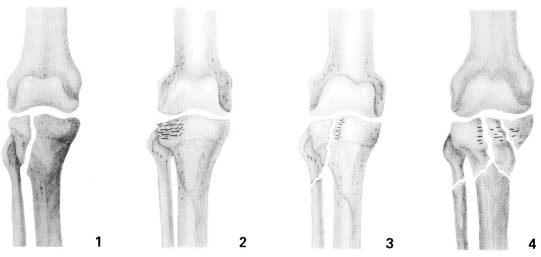

1   2   3   4

PRE - OPERATIVE

Indications

There is much disagreement in the literature as to the place of open reduction and internal fixation in the treatment of these fractures. It is therefore difficult to lay down firm criteria for operation, as in many instances it will depend not only on the surgeon's attitude and approach to operative treatment, but also on the patient's age, general and local condition, associated injuries, and the quality of knee function required by the patient. In contrast to the treatment of ankle fractures, there is no firm evidence to support an anatomical reduction in every case, although in principle it would seem to be desirable. Some degree of angular deformity, particularly on the lateral side, may be tolerated without inevitable late deterioration of the joint (Apley, 1956); although, if this exceeds 10°, osteo-arthrosis is more likely to develop (Rasmussen, 1973). There have been few comparative studies of operative and non-operative treatment. Most have had too few cases to justify any clear-cut conclusions. Courvoisier (1973), in his extensive study, found that the final result depended on the care taken to reach an exact diagnosis and to apply the selected technique of treatment, whether operative or non-operative. Schatzker (1977), emphasized the benefits to be obtained from operation, particularly the institution of early joint movement, which is essential if a poor result is to be avoided. However, operative treatment may be extremely difficult, particularly as the degree of damage is always greater than expected, and poor operative treatment may lead to a worse result than poor non-operative treatment.

Hohl (1975) has described the detailed indications in each of the various fracture types. The presence of an intact fibula is an important stabilizing influence and if a fracture of the neck of the fibula is present, loss of position following reduction is more likely to occur. If, after reduction, there is more than 4 mm of separation of the fragments, operative treatment should be strongly considered. Compression of the cancellous bone cannot be reduced by closed means and if depression of a major part of the articular surface exceeds 6–8 mm, elevation should be carried out (Barr, 1940). In younger patients when stress testing demonstrates more than five additional degrees of valgus deformity, despite lesser amounts of articular depression, open reduction should be recommended. Rasmussen (1973) emphasized the importance of knee joint stability and operation should be performed to correct any significant instability.

Complete rupture of the collateral ligaments should be repaired. It is, however, often difficult to diagnose this accurately until after fixation of the bony fragments.

Pre-operative preparation

An ample wool and crêpe bandage should be applied to the knee and the limb supported in a foam gutter. If the closed reduction has been unsuccessful, or the degree of displacement or depression too great, operation should be carried out immediately if the skin condition is satisfactory. If other associated injuries cause delay in treatment for more than 24 hr, it is usually advisable to delay open reduction for 5–7 days until the swelling and soft tissue oedema have decreased. The fracture should therefore be immobilized in plaster-of-Paris, or the position maintained with skeletal traction. In any event open reduction and internal fixation should be carried out within 14 days as it may be difficult to obtain a satisfactory reduction and fixation after this time.

Anaesthesia

Operation should be carried out under general anaesthesia with the use of a pneumatic tourniquet applied to the mid-thigh over a layer of wool. Exsanguination of the limb is carried out with an Esmarch bandage and the tourniquet is inflated to a pressure of 400 mmHg for a maximum of 2 hr. In older patients it may be advisable to restrict the use of the tourniquet.

Position of patient

The patient is positioned prone on the operation table and the fractured knee is supported in a position of 45° of flexion by means of a foam triangle placed under the thigh. Alternatively, the knee is positioned at a break in the operating table so that the knee can be flexed if desired. The area surrounding the knee is shaved and the skin prepared with at least three applications of a suitable antiseptic. Sterile towelling is applied to the limb so that it is free and an adhesive plastic such as Op-site applied to the area of the incision. The opposite iliac crest is prepared in order to take a corticocancellous bone graft.

THE OPERATION

The incision

5

A number of approaches have been described for these fractures. The incision chosen must depend on the type of fracture and the means of internal fixation to be used. It is important that adequate exposure of the joint surface and tibial condyle is obtained. The anterior lazy S incision starts in front of the lateral or medial femoral condyle and runs downwards, curving forwards at the level of the joint line, then bending downwards to run longitudinally along the anterior crest of the tibia. The incision may be used on either the medial or the lateral side and either the upper or the lower part of the incision can be curved outwards to give appropriate access as required.

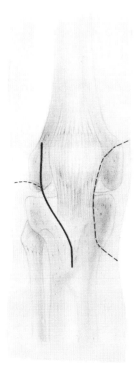

5

6

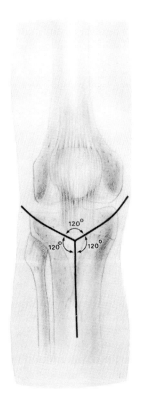

6

In comminuted fractures where it is necessary to approach both the medial and the lateral sides of the joint, the Y-shaped triradiate incision gives excellent access. There should be 120° between each limb of the incision and they should meet over the middle of the patellar tendon, rather than over the tibial tubercle. Great care must be taken with this incision to avoid skin edge necrosis. The skin flaps should be elevated as deeply as possible, at the level of the capsular plane in order to preserve the blood supply, and meticulous skin suturing is necessary using fine subcuticular or mattress sutures.

7

Exposure of the fracture

The incision is deepened through the subcutaneous tissue and the fibres of the iliotibial band may be split near the joint line and reflected distally to expose the capsule. Elevation of the skin flaps should be carried out with great care and it is advisable to use skin retraction sutures. A longitudinal incision is made in the capsule at the side of the patellar tendon, with a transverse extension at the level of the joint line. The capsular attachments are elevated as far as the collateral ligament. The meniscus itself is frequently found to be undamaged or sometimes only peripherally detached and therefore should be preserved. The coronary ligaments holding the meniscus to the tibia are divided with the capsule so that the meniscus is elevated to permit visualization of the tibial condyle. Thorough inspection of the articular surface should be carried out in order to identify any central or posterior compression fractures.

The separated peripheral fracture is then exposed by elevating the muscles on the lateral side, care being taken to preserve as much of the soft tissue attachments as possible. On the medial side, the periosteum is elevated a short distance from the fracture edges so that an adequate reduction can be obtained.

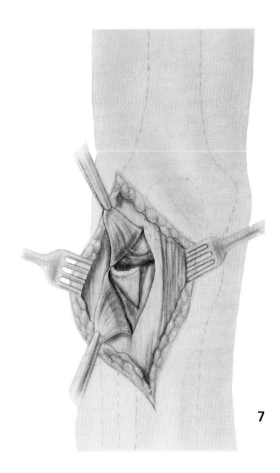

7

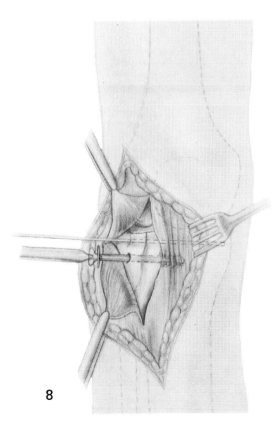

8

8

Reduction of the fracture

Once exposure of the bony lesion has been carried out and the full extent of the articular injury identified, the main fracture fragments are separated using a bone hook and the fracture surfaces cleaned with a small curette. Loose bone fragments, soft tissue and haematoma are removed to allow an anatomical reduction of the fracture to be carried out. Fractured articular fragments may need to be elevated first before reduction of the peripheral fragment. The reduction is held in position with temporary Kirschner wires while preparation is made for the definitive fixation. There is no set order of sequence since no two lesions are ever exactly the same.

9

Elevation and cancellous bone grafting

When dealing with a pure compression fracture, it is necessary to make a window in the anterior cortex of the tibia, approximately 1 cm below the edge of the tibial margin. This permits introduction of an instrument which can be used to elevate the fracture. In comminuted and compression fractures there is always loss of cancellous bone substance and in order to maintain the stability of the articular surface, it is necessary to pack the defect with corticocancellous bone obtained from the iliac crest. The bone fragments are packed into the cavity and it is advisable to over-correct the articular surface by elevating it 2 – 3 mm above the correct level. The forces acting through the knee in the simple assisted non-weight-bearing exercises are sufficient to impact the fragments to the correct level.

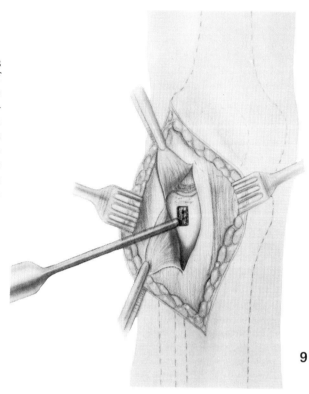

9

10

10

Fixation of the fracture

When treating a pure separation fracture with good quality bone with no compression of the cancellous surfaces, fixation can be carried out with cancellous lag screws. When the fracture is accompanied by compression, there is often a deficiency of the cortical margins and a small T-plate should be used as a buttress in addition to the interfragmentary screws. An alternative technique is the use of bolts which go across the tibia from medial to lateral side. When treating a severe comminuted fracture, a variety of techniques may be required and it is often necessary to use a buttress plate on both medial and lateral sides of the tibia held together by wire or bolts.

The articular soft tissues

Preservation of the meniscus should be attempted if at all possible. However, if there is a substantial tear then meniscectomy should be performed, though a peripheral detachment can be repaired. Associated ruptures of the collateral ligaments should be repaired and this may necessitate a separate incision on the other side of the joint. Peroperative radiographs should be taken after fixation of the fracture together with stress views to confirm that a satisfactory reconstruction has been carried out and to exclude associated ligamentous injury. Rupture of the cruciate ligaments should be repaired wherever possible, although in most instances this is less important than repair of the collateral ligaments.

Wound closure

The wound and knee joint should be thoroughly irrigated with Ringer's Polybactrin solution prior to closure. The synovium and capsule are repaired with polyglycolic acid (Dexon) sutures and a suction drain is placed under the subcutaneous layer which is closed with interrupted sutures. The skin is closed with interrupted 3/0 nylon sutures and a meticulous technique is necessary, particularly when the triradiate incision has been used, in order to reduce wound problems and allow safe early mobilization. The use of the Donati-Allgöwer subcuticular mattress suture helps to protect the vascularity of the skin edges. The wound is covered with a sterile dressing and a compression bandage applied with the knee in 90° of flexion. A further wool and Domette Robert Jones bandage is applied and the tourniquet is then released.

POSTOPERATIVE CARE

The limb is elevated and can be readily held in the 90/90 position with an evacuation splint. The compression dressings are removed daily and the leg extended fully so that quadriceps activity can be commenced for increasing periods each day. The suction drain is removed at 48 hr and by the end of the first week an adequate range of flexion will have been established and the limb is then rested in the extended position. If there is any doubt about the wound, or the stability of the fracture is insufficient to allow early function, then the knee should be splinted in the extended position. In any event immobilization of the joint should not be continued for longer than 3 weeks as the end result becomes less satisfactory (Hohl, 1975). The stitches are removed when the wound has healed, usually at the fourteenth to sixteenth day and it is then possible to allow hydrotherapy in addition to the programme of static and active exercises. The patient may be allowed to get up non-weight-bearing in the second week if progress is satisfactory. Care must, however, be taken to avoid dependent oedema.

The time that weight-bearing is introduced varies considerably depending on the precise fracture type and the degree of stability obtained, although this will usually be between the fourth and tenth week. A functional brace consisting of a plastic quadrilateral socket and knee hinges can be used to supplement the internal fixation. This is applied when wound healing is complete, usually in the third week and allows weight-bearing to be commenced at an earlier stage. In fractures with any significant degree of compression, unrestricted weight-bearing should not be allowed until the third to the fifth month when revascularization of the bone graft will have occurred and the area of cancellous bone will be sufficiently consolidated.

Removal of the metal is often necessary because of discomfort under the skin. In any event plates should generally be removed at between 12 and 18 months in order to allow the bone to return to its normal structure.

References

Apley, A. G. (1956). 'Fracture of the lateral tibial condyle treated by skeletal traction and early mobilisation.' *J. Bone Jt Surg.* **32B,** 699

Barr, J. S. (1940). 'The treatment of fracture of the external tibial condyle.' *J. Am. med. Ass.* **115,** 1683

Courvoisier, E. (1973). *Fracture of the Tibial Tables.* AO Bulletin. Swiss Association for the Study of Internal Fixation

Hohl, M. (1967). 'Tibial condylar fractures.' *J. Bone Jt Surg.* **49A,** 1455

Hohl, M. (1975). 'Fractures about the knee.' In *Fractures,* Edited by C. A. Rockwood and D. P. Green, Chapter 16, p. 1157. Philadelphia, Toronto: Lippincott

Palmer, Ivor (1951). 'Fractures of the upper end of the tibia.' *J. Bone Jt Surg.* **33B,** 160

Schatzker, I. (1977). *Comparative Study in Tibia Plateau Fractures.* 24th AO Course, Davos

Rasmussen, P. S. (1973). 'Tibial condylar fractures.' *J. Bone Jt Surg.* **55A,** 1331

[The illustrations for this Chapter on Fractures of the Tibial Condyles were drawn by Miss S. Barker.]

Fractures of the Tibial Shaft

Christopher E. Ackroyd, M.A., F.R.C.S.
Clinical Reader, Nuffield Department of Orthopaedic Surgery,
University of Oxford

PRE-OPERATIVE

Indications

Much controversy surrounds the treatment of tibial shaft fractures. Nicoll (1964) and Edwards and Nilsson (1969) in their large surveys have clearly identified the severity of the injury as one of the most important factors in determining the behaviour of the fracture and the end result. There have, however, been several large reviews of severe tibial shaft fractures treated by immediate weight-bearing in long-leg or below-knee total contact plaster-of-Paris casts with excellent results and little difference in behaviour between fractures of differing types and severities (Dehne et al., 1961; Sarmiento, 1967; Brown and Urban, 1969; Burkhalter and Protzman, 1975). Other authors have reported similarly large series of tibial fractures, treated by rigid internal fixation and early functional treatment with good results (Hicks, 1971; Burwell, 1971; Solheim, 1973). Internal fixation of closed fractures is always complicated by a small incidence of deep infection, although the rate for open fractures may not be very different from that occurring with non-operative treatment. Olerud and Karlström (1972) drew attention to the fact that healing of the fracture could be delayed following internal fixation, although other authors reported rates of healing which differ little from those after non-operative treatment (Thunold, Varhaug and Bjerkest, 1975; Ruedi, Webb and Allgöwer, 1976). The advantage which is obtained from the use of rigid internal fixation is a reduction or elimination of external splintage so that active functional treatment of joints can be instituted at an early stage. This is reflected in the end results with greater than 90 per cent of good and excellent results. (Olerud and Karlström, 1971; Ruedi, Webb and Allgöwer, 1976).

The exponents of both methods admit that there is an area of common ground and it is thus possible to lay down some firms guiding principles. Undisplaced fractures, or those that can be reduced into a stable position with good alignment, achieve excellent results with closed methods. Unstable fractures in which a satisfactory position has been achieved and maintained by manipulative reduction may also be treated very satisfactorily by closed methods. More difficulty arises when there is extreme comminution, a segmental fracture or difficulty in maintaining an adequate reduction, particularly when there has been skin contusion or an open fracture. When the skin condition is poor, or when there is a Grade 2 or 3 open fracture, the use of rigid external skeletal fixation devices have simplified the management considerably. There is a small group of patients in whom multiple injuries, and particularly other injuries in the same limb, may form the indication for primary or delayed primary internal fixation. Thus, in general, internal fixation of tibial fractures is seldom necessary as a primary treatment and is probably best reserved for those cases in which a satisfactory position of the fracture cannot be obtained, or where delayed healing is anticipated and prolonged immobilization of joints may otherwise be necessary.

In deciding whether internal fixation should be carried out it is important to consider the whole patient, particularly the age and any specific factors such as the skin condition. Internal fixation of the tibia should be regarded as a planned procedure carried out in optimum conditions, to fit in with the management of other injuries so as to produce a definite advantage for the patient. Many of the indications for operation are relative and will depend upon the precise criteria for shortening, angulation and rotation that are accepted by the patient and his surgeon.

Pre-operative preparation

Delayed primary internal fixation is favoured in many centres and temporary os calcis traction, with a firm gutter support or plaster back splint, will immobilize the fracture sufficiently to relieve pain. Operation should be delayed until the soft tissue swelling has decreased and skin contusion or abrasions have healed. The limb should be elevated to reduce the swelling and a careful check kept on the circulation of the foot and the integrity of nerve and muscles to identify compartmental compression and impending ischaemia (Owen and Tsimboukis, 1967; Matsen and Clawson, 1975). If primary fixation is being performed, it should be carried out within 12 hr before significant swelling has occurred.

The area of skin over the site of incision should be lightly shaved and an appropriate antiseptic applied.

Anaesthesia

The operation is carried out under general anaesthesia and the use of a tourniquet considerably improves the operative field. The limb is exsanguinated with an Esmarch bandage, although if there is significant soft tissue damage, then the part of the limb distal to the fracture is not included. A pneumatic tourniquet applied over a layer of wool is inflated to 400 mmHg and can be left in position for up to 2 hr.

Position of patient

The patient should be placed supine on the operating table and the area of the incision prepared with at least three applications of a suitable antiseptic. Sterile towelling is applied to the limb and the site of incision may be covered with adhesive plastic.

Means of fixation

An intramedullary nail is eminently suitable for transverse or short oblique fractures. However, this technique will not be discussed in this chapter. A single long oblique fracture may be adequately stabilized with three interfragmentary screws if its length is more than two-and-a-half times the diameter of the shaft. Interfragmentary screws should be placed across the fracture wherever possible in order to improve the torsional stability and a neutralization plate will be necessary to resist bending strains. Stabilization of segmental fractures will usually necessitate the use of two plates, although in this situation, or when there is severe comminution, the use of external skeletal fixation may be preferable.

THE OPERATION

1&2

The incisions

The tibia may be approached by an anterior, posteromedial or posterolateral incision. The anterior incision is favoured most commonly because of the ease of access to the medial subcutaneous surface of the tibia and access to the lateral surface. However, skin healing may be a problem with this incision, particularly if the skin is contused as a result of the injury, and great care is necessary in the manipulation of the soft tissues. The skin of the anteromedial surface of the leg is supplied by segmental vessels that emerge through the deep fascia on the lateral and medial sides of the subcutaneous surface at three or four levels (Manchot, 1895). These vessels anastomose in the region of the anterior tibial border. A knowledge of the blood supply to the skin in this area is important; in planning the incision care should be taken to avoid damage to these perforating vessels.

Wherever possible, application of a plate should be to the tension surface of a bone so that there is a greater resistance to the bending strains that may be applied during functional loading. Ease of access to the anteromedial border has made this a common site for plate application, although the plate necessarily lies directly under the skin. The biomechanical studies of Minns, Bramble and Campbell (1977) have suggested that the anterolateral surface of the tibia is mainly in tension during physiological loading and that the plate should be applied on this surface whenever possible, particularly as there is the additional advantage of being able to cover it with muscle. Access is, however, limited at the upper and lower aspects of the anterolateral surface.

The anterior incision should be straight, made 1 cm lateral to the crest of the tibia. The incision may be extended downwards and medially if there is a fracture of the lower tibia and the medial malleolus is to be exposed. This incision may also be extended upwards, either medially or laterally, to approach the tibial plateaux.

The posteromedial incision is placed just posterior to the medial border of the tibia, care being taken to avoid the long saphenous nerve and vein. The posterolateral incision (Harmon, 1945), is made overlying the line of the fibula in the posterolateral aspect of the calf. This incision is rarely required, the main indication being when bone grafting is being carried out and the skin on the anteromedial surface is defective or of poor quality.

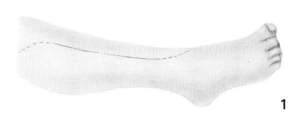

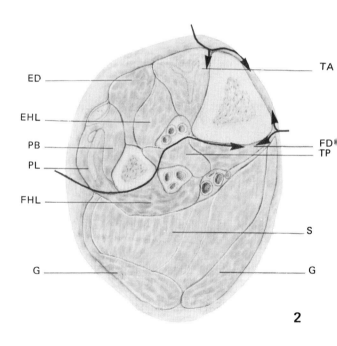

ED = extensor digitorum; EHL = extensor hallucis longus; PB = peroneus brevis; PL = pollucis longus; FHL = flexor hallucis longus; G = gastrocnemius; TA = tibialis anterior; FDL = flexor digitorum longus; TP = tibialis posterior; S = soleus

3

Exposure of the fracture — anteromedial approach

The incision is deepened through the subcutaneous tissue and the skin flap elevated leaving the periosteum of the tibia intact. The deep fascia and periosteum over the anterior border of the tibia at the level of the fracture are incised to expose the fracture ends. These are gently retracted with a small bone hook, the haematoma removed and the bone ends cleaned with a curette. Care is taken to avoid stripping of the periosteum although it is usually necessary to clear it 1–2 mm from the edge of the fracture. If there is a butterfly fragment with soft tissue attachment, this should be preserved at all costs. When it is necessary to approach the lateral surface of the tibia, the origin of the tibialis anterior muscle is separated from the periosteum of the lateral surface.

When delayed internal fixation is being carried out, the periosteum is often adherent to muscle and subcutaneous tissue and in these circumstances it is much less damaging to elevate the periosteum over the area of bone required. However, excessive stripping of the periosteum should be avoided if possible by relieving incisions.

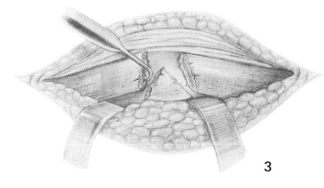

3

4

Reduction of the fracture

When the fracture ends have been cleaned and the wound washed out with Ringer's Polybactrin solution, reduction can be carried out. This is achieved using bone hooks and by traction on the foot. Medium-sized reduction clamps are applied to hold the reduction, or alternatively, a temporary circlage wire may produce less damage to the soft tissue and bone.

Careful consideration must now be given to the precise technique of fixation. Screws alone may only be used in a long spiral fracture when it is possible to insert three screws between proximal and distal main fragments. Care must always be taken to identify any secondary fractures which are not visible on the radiograph and may dictate the use of a neutralization plate. Short oblique fractures should be fixed with an interfragmentary screw supplemented by a neutralization plate. The screw may be incorporated into the plate, or applied separately, depending on the exact line of the fracture.

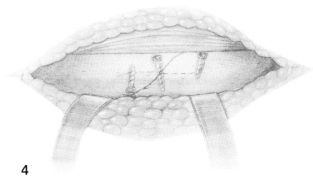

4

5

Fixation of the fracture

Fractures without comminution pose no great problem for internal fixation. However, tibial fractures commonly have a butterfly fragment. When this is in the anterior or anterolateral position, it is relatively easy to deal with. If there is sufficient bone contact between each of the three surfaces, each may be fixed with an interfragmentary screw and the fixation supplemented with a neutralization plate. If there is poor contact between any of the three fracture surfaces, then this screw is omitted although the use of the smaller 3·5 mm screw may be necessary for smaller fragments. The posterolateral or posteromedial butterfly fragment is much more difficult to deal with and it is usually necessary to incorporate the interfragmentary screws in the plate (Müller, Allgöwer and Willenegger, 1970).

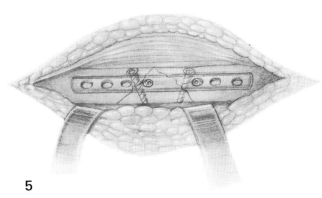

5

6

Application of the plate

The plate should be applied to the surface of the tibia on which it can most easily be positioned, producing as little soft tissue damage as possible and taking into account factors such as, the direction of the fracture, the position of a butterfly fragment and condition of the overlying skin. When reduction has been achieved and interfragmentary screws inserted, positioning and contouring of the plate can be carried out with the aid of a malleable template. The appropriate length of plate is chosen to ensure at least five cortices grip both proximal and distal main fragments. Contouring of the plate is important as it should be exactly the shape of the underlying bone and preferably a little under-bent so that when the ends of the plate are in contact, there is a small gap between the plate and the bone at the centre of the fracture site. If the plate is over-bent this will lead to opening of the fracture at the opposite side. The lower third of the medial surface of the tibia has a twist to it and a torsional bend should be applied to the plate so that it conforms exactly to the bone contours.

When interfragmentary screws have been used to fix the main fracture surfaces, the dynamic compression plate is applied as a neutralization plate and the screws are inserted from the centre outwards, using the green neutral drill guide. If it is necessary to apply compression at the fracture site, then the first screw is inserted 1 cm from the fracture edge on one main fragment, and the second screw is applied to

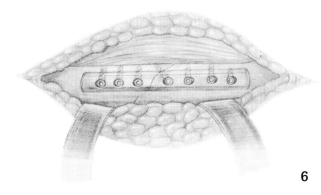

6

the first convenient screw hole in the other main fragment, utilizing the yellow load guide which will ensure that compression occurs at the fracture site when the screws are tightened. If there is a gap of more than 1 mm at the fracture site after reduction then the screws on both sides of the fracture should be inserted in the load position so that more compression is obtained.

In comminuted fractures of the tibia, it may not be possible to stabilize all bone fragments adequately with interfragmentary screws. In this case, small loose fragments that no longer have any soft tissue attachment should be discarded and if this results in a cortical bone defect, the defect should be filled with a cancellous bone graft.

7

Wound closure

When the fixation has been completed, the wound should be thoroughly washed with Ringer's Polybactrin solution and closed with interrupted polyglycolic acid sutures to the subcutaneous tissue. It is generally not necessary to close the deep fascia as this helps to decompress the anterior muscle compartment. Great care should be taken with wound closure in this area, and when vascularity of one side of the skin is reduced, interrupted 3/0 nylon sutures, inserted by the Donati-Allgöwer technique, reduces the constricting effect on the skin. When the skin edges are of good quality and the dermis of reasonable thickness, continuous 2/0 subcuticular nylon sutures may be used. The use of a suction drain should prevent haematoma formation and the wound is covered with the sterile dressing, and a compression wool and crêpe bandage. Fractures near the ankle joint, or where there has been considerable soft tissue damage, are best supported in a plaster back splint for the first few postoperative days.

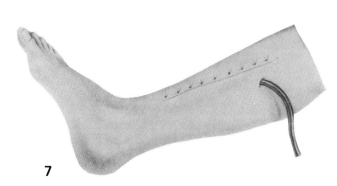

7

POSTOPERATIVE CARE

After the tourniquet has been removed, and circulation to the foot re-established, the limb should be elevated at 45° on a foam gutter splint. Circulation, sensation and movement of the toes should be checked at regular intervals during the first 48 hr and the presence of excessive postoperative pain should alert the surgeon to the possibility of a compartmental compression syndrome. The wound should be inspected on the fifth postoperative day and if this is satisfactory, active movements of the anke joints can be commenced. A back splint should be used at night in order to rest the ankle in the neutral position. When wound healing is complete, the patient may start to mobilize with crutches without weight-bearing. If fixation is satisfactory and the patient reliable, no additional external splintage is necessary and graded weight-bearing can be commenced at between 4 and 6 weeks depending on the type of fracture and its fixation. If there is any doubt about the fixation, or the reliability of the patient, a below-knee walking plaster should be applied when the wound has healed and satisfactory ankle joint movement has returned. This may usually be discarded at between 4 and 6 weeks from operation.

After anatomical reduction and rigid internal fixation the fracture line is seldom visible and assessment of union is therefore difficult. Primary bone healing produces little visible periosteal or endosteal callus, although careful observation of the cortices usually shows some evidence of cortical remodelling or new bone formation. In most instances, full weight-bearing is achieved by the twelfth week, although when there is extensive necrosis of the fracture ends, healing may take many months. Care should be taken to observe for the warning signs of instability of the fixation which will require protection, either by restriction of weight-bearing, or additional external splintage. The signs of instability of the fixation are pain at the fracture site, swelling, warmth and tenderness, and may be accompanied by radiological signs of thin callus formation in the region of the periosteum — the so-called 'cloudy irritation callus'. These signs indicate that there is some movement at the fracture site which is stimulating new bone formation. The amount of force which is transmitted through the limb should therefore be restricted until firm union has occurred. Occasionally fatigue failure of a plate may occur with little evidence of healing. This indicates that the forces exerted on the plate have been too great, sometimes for biomechanical reasons or that healing has been unduly prolonged.

The bone underneath the plate undergoes resorption, producing stress protection osteoporosis; for this reason it is usually advisable to remove diaphyseal plates in weight-bearing bones so that the normal bony architecture can be restored. The tibial plate should be removed at between 18 and 24 months to avoid the risk of refracture. Careful study of good quality radiographs taken in several planes will enable examination of the cortical bone in the area of the fracture and it is usually possible to identify the subtle changes that occur as a result of cortical remodelling. When the cortex remains dense and sclerotic with no evidence of remodelling, the plate should be left *in situ* for longer. As a result of the stress protection osteoporosis, the underlying bone is structurally weaker and thus activity should be restricted for several months after removal of the plate in order to allow remodelling to occur.

References

Brown, P. W. and Urban, J. G. (1969). 'Early weight-bearing treatment of open fractures of the tibia. An end-result study of 63 cases.' *J. Bone Jt Surg.* **51A**, 59

Burkhalter, W. E. and Protzman, R. (1975). 'The tibial shaft fracture.' *J. Trauma* **15**, 785

Burwell, H. N. (1971). 'Plate fixation of tibial shaft fractures.' *J. Bone Jt Surg.* **53B**, 258

Dehne, E., Metz, C. W., Deffer, P. A. and Hall, R. M. (1961). 'Non-operative treatment of the fractured tibia by immediate weight-bearing.' *J. Trauma* **1**, 514

Edwards, P. and Nilsson, B. E. (1969). 'The time of disability following fracture of the shaft of the tibia.' *Acta orthop. scand.* **40**, 501

Harmon, P. H. (1945). 'A simplified surgical approach to the posterior tibia for bone-grafting and fibular transference.' *J. Bone Jt Surg.* **27**, 496

Hicks, J. H. (1971). 'High rigidity in fractures of the tibia.' *Injury* **3**, 121

Manchot, C. (1895). *Die Hautarterien von den Körpern.* Leipzig: Verlag von Vogel

Matsen, E. A. and Clawson, D. K. (1975). 'The deep posterior compartmental syndrome of the leg.' *J. Bone Jt Surg.* **57A**, 34

Minns, R. I., Bremble, G. R. and Campbell, J. (1977). 'A biomechanical study of internal fixation of the tibial shaft.' *J. Biomechanics* **10**, 569

Müller, M. E., Allgöwer, M. and Willenegger, H. (1970). *Manual of Internal Fixation.* Berlin, Heidelberg, New York: Springer-Verlag

Nicoll, E. A. (1964). 'Fractures of the tibial shaft: a survey of 705 cases.' *J. Bone Jt Surg.* **46B**, 373

Olerud, S. and Karlström, G. (1972). 'Tibial fractures treated by AO compression osteosynthesis: experiences from a five-year material.' *Acta orthop. scand.,* suppl. 140

Owen, R. and Tsimboukis, B. (1967). 'Ischaemia complicating closed tibial and fibular shaft fractures.' *J. Bone Jt Surg.* **49B**, 268

Ruedi, T., Webb, J. K. and Allgöwer, M. (1976). 'Experience with the dynamic compression plate (DCP) in 418 recent fractures of the tibial shaft.' *Injury* **7**, 252

Sarmiento, A. (1967). 'A functional below-the-knee cast for tibial fractures.' *J. Bone Jt Surg.* **49A**, 855

Solheim, K. (1973). 'Tibial fractures treated according to the AO method.' *Injury* **4**, 213

Thurnold, J., Varhaug, J. E. and Bjerkest, T. (1975). 'Tibial shaft fractures treated by rigid internal fixation: The early results of a 4-year series.' *Injury* **7**, 125

[*The illustrations for this Chapter on Fractures of the Tibial Shaft were drawn by Miss S. Barker.*]

Fractures of the Ankle

Christopher E. Ackroyd, M.A., F.R.C.S.
Clinical Reader, Nuffield Department of Orthopaedic Surgery,
University of Oxford

PRE - OPERATIVE

Classification

Fractures of the ankle have been classified in many different ways. A great advance in understanding the mechanism of injury was made when Lauge-Hansen (1950) introduced his genetic classification. This was based on the concept that each of the various patterns of fracture-dislocation of the ankle was the end-result of the sequence of bony and ligamentous failure resulting from a deforming force. This has been slightly modified by Colton (1976) and has been particularly useful in understanding the mechanism of injury which is important when carrying out a closed reduction and plaster-of-Paris fixation. This system of classification is of less practical use when carrying out open reduction and internal fixation.

1a, b & c

A simpler system has been devised by Danis (1949), and further modified by Weber (1966) into three types. This classification centres around the integrity of the tibiofibular syndesmosis, which is important in maintaining the stability of the ankle mortice.

Emphasis is placed on the correct recognition of both bony and ligamentous injuries. Type A fractures occur at the level of the ankle joint, or below, and ligamentous injuries are rarely seen. Type B injuries occur through the area of the syndesmosis, with varying degrees of damage to the three component parts. They may be associated with bony or ligamentous injury on the medial side. Type C fractures involve injury to the fibula above the level of the syndesmosis with associated ligamentous or bony injury on the medial side. The fibular fracture may be low, running into the substance of the syndesmosis, higher up the shaft of the fibula, or the Maisonneuve fracture of the neck of the fibula.

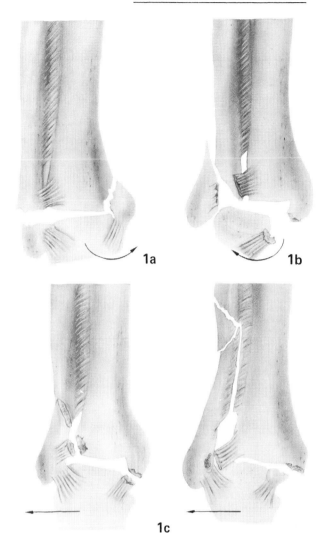

1a

1b

1c

Indications

The most important and fundamental consideration in the treatment of ankle injuries is the restoration of the normal anatomy. Authors of all major reviews of the subject emphasize the importance of achieving and maintaining as near a perfect reduction as possible (Burwell and Charnley, 1965; Klossner, 1962; Solonen and Lauttamus, 1968). This factor alone has a major influence on the long-term results and the degree of initial displacement and medial ligament damage have a less important effect (Joy, Patzakis and Harvey, 1974).

In Type A fractures it is usually the degree of displacement which determines the need for operation. If a perfect reduction cannot be obtained by closed manipulation, open reduction should be carried out. In Type B injuries, subluxation or dislocation of the ankle with displacement of the lateral malleolus and talus of more than 1—2 mm, implies some ligamentous damage to the syndesmosis. Displacement of this degree often requires open reduction and rigid fixation, particularly in the young and middle age groups. This allows the added advantage of earlier weight-bearing and joint function. Closed reduction and plaster-of-Paris fixation may be carried out in some cases although care must be taken to achieve and maintain a perfect anatomical alignment. Type C fractures, with more than 1—2 mm of displacement of the talus, have major disruption of the syndesmosis. These are best treated by primary open reduction and internal fixation (Colton, 1976; Müller, Allgöwer and Willenegger, 1970).

The age of the patient, quality of bone, degree of comminution, and general medical condition, will also play a part in deciding whether to embark on operative treatment. Poor quality skin, severe soft tissue swelling and contaminated open fractures are contra-indications to operation. Less than a perfect reduction may be accepted in the elderly. However, persistent lateral displacement of the talus of more than 2 mm may lead to a poor result. Loss of position after initial reduction and closed treatment is an indication for operation and should be recognized within the first 2 weeks. After this time the operation becomes much more difficult and it may be necessary to break down the uniting fracture in order to achieve an adequate reduction.

The fractured posterior malleolar fragment bears the attachment of the posterior inferior tibiofibular ligament, and reduction and fixation may be required to restore stability of the syndesmosis. When the fragment is greater than 20—25 per cent of the articular surface of the ankle, it should be held in an anatomical position to prevent posterior subluxation of the talus which may otherwise result (Wilson, 1975). After fixation of the lateral complex, dorsiflexion of the foot may reduce the fragment satisfactorily. However, in order to allow early active movement of the joint rigid fixation is necessary.

Pre-operative preparation

The limb should be immobilized in a temporary splint at the earliest possible moment after reducing any obvious deformity likely to compromise skin or arterial supply. Elevation at 45° delays the onset of swelling. Provisional reduction may be carried out with the use of Entonox or titrated doses of intravenous analgesic. Open fractures should be covered with a sterile dressing as soon as possible and the wound should not be disturbed until the patient has reached the operating theatre. Operation should be carried out as soon as possible and in any event within 24 hr, before significant soft tissue swelling has occurred. After this time it is preferable to delay operation for 5—7 days when the swelling will have significantly reduced. Complete radiological assessment of the injury is essential prior to operation and the addition of an oblique view is often helpful.

Anaesthesia

Operation should be carried out under general anaesthesia although epidural anaesthesia may be indicated in some cases. Preliminary skin preparation should be carried out prior to application of the tourniquet with a suitable antiseptic. The limb is exsanguinated with an Esmarch bandage, although if there is severe soft tissue damage the foot may be omitted. A pneumatic tourniquet is applied to the thigh over a layer of wool and inflated to 400 mmHg for a maximum of 2 hr.

Position of patient

The patient is positioned supine on the operating table with a sandbag placed under the appropriate buttock. The skin is prepared with at least three applications of antiseptic solution and the limb is draped with sterile towelling. The foot may be covered with a surgeon's glove or sterile plastic sheeting. The skin of the operating area may be protected by application of adhesive plastic. The surgeon and assistant should assume a comfortable sitting position.

THE OPERATION

LATERAL COMPLEX

2

The incision

The approach to each fracture should be carefully planned in advance, based on information from the pre-operative radiographs and the known characteristics of the fracture type in question. It is usually necessary to approach the lateral side first, in order to re-establish the length of the fibula. An antero-lateral or posterolateral incision is chosen and care taken to avoid the sural nerve. As the incision is deepened through the subcutaneous tissues, superficial veins are divided and tied. When the deep fascia covering the lateral malleolus is reached, the skin flaps are elevated and retracted using sharp dissection.

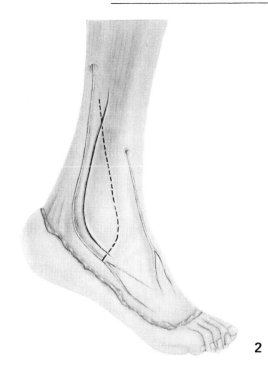

2

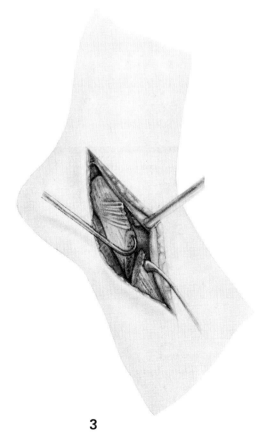

3

3

Exposure of the fracture

The deep fascia making up the extensor retinaculum is divided to expose the fracture. The fracture ends are distracted with a small bone hook and haematoma and bone fragments removed with a small curette. The periosteum at the fracture edge is gently scraped back 1–2 mm so that it is clear of the fracture and will not interfere with the reduction. When operation has been delayed by a week or more, the haematoma will have become organized and more vigorous action will be required to clean the fracture ends, perhaps with a small periosteal elevator.

4

Reduction of the fracture

The fracture is now reduced using one or two bone hooks. The assistant may help by manipulating the foot with traction and internal rotation. Difficulty in reduction may occur as a result of several problems.

The medial complex may block reduction and rarely the tibialis posterior tendon may be trapped in the ankle joint. The presence of bone fragments, either the posterior malleolus or the anterior Tillaux fragment may block reduction. Reduction is held temporarily with reduction clamps, circlage wire or Kirschner wires. Depending on the characteristics of the fracture, the final decision must now be made on the method of achieving fixation. Long oblique fractures can be fixed with two interfragmentary screws. It is usually more satisfactory to choose the 3·5 mm screw size. The proximal cortex is over-drilled to 3·6 mm and the distal cortex is drilled out to 2 mm prior to tapping the screw threads (Müller, Allgöwer and Willenegger, 1970).

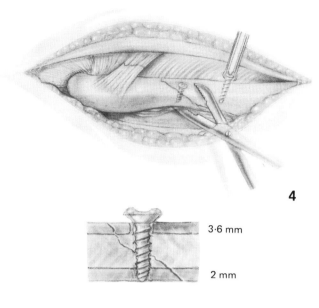

4

3·6 mm

2 mm

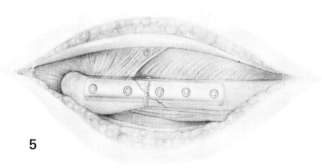

5

5

Short oblique and transverse fractures

For short oblique fractures, a single interfragmentary screw will not produce sufficient stability and a neutralization plate must be applied using a four- or five-hole one-third tubular plate. Alternatively, the small plate may be used as a buttress against the obliquity of the fracture. Transverse fractures may be fixed by a plate, tension band wiring or a single intramedullary screw. Care must be taken with the latter to prevent rotational instability.

6a & b

The tibiofibular syndesmosis

Once the fibular fracture has been stabilized, and the length of the fibula re-established, it is necessary to determine the stability of the inferior tibiofibular joint. In Type B fractures, the anterior ligament is invariably ruptured and this should be repaired with Dexon sutures. If there is avulsion of a bony fragment from either end, this can be stabilized with an inter-fragmentary screw, usually of the 4 mm cancellous type. If the posterior fragment and attached ligament are not to be stabilized and excessive movement between the fibula and tibia remains, then a transfixion diastasis screw should be inserted. This is invariably necessary in the Type C fractures. This screw acts as a spacer, holding the fibula loosely against the tibia and should be inserted with the ankle in full dorsiflexion so that the fibula lies correctly in the notch of the tibia. Whichever size of screw is chosen, at least three cortices should be tapped so that when the screw is tightened, the fibula is not forced against the tibia but held in correct apposition to allow healing of the interosseous syndesmosis ligament.

A peroperative 20° internal rotation and lateral radiograph is now obtained to ensure there is correct anatomical alignment of the ankle mortice. Lateral stressing of the syndesmosis may also be carried out at the same time. The beak of bone on the medial side of the lateral malleolus should form a smooth curved line with the subchondral bone of the tibia. This indicates the correct relationship between the tibia and fibula.

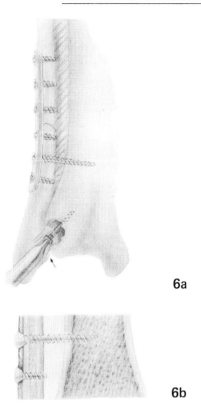

6a

6b

7

The posterior malleolus

The posterior inferior tibiofibular ligament is attached to the posterolateral aspect of the tibia and a large piece of bone with its attachment may be avulsed from the tibia making up the posterior malleolus. If there is greater than 20–25 per cent of the articular surface, then it should be fixed back into position and held rigidly with one or two screws. This then contributes to the stability of the syndesmosis and may obviate the need for a transfixion screw. If the fragment is smaller than this, and is shown to be reduced satisfactorily in the lateral check radiograph after fixation of the fibular fracture, then it may be left free. The direct approach is through an enlarged posterior lateral incision between the peroneal tendons and flexor hallucis longus. After reduction, the fragment is held with temporary Kirschner wires and the small or large cancellous screw is inserted to produce interfragmentary compression. When the fragment is large in size, approach from a posteromedial incision may give better access. It is possible to insert the screw in a retrograde fashion so that direct exposure of the fragment is not necessary. A short threaded cancellous screw is inserted through a separate anterior incision and will pick up the posterior fragment producing interfragmentary compression.

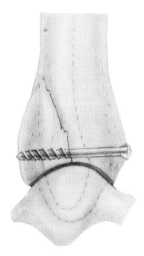

7

THE MEDIAL COMPLEX

8

The incision

The sandbag is then removed from under the buttock in order to give good access to the medial malleolus. This may be approached by either vertical or horizontal incisions. Care should be taken to avoid the long saphenous nerve, and it may be necessary to tie the long saphenous vein.

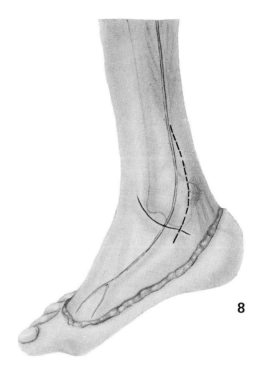

8

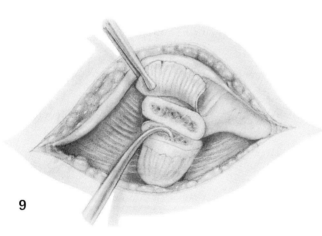

9

9

Exposure of the fracture

The incision is deepened through the deep fascia to expose the periosteum of the medial malleolus and the fracture site. There is often a large flap of periosteum lying between the fracture surfaces. This is lifted out and the fractured surfaces are cleaned with a small curette and the periosteum carefully scraped back 1—2 mm from the fracture edge. The fractured medial malleolus is retracted with a small bone hook and a good view is obtained of the medial side of the ankle joint. All haematoma and bone or cartilaginous debris should be removed from the joint and irrigation carried out with Ringer's Polybactrin solution. Inspection of the articular surface of the talus and tibia is carried out and the degree of damage recorded.

10

Reduction and fixation of the fracture

The fracture is now reduced anatomically and held in position by a temporary Kirschner wire and a reduction clamp. The usual method of fixation is with a malleolar screw which has a smooth shank to allow sliding of the proximal fragment and therefore compression at the fracture line. Alternatively, the tension band wiring technique may be used, or in vertical shear abduction fractures two 4 mm cancellous screws produce excellent fixation. The periosteum is cleared from the tip of the medial malleolus at the site of screw insertion and the proximal cortex is drilled with a 3·2 mm drill. The screw should be directed so that it crosses the fracture line at right angles to it in both planes. The screw length can be obtained with the use of an awl or a Kirschner wire so that the screw tip lies just short of the opposite cortex of the tibia. An appropriate malleolar screw is chosen ensuring that the smooth shank is greater than the thickness of the proximal fragment. This screw is self-drilling and self-tapping and can be inserted directly into bone without previously tapping the thread. If there is any rotational instability, the Kirschner wire can be bent over and left in position, or a second small cancellous screw may be inserted.

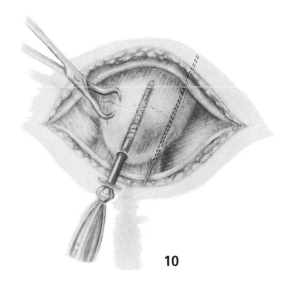

10

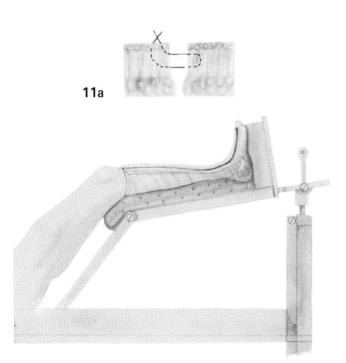

11a

11b

11a & b

Wound closure

The wounds are closed using interrupted fine Dexon sutures to the deep fascia and subcutaneous tissue and interrupted 3/0 nylon sutures to the skin. Small suction drains may be inserted under the skin flaps to prevent haematoma formation. Care should be taken to ensure there is no tension on the wound edges and use of the Donati-Allgöwer mattress suture may help to protect poorly vascularized skin edges. A sterile dressing is applied to the wounds and plaster wool applied to the limb. The ankle is immobilized in a U-plaster-of-Paris back-splint, the tourniquet released and the limb elevated at 45° on a frame.

POSTOPERATIVE CARE

Elevation of the limb is maintained for at least 5 days and the suction drains are removed at 48 hr. On the fifth day the plaster is removed and the wounds inspected. If they are satisfactory then active ankle movements are commenced. These should start as a programme of several hours exercise a day and gradually increase so that the ankle can be left unsupported for the entire day. At all other times, the ankle should be rested in a back-splint to prevent development of an equinus deformity. During this period the patient may start to get up with crutches and walk without weight-bearing. The skin sutures are removed when the wound has healed at approximately the tenth to the fourteenth day. If a satisfactory fixation has been obtained, partial weight-bearing may be commenced, support to the soft tissues being provided by a crêpe bandage. If an adequate fixation has not been obtained or other factors suggest that

additional external splintage would be advisable, a below-knee walking plaster should be applied for a further 2—4 weeks. A check radiograph is obtained prior to discharge from hospital and at 6 weeks, when it should be possible to discontinue external splintage. The introduction of weight-bearing will vary to some extent from patient to patient and factors such as pain, swelling and warmth around the ankle indicate that a more cautious programme should be advised.

In Type C fractures, when a diastasis screw has been inserted for tibiofibular stability, full weight-bearing should be restricted until ligamentous healing has occurred and the screw has been removed. This should be carried out at between 6 and 8 weeks. In general, the implants should be removed at between 9 and 12 months, particularly if there are pressure symptoms beneath the skin. Isolated screws may, however, be left *in situ* indefinitely provided they give rise to no symptoms.

References

Burwell, H. N. and Charnley, A. D. (1965). 'The treatment of displaced fractures at the ankle joint by rigid internal fixation and early joint movement.' *J. Bone Jt Surg.* **47B**, 634

Colton, C. L. (1976). 'Injuries of the ankle.' In *Watson-Jones Fractures and Joint Injuries,* 5th Edition. Edited by J. N. Wilson. Edinburgh, London, New York: Churchill Livingstone

Danis, R. (1949). *Theorie et Practique de L'Osteosynthese.* Paris: Masson

Joy, G., Patazakis, M. J. and Harvey, J. P. (1974). 'Precise evaluation of the reduction of severe ankle fractures.' *J. Bone Jt Surg.* **56A**, 979

Klossner, O. (1962). 'Late results of operative and non-operative treatment of severe ankle fractures.' *Acta chir. scand.,* Suppl. 293

Lauge-Hansen, N. (1950). 'Fractures of the ankle II. Combined experimental-surgical and experimental-roentgenologic investigations.' *Archs Surg.* **60**, 957

Müller, M. E., Allgöwer, M. and Willenegger, H. (1970). *Manual of Internal Fixation.* Berlin, Heidelberg, New York: Springer-Verlag

Solonen, K. A. and Lauttamus, L. (1968). 'Operative treatment of ankle fractures.' *Acta orthop. scand.* **39**, 223

Weber, B. G. (1966). *Die Verletzargen des oberen Sprunggelenkes; Aktuelle Probleme in der Chirurgie.* B.3. Bern and Stuttgart: Huber

Wilson, F. C. (1975). 'Fractures and dislocations of the ankle.' In *Fractures,* Edited by C. A. Rockwood and C. P. Green. Philadelphia, Toronto: Lippincott

[*The illustrations for this Chapter on Fractures of the Ankle were drawn by Miss S. Barker and Mrs. P. Dewhurst.*]

Display, Correction and Fixation of Stove-in Hip Joints

E. Letournel, M.D.
Professor of Orthopaedic Surgery and Traumatology,
Centre Medico-Chirurgical de la Porte de Choisy, Paris

PRE - OPERATIVE

A stove-in hip is associated with different types of acetabular fracture.

To give the hip its original appearance and arrangement the central dislocation of the head has first to be corrected and then to be prevented by reconstructing the acetabulum, restoring perfect articular congruency and stability gives the patient the best chance of avoiding post-traumatic osteo-arthrosis.

1a,b&c

In order to gain a clear understanding of the fracture lines disrupting the iliac bone, four radiographic views are essential:

(*1*) the anteroposterior view of the whole pelvis in case there are fractures on both sides;

(*2*) the standard anteroposterior radiograph of the injured hip;

(*3*) the obturator oblique view, with the patient supine but rolled 45° away from the side of the injury;

(*4*) the iliac wing oblique view with the patient supine but rolled 45° *towards* the affected site.

The typical landmarks are studied carefully in each view.

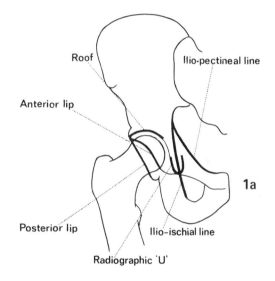

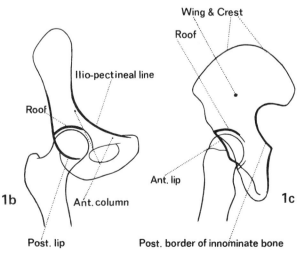

Indications for surgery

All the displaced fractures of the innominate bone resulting in a stove-in hip should be treated surgically. This applies whether the incongruity is shown by three, two or only one x-ray view. Even if the head can be reduced under a remaining part of the roof, surgical fixation offers the only possibility of restoring complete articular congruency.

One exception can be accepted: in some cases, among the most complex fractures, the different parts of the articular crescent are shown, by all three x-ray views, to be congruent with the centrally displaced head. In these cases bed rest and active exercises may lead to a good result, but the hip is never perfect and it remains displaced. Thus, if there is no contra-indication, operation is advised in order to restore a congruent hip in its normal place. The choice must depend on the surgeon, who must be confident of restoring an accurately fitting and correctly placed hip.

Time of operation

It is never an emergency, and the operation is perhaps easier when performed after 3–5 or 6 days when bleeding from pelvic veins disrupted at the time of injury has stopped.

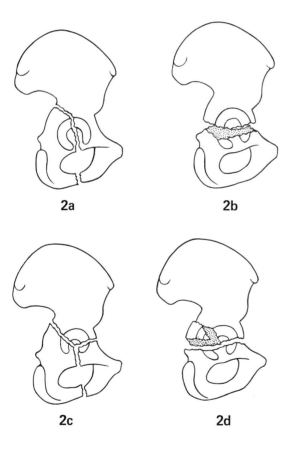

2a

2b

2c

2d

The approach

This depends on the type of acetabular fracture associated with the stove-in hip.

2a-d

(*a*) If the centrally dislocated head is associated with:

(*i*) a posterior column fracture (*a*);

(*ii*) or any type of transverse fracture (*b*);

(*iii*) or a T-shaped fracture (*c*);

(*iv*) or an associated transverse and posterior fracture (*d*), good access is gained through a posterior or Kocher-Langenbeck type of incision.

3a,b&c

(*b*) If the associated fracture is either

(*i*) an anterior wall (*a*) or an anterior column fracture (*b*);

(*ii*) or a combination of anterior and transverse fractures (*c*), the ilio-inguinal, anterior approach has to be used.

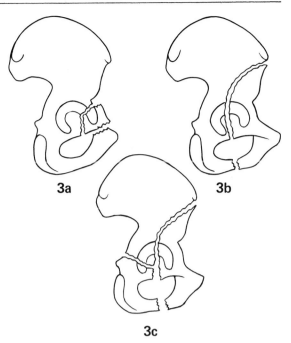

3a　　　　　**3b**

3c

4a&b

(*c*) If the fracture affects the whole of both columns, the whole articular crescent of the acetabulum is detached in several pieces, so that only the back part of the ilium remains connected to the sacrum.

A posterior approach may be used if the uppermost fracture-line extends to the anterior edge of the iliac bone (*a*), but when, as most often happens, the uppermost fracture-line reaches the crest (*b*), the ilio-inguinal anterior incision has to be used.

Some cases require the two approaches for the one operation. A more recently described lateral approach may be advisable in some cases.

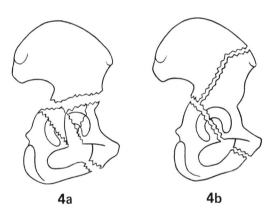

4a　　　　　**4b**

Anaesthesia

Any form of general anaesthesia can be used, but good relaxation is particularly useful during an anterior approach.

The equipment

5

Screws

Cortical screws from 22 to 120 mm long are most useful, but cancellous bone screws and Venable screws are needed from time to time.

Plates

Straight Sherman's vitallium plates, with equidistant holes, or Letournel's vitallium curved acetabulum plates with 6 to 12 holes are used.

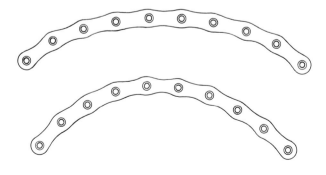

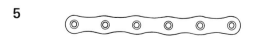

5

THE OPERATION

POSTERIOR APPROACH

The position of the patient, the equipment and the Kocher-Langenbeck approach are described in the Chapter on 'Replacement and Fixation of Posterior Lip of Acetabulum', pages 188–193.

Because the fracture lines divide the posterior column the hip's capsule is more or less torn and gives access to the inside of the joint. This access may be improved by a capsulotomy along either the posterior wall or the lateral lip of the roof, depending on the existing damage. The joint is cleared of clots and loose fragments, so that the intra-articular track of the fracture lines can be identified.

REDUCTION AND FIXATION

Principles

The centrally dislocated head is extracted with the aid of traction allowed by the orthopaedic table and supplemented by a big hook placed around the femur just under the neck.

6a&b

The fragments are then set in place by direct manipulation, taking care to disturb their soft tissue attachments as little as possible. Replacement is sometimes difficult to achieve or to maintain and it may be advisable to use forceps to grip one or two temporary screws, which must be inserted away from the intended site of the plate.

The procedure adopted depends on whether or not part of the roof of the acetabulum remains intact and undisplaced.

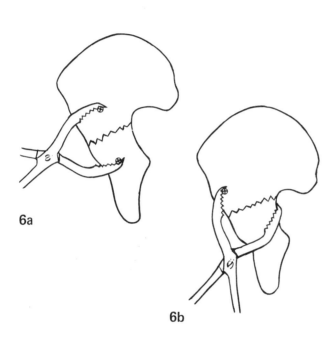

6a

6b

7

If part of the roof remains undisturbed under the blade of the ilium the head is replaced under it, taking care to get a perfect fit. The head is kept in place by traction or in some cases by temporary transfixion.

The means of reduction and fixation of the fragments depend on the type of the fracture.

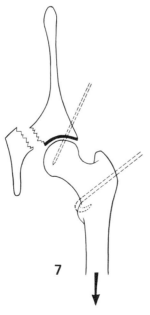

7

8

Posterior column fracture

The big fragment is manipulated by forceps with one jaw inside the greater sciatic notch, the other taking hold of the outer aspect of the ilium or on a temporary screw. A plate is shaped so as to lie perfectly on the posterior aspect of the column from the upper pole of the ischial tuberosity up to the blade of the ilium, with at least three screws above the fracture-line. One must be careful to avoid leaving the column twisted out of line; this is done by control exercised from inside the pelvis, working through the greater sciatic notch.

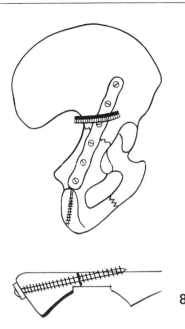

8

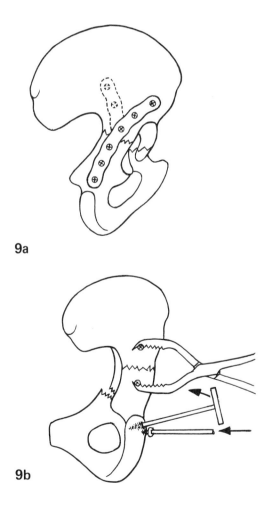

9a

9b

9a & b

Transverse fracture

The inferior part of the innominate bone is manipulated and plated as above, but there is often difficulty in dealing with the anterior part of the fracture at the level of the iliopectineal line. A finger introduced through the greater sciatic notch helps the manipulation, which can be further aided either by pushing the ischial tuberosity inwards or by inserting a femoral head extractor into it to act as a temporary handle. A 10–12 cm screw may be driven across the fracture-line to reach the superior aspect of the iliopectineal line.

10a&b

Associated transverse and posterior acetabular fractures

The transverse component is dealt with as above and fixed by a plate which is placed near the greater sciatic notch and passes under the gluteal muscles to be screwed into the posterior part of the ilium.

A large posterior acetabular fragment is fixed by isolated screws or, more safely, by a curved plate, as already described for this fracture on its own (*see Illustration 9a and b*).

11a&b

T-fractures

The head is placed and held under the roof and the fragment of the posterior column is set in place and plated as above, but one must avoid long screws which could reach the still displaced fragment of the anterior column.

Working through the greater sciatic notch, it may be possible to replace the anterior column and then to fix it with at least two long screws inserted from behind. If this is not possible this component must be approached from in front, using the appropriate incision (*see Illustration 11b*).

12

If none of the roof of the acetabulum remains attached to any part of the ilium that is still connected to the sacrum the operation is more difficult. This is the pattern that affects the whole of both columns.

First the head is extracted from the pelvis and maintained by traction in a position which allows the surgeon to reduce the posterior column fragment.

The placement of the posterior column fragment must be perfect and should be controlled both from inside the pelvis and on the outer aspect of the bone because if one accepts a small imperfection at this stage, it will be impossible to deal accurately with the other fracture-lines and the error will increase from step to step. The posterior column fracture is plated as if it were an isolated fracture of this part but avoiding screws long enough to reach and fix the displaced anterior column before it has been correctly replaced.

Then by freeing the inferior part of the ilium, up to its anterior border if necessary, the upper part of the anterior column fragment is replaced either by using forceps to take hold of a temporary screw or by a lever introduced into the fracture-line.

A curved acetabular plate fixes the upper part of the anterior column to the posterior one; it should, if possible, cross the inferior angle of the iliac fracture-line.

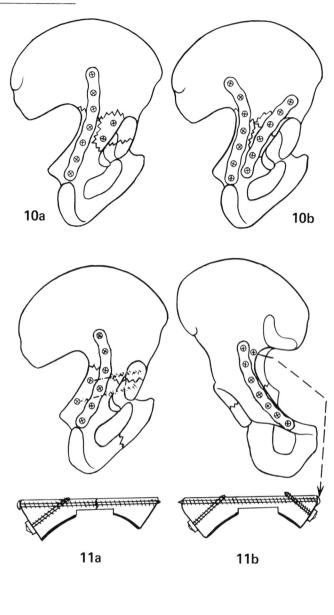

10a   10b

11a   11b

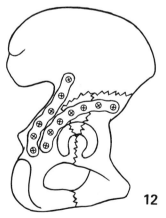

12

18

Medial to th
the transvers
space is ente
 The vesse
order not t
great vessels
 When nec
can be divide

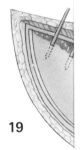

19

20

In most cas
from the pe
while assem
performed i
done by mak
gluteus medi
head extrac
inserted, an
the femur a
or a device a

ILIO-INGUINAL APPROACH

Position of patient

The patient is supine on an orthopaedic table, unless there is a vertical anterior fracture-line of the opposite innominate bone, in which case traction would push upwards the two pubes and would prevent complete replacement.

13a & b

Towelling

The operative field has to extend: (*a*) upwards for three fingers' breadth above the iliac crest; (*b*) inwards for three to four fingers' breadth beyond the mid-line; (*c*) inferiorly from the level of the superior border of the symphysis, sideways to the femoral vessels and then obliquely to the greater trochanter; and (*d*) laterally to just behind the line of the femur.

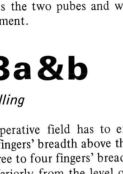

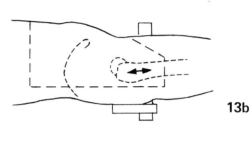

13a

13b

The approach

14 & 15

An incision is made along the anterior two-thirds of the iliac crest and then from its anterior superior spine towards the mid-line two fingers' breadth above the pubic symphysis.

Along the iliac crest the anterior abdominal muscles are detached and stripped in continuity with the iliacus from the inner aspect of the iliac wing. Beyond the fracture the rugine reaches the brim of the true pelvis. The iliac fossa is packed with a large swab.

The external oblique aponeurosis is incised 2 cm above the superficial inguinal ring and the inguinal canal is opened; the spermatic cord is then isolated and a tape is passed round it.

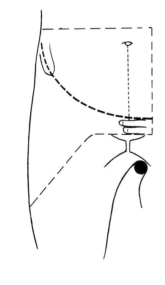

14a

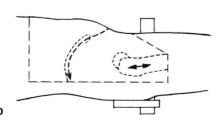

14b

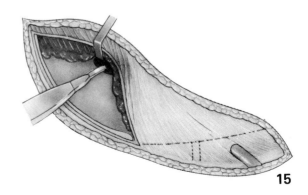

15

Replacement and fixation of fracture

If there is still a part of the articular crescent in its right place and attached to the wing it consists of the whole or a part of the posterior wall and a more or less important part of the roof, the fracture is of the anterior column type, either isolated or associated with a transverse fracture of the posterior column.

The head is replaced against the remaining part of the articular crescent, aided by both longitudinal and lateral traction.

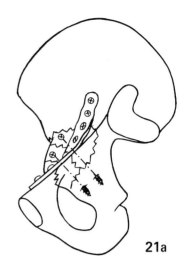

21a

21a, b & c

The fragments of the anterior column are then manipulated by means of forceps, or pushed directly into their normal position; a lever inserted in a fracture-line may facilitate this. A large fragment of the anterior column may be seized by a forceps astride either the crest of the ilium or the anterior border of the ilium between the anterior spines.

The correction achieved, a few screws are inserted from the anterior fragments to the intact posterior part of the roof or to the posterior column. Then the plates must be shaped. The anterior column may be fixed by one or more plates screwed along the superior or inner aspect of the iliac crest, in the iliac fossa, or along the superior aspect of the iliopectineal line from the sacro-iliac joint to the pubic symphysis if necessary.

If a fracture-line divides the posterior column, the reduction of its inferior fragment is achieved by direct manipulation of the fragment deep to the brim of the true pelvis, between the vessels and the iliopsoas muscle. Two 90—110 mm long screws are used to fix the fragment; they run parallel to the inner aspect of the bone and they may be used without a plate or to hole one of the plates in place.

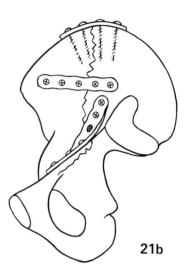

21b

If the whole articular crescent is broken and detached from the wing the fracture is a combination of both the anterior and posterior column types.

Combined lateral and longitudinal traction extracts the stove-in hip and keeps the head in approximately the right place; slight over-traction does not matter.

Then the fragments of the anterior column must be assembled as in the case just described.

Very often replacement is achieved by gripping the anterior column with forceps and using a lever in the fracture-line to restore the displaced pieces of bone to their proper relationship.

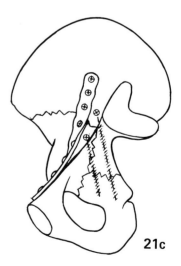

21c

22

The first steps in fixation are achieved by isolated screws, but it is nearly always necessary to use plates as well. One must at this stage take care not to insert screws that can reach the still displaced posterior column and so hold it out of place. When traction is released the head should be in perfect contact with the reconstructed anterior column and the roof.

When this is done, in most cases the posterior column remains displaced but its displacement has been lessened and, by working either between vessels and muscle or between vessels and cord, the posterior column can be pushed outwards and downwards and set perfectly or nearly perfectly in place. Screws to fix the posterior column can be inserted through the plate or apart from it. They need to be 90—120 mm long from the iliac fossa or the pubic ramus either parallel to the inner aspect of the bone, reaching the posterior aspect of the posterior column, or obliquely, to reach the quadrilateral surface.

By moving the hip before closure one can ensure that there are no screws in the joint.

If a satisfactory position of the posterior column is impossible to achieve, the anterior incision is closed. The patient must then be placed prone, but this must not be done until the circulation has been stabilized by the replacement of any lost blood. The posterior column is then exposed and fixed from behind in the way that has already been described.

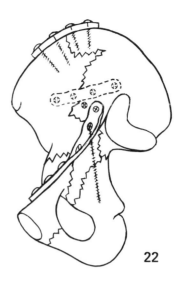

22

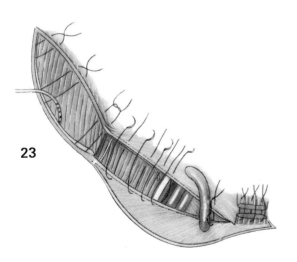

23

23

Closure of the ilio-inguinal incision is anatomical and straightforward, but it must be done with care. Suction drains are inserted into the retropubic space and into the iliac fossa. The abdominal muscles are re-attached. If divided, the anterior sheath of rectus abdominis, the conjoint tendon and the transversalis fascia are sutured. The tapes are removed, and one must see that the artery still pulsates and that the nerves are undamaged. The origins of the internal oblique and transversus abdominis are sutured to the inguinal ligament, using a fish hook type of needle. The spermatic cord is put in place and the external oblique repaired. The inguinal canal, which has been so widely opened is thus securely repaired.

THE LATERAL APPROACH

24

This is performed with the patient on his side on an orthopaedic table. The pelvic support inserted between the thighs of the patient can be moved downwards and upwards and this adjustment, combined with longitudinal traction, allows one to extract the head from the pelvis and keep it in the right position while rebuilding the acetabulum.

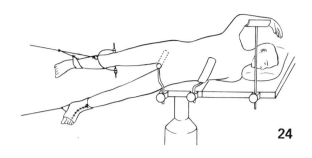

24

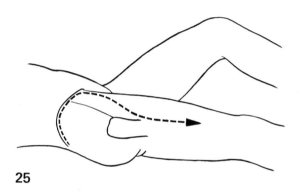

25

25

The skin incision is J-shaped and runs along the whole length of the iliac crest from the posterior superior spine and then downwards from the anterior superior spine to the middle of the thigh in the direction of the lateral side of the patella.

26

The gluteus muscles and the tensor fasciae latae are stripped from the outer aspect of the ilium, but from the anterior superior spine one should work within the sheath of the tensor, along the anterior border of the muscle, in order to avoid most of the branches of the lateral cutaneous nerve of the thigh. The fascia lata is split down to the end of the incision.

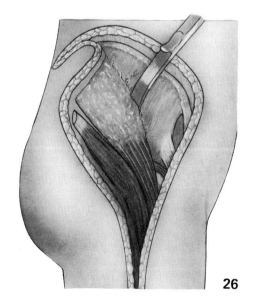

26

27

As the stripping of the gluteus muscles from the ilium progresses the articular capsule is reached along its anterior and superior aspects; these are also stripped, giving access to the anterior border of the greater trochanter. The tendon of gluteus minimus is then cut close to the greater trochanter, followed by the tendon of gluteus medius, which is cut close to the lateral aspect of the greater trochanter. This makes a large, thick flap containing the three gluteus muscles, the tensor fasciae latae, their blood and nerve supplies. The flap is retracted backwards to give access to the posterior part of the hip joint, which is covered by the external rotators. Piriformis and obturator internus are cut and marked by a stitch, as in a posterior approach, and the special retractor can then be inserted into either sciatic notch.

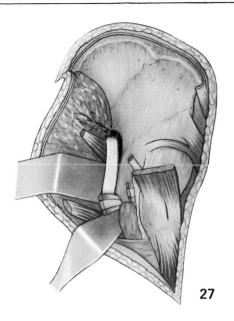

27

28

This approach gives access to the entire blade of the ilium, the whole posterior column up to the upper pole of the ischial tuberosity and to the anterior column, but not beyond the body of the pubis. One can strip the iliacus and gain access to the iliac fossa up to the iliopectineal line, but it is not easy to work there.

The approach is advisable for:

(1) transverse fracture passing through the roof of the acetabulum;

(2) transverse fractures associated with fractures of the anterior column and;

(3) some fractures of both anterior and posterior columns.

It is particularly useful in mal-united cases when it is decided not to rebuild the inferior part of the anterior column.

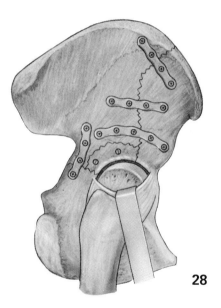

28

Closure

The wound is closed by re-attaching the gluteal muscles and two or three suction drains should be used.

POSTOPERATIVE CARE

The patient stays in bed for 10–15 days.

Passive exercises of the reconstructed hip begin on the third day.

Antibiotics are given for 2 days before and 8 days after an ilio-inguinal approach.

Anticoagulants are used in all cases.

Walking without weight-bearing is allowed from the fifteenth day.

The return to full weight-bearing usually requires 75–90 days according to x-ray appearances.

[*The illustrations for this Chapter on Display, Correction and Fixation of Stove-in Hip Joints were drawn by Mr. F. Price.*]

Replacement and Fixation of Posterior Lip of Acetabulum
(following Posterior Fracture-Dislocation)

E. Letournel, M.D.
Professor of Orthopaedic Surgery and Traumatology,
Centre Medico-Chirurgical de la Porte de Choisy, Paris

PRE-OPERATIVE

Indications

The replacement and fixation of a fracture of the posterior lip of the acetabulum is advisable because the restoration of the articular crescent restores the stability of the joint and allows a natural distribution of intra-articular pressure, thereby preventing post-traumatic osteo-arthrosis.

Furthermore the surgical correction allows one to clear the joint of any small fragments which are not visible with x-rays and can give troubles later on. It enables the surgeon to recognize the fractures in which the external part of the posterior wall is separated into one or more fragments, whereas the inner part is impacted into the underlying cancellous bone and has to be dislodged and replaced in contact with the femoral head. Good fixation allows early walking without weight-bearing and avoids all kinds of postoperative immobilization.

The only contra-indication is small fragments that are too small to be screwed.

Time of operation

The dislocation must be reduced as soon as possible after injury. Usually the femoral head is stable, but the fragments remain displaced. Rest in bed with slight external rotation of the limb avoids recurrent dislocation; traction is not necessary.

If the hip cannot be reduced (because, for example, of a big intra-articular fragment) or is unstable after reduction because of the extent of the fracture, operation should be carried out as an emergency.

Provided that the reduced head remains in the joint, replacement of the posterior fragment can be easily performed during the first 6 or 8 days after injury, so there is plenty of time in which to prepare the patient.

Anaesthesia

General anaesthesia is necessary and blood for transfusion should be available.

1

Position of patient

The patient is placed prone on an orthopaedic table.

To relax the sciatic nerve and avoid damaging it during the posterior approach, the knee should be flexed about 45° and a transcondylar Steinmann pin allows traction on the limb.

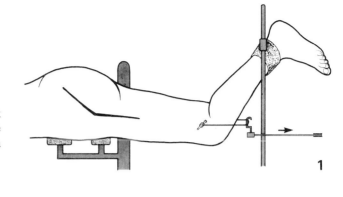

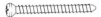

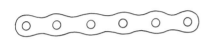

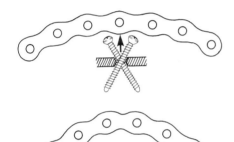

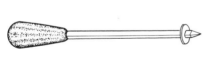

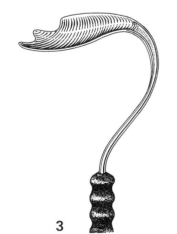

2

The device

Screws are used; plates may also be necessary.

The plates do not need to be very thick and wide and they must be capable of being shaped to lie perfectly on the reconstructed posterior wall. Vitallium Sherman's plates are satisfactory because they can be easily shaped in all directions. There are also curved Vitallium Letournel acetabular plates with 6, 8 or 10 holes and two curvatures.

To give them the desired shape one can use special benders or, more commonly, two big forceps grasping the plate at the right places. It is essential to shape the plate to follow perfectly the contours of the posterior column where it must lie; it is easy to make it too much or too little curved and so to spoil the position of the fragment(s) when the screws are driven home.

3

Special tools

It is helpful to have an instrument to push fragments into place and it should be protected by a shield 4 mm from its end.

A special retractor may be inserted in either sciatic notch; it takes a good hold because of its distal hook, and it presents a concave surface to the nerve, but it must be kept closely against the bone (sciatic spine upwards, ischial tuberosity downwards) in order to avoid compression of the nerve by one or other side of its hook.

THE OPERATION

4a&b

Kocher-Langenbeck approach

The skin incision has two limbs centred on the superior part of the greater trochanter; the upper runs two-thirds of the way towards the posterior-superior iliac spine and the lower passes down the lateral aspect of the thigh.

The gluteus maximus and the fascia lata are split in the line of the incision. The gluteus maximus is split only as far as the first important vascular pedicle.

The tendon of piriformis is divided, lifted up and attached by a stitch to the internal lip of the incision. Lifting the muscle exposes the sciatic nerve and gives access to the greater sciatic notch and to the neuro-vascular pedicle of the gluteal muscles.

The obturator internus and the gemelli are also divided through their terminal tendons, secured with a stitch and freed carefully from the bone. The underlying synovial bursa is opened and gives access to the lesser sciatic notch, into which the special retractor can be inserted and where it will remain separated from the nerve by the obturator tendon. The whole of both sciatic notches must be reached and exposed.

The upper pole of the ischial tuberosity has to be cleared of muscular insertions but it is not always necessary to divide the quadratus femoris.

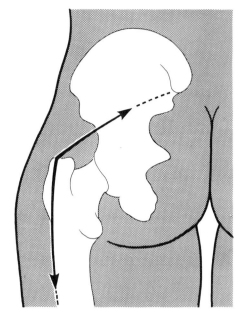

4a

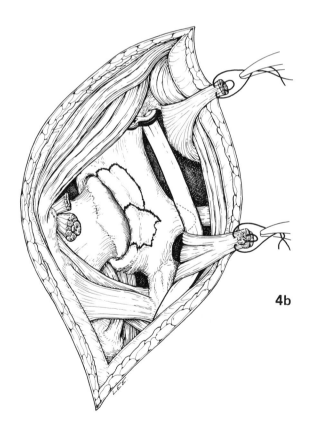

4b

5a&b

Posterior wall fracture

The posterior wall fracture can then be displayed. It varies from case to case. The most typical is separate fragments with a part of the articular surface and a part of the retro-acetabular surface; these fragments may or may not remain attached to the capsule and other soft parts. Fragments are often embedded in the underlying cancellous bone and must be carefully looked for. Sometimes there are isolated fragments of the articular or of the posterior cortical surface. Both the extent of the posterior wall avulsion and the number of fragments vary greatly from one case to another. The displaced fragments and the tear of the capsule allow access to the joint. Although it is difficult to avoid some stripping of the soft tissues from these fragments, such dissection should be kept to a minimum.

Clearing the joint

The joint must be cleared of any fragments that are in the acetabular fossa and one must not forget to remove the fragment that is sometimes attached to the ligamentum teres, which generally remains attached to the head.

With the aid of traction one gains an excellent view of the joint and should easily recognize both free and impacted fragments.

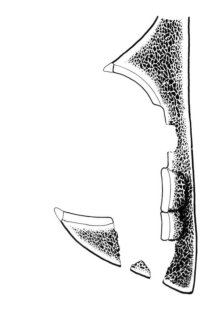

5a

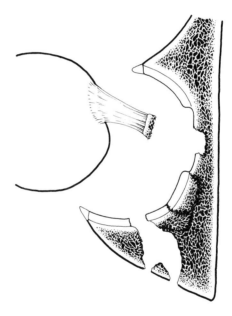

5b

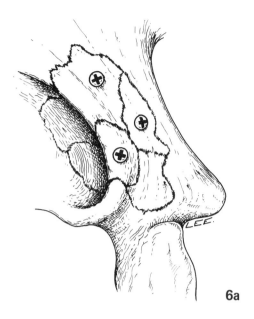

6a

6a&b

The reduction

When traction is released the head takes its place under the roof and the anterior part of the articular crescent, but one must ensure that the contact is perfect. The fragments are then replaced. First, any impacted fragments are gently mobilized with a chisel or a lever, trying to keep their cancellous part intact and they are set in place upon the head of the femur. The posterior fragments are then replaced. It is easy when there is only one fragment, it is more difficult when there are several pieces, which have to be put in their right places as carefully and perfectly as the pieces of jigsaw puzzle. This takes time and may require many trials and errors. When there is a combination of separated and impacted fragments there may be found to be a gap after they have been re-assembled as best one can; if this is likely to impair the stability of the reconstruction it should be filled with cancellous bone from the ilium or from the greater trochanter of the femur.

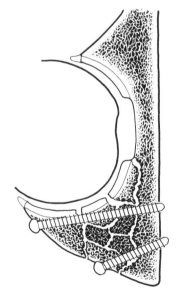

6b

7a,b&c

Fixation

In the case of small fragments two or three isolated screws may suffice; this is most likely to be so when the fragments bear a small portion of articular surface. A single big fragment may be fixed by several screws inserted in different directions. These screws are inserted into the posterior aspect of the fragment and are directed to the quadrilateral surface of the iliac bone where they obtain a good hold. One must always take care to avoid the joint and the head and it is wise to test the movement of the head in its socket so as to be sure that there is no grating. A finger passed through the great sciatic notch tests the length of the screws.

In most cases plates are needed as well as screws. Two or three screws are used to hold the fragments in place. Then a plate has to be fitted to the posterior column, from the upper pole of the ischial tuberosity to the posterior part of the wing or above the roof of the acetabulum, depending on the size and the exact site of the posterior fracture(s). The plate follows the long axis of the articular fragments. Whether straight or curved, the lower end of the plate is given a sharp bend to follow the contour of the 'infra-acetabular groove'. The rest of the plate is shaped to follow exactly the contours of the posterior column so as to be in perfect contact with the bone. The pedicle of the gluteal muscles is very carefully freed from the bone if it is necessary to insert the plate under it. The plate is then screwed down, taking care not to enter the joint. The lowest screw is inserted into the ischial tuberosity, where it finds a very strong hold and may be 40 or 45 mm long. The screws over the roof may be 30–40 mm and those into the posterior part of the wing, 25–35 mm. The intermediate screws, like the separate ones, take hold of the quadrilateral surface. If possible, one should insert two screws beyond each extremity of the fracture site.

One must always test the freedom of the joint after plating.

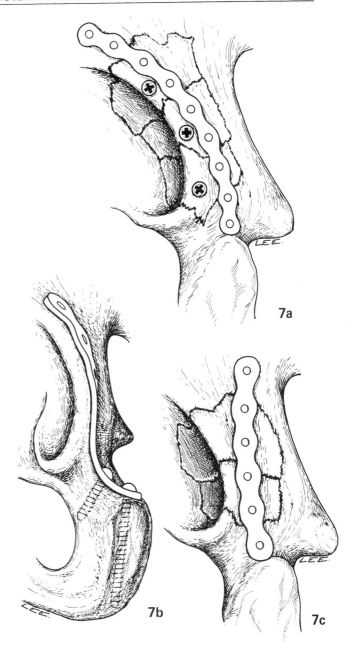

7a

7b

7c

Closure

Piriformis and obturator internus are re-attached to their tendons and sewn together side to side in order to provide a muscular pad between the sciatic nerve and the plate.

One or two suction drains are required.
Gluteus maximus is sutured and the skin closed.
The transcondylar traction pin is removed.

POSTOPERATIVE CARE

No plaster, splint or traction is required, only bed rest.
The patient is allowed to move his limb.
Passive exercises begin on the second or third day.
Suction drains are removed after 5 or 6 days.
Walking without weight-bearing is allowed on the eighth to the tenth day.
Full weight-bearing is allowed after 75 days.

[The illustrations for this Chapter on Replacement and Fixation of Posterior Lip of Acetabulum (following Posterior Fracture-Dislocation) were drawn by Mrs. G. Lee.]

Exposure and Fixation of Disrupted Pubic Symphysis

E. Letournel, M.D.
Professor of Orthopaedic Surgery and Traumatology,
Centre Medico-Chirurgical de la Porte de Choisy, Paris

PRE-OPERATIVE

Indications

It is often worthwhile attempting to restore the shape and stability of a fractured pelvis; even though there may appear to be merely disruption or overlapping of the symphysis pubis there is usually sacro-iliac damage as well, but this can be corrected if the pubis is fixed in place.

Operation is advisable: (*1*) when the pubic bones overlap; (*2*) when the pubic interval is greater than 1 cm; thus, only very small disruptions are treated conservatively.

Furthermore, this surgical treatment avoids all kinds of postoperative immobilization and allows walking with crutches sometimes only 10 days after operation.

Time of operation

This is not an emergency and delay of a few days allows: (*1*) the spontaneous arrest of bleeding from pelvic veins disrupted at the time of injury and (*2*) preparing the skin for incision through the pubic hair.

Anaesthesia

General anaesthesia is used.

The urinary bladder has to be evacuated either spontaneously or by catheter.

Position of patient

The patient may be placed upon an ordinary operating table, but an orthopaedic table may be useful to facilitate the reduction of the more severe disruptions by allowing asymmetrical traction on the limbs and internal rotation of both hips. The patient should be so placed that the hips can be hyperextended by suitable adjustment of the table.

1

The apparatus

There is no special device. One can use a vitallium modified Sherman plate with equidistant holes. If it is to be applied on the superior aspect of the pubic bones it has to be bent along its long axis in two directions, posteriorly and superiorly.

A plate of four or six holes is used. Thick and wide plates are not suitable; Sherman's are adequate as they can be shaped so as to lie perfectly on the bone.

To give the plate its posterior concavity one can use any bending apparatus, but two strong forceps grasping the plate on either part of the mid-line and taking hold of short screws inserted into the outer holes allow one to obtain the desired amount of posterior curvature.

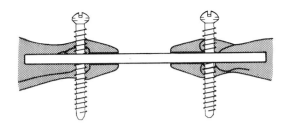

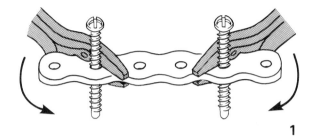

1

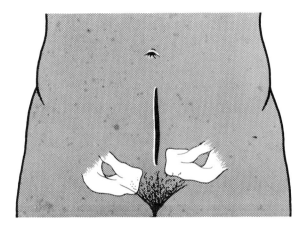

2a

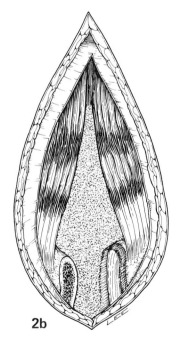

2b

THE OPERATION

2a&b

The exposure

In a case of simple disruption of the pubic symphysis, a vertical median incision is adequate. It should be 10–12 cm long and extend distally to the level of the superior border of the symphysis, i.e. crossing the pubic hair area.

The recti abdominis are separated along the linea alba.

Retzius's space is opened, the bladder is pushed back, and the posterior surfaces of the pubes are exposed.

The tear of a pubic symphysis is always asymmetrical.

On one side the bone has been cleared of all its muscular and ligamentous insertions, and the rectus itself is attached only to the prepubic soft parts. On the other side the rectus is normally attached, and the capsule and the cartilage remain attached to the bone; the anterior and inferior symphysis ligaments are torn in all cases.

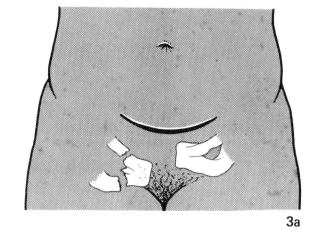

3a

3a&b

In some cases, a disrupted symphysis is associated with a vertical fracture through one obturator foramen that also crosses the pubic and ischiopubic rami. If this fracture is displaced it is necessary to reduce the displacement and plate it at the same time as the symphysis. In this case a vertical incision is not suitable and a horizontal approach such as a Pfannenstiel incision is more appropriate. If necessary, one rectus abdominis is cut transversely near its pubic insertion and repaired later on.

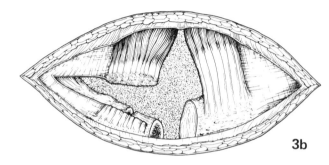

3b

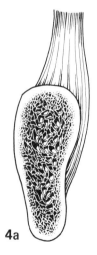

4a

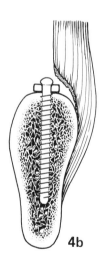

4b

4a&b

In any case it is necessary to free the superior aspect of the pubic rami where the plate will be inserted. As a rule, one side is already freed by the injuring force; on the other side the superior aspect has to be cleared from back to front, but the rectus must remain attached to the anterior border of that surface.

Removing the cartilage makes it easier to obtain a perfect correction of the displacement.

5a & b

The reduction

Internal rotation of both lower limbs, axial traction and hyperextension of the hip, allowed by the orthopaedic table, facilitate the reduction but a direct action on the pubic bones is always necessary. The author uses Faraboeuf's forceps, whose jaws take hold of the anterior aspect of the pubic angle, or, better, are inserted into the obturator foramina (*see Illustration 6a*).

Often the reduction is not achieved in one stage; when several stages are needed allow a few minutes between successive stages.

The symphysis must fit in all directions and not only its superior aspect; a possible twist of the ilium has to be corrected to align the posterior aspects of the pubic bones correctly.

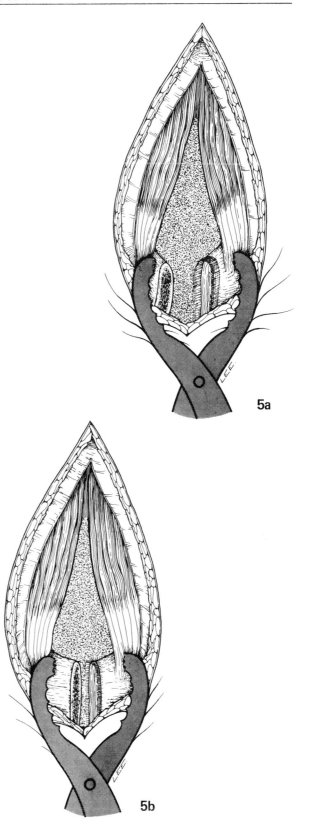

5a

5b

The fixation

6a&b

As the reduction is achieved a four or six hole plate is shaped to lie perfectly on the superior aspect of each pubic ramus.

Two screws can be inserted in the body of each pubis. These screws should be parallel to the posterior surface of the pubis, that is to say directed obliquely backwards and downwards. From in front they look vertical and parallel or slightly divergent. Thirty-five or forty-five millimetre screws should be used.

If a six hole plate is used, the outer screws will be inserted into the superior pubic rami; they have to be shorter and must avoid the obturator vessels, but being screwed into two cortices they have a firm grasp.

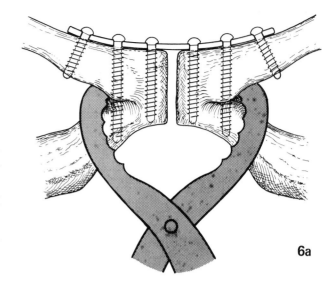

6a

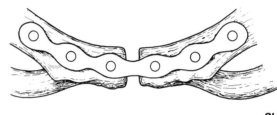

6b

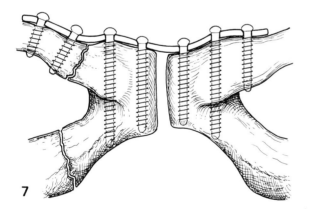

7

7

If it is necessary to span a disrupted symphysis and a fracture into the obturator foramen, the problem is more difficult and it is more important to understand the objective than to describe the procedure in detail. It may be best to start by fitting the symphysis accurately together, sometimes one should start with the fracture and hold it with a single screw. A long enough plate must be used to allow each fragment to be gripped by two screws and it must be made to fit all fragments accurately while they are accurately in place.

Closure of the wound

One or two suction drains are inserted, one in front, one behind the repaired symphysis.

If the rectus has been cut across it is repaired carefully.

The linea alba is sutured.

The skin incision is closed.

POSTOPERATIVE CARE

Prophylactic antibiotics may be used as the pubic hair area has been cut through.
Suction drains are removed after 4–6 days.
The patient remains in bed without any type of immobilization.
Walking with partial weight-bearing and crutches is allowed after 14 days.
Full weight-bearing is allowed after 6 weeks.

[*The illustrations for this Chapter on Exposure and Fixation of Disrupted Pubic Symphysis were drawn by Mrs. G. Lee.*]

Fractures in Children

A. G. Pollen, F.R.C.S.
Consultant Orthopaedic and Traumatic Surgeon,
Bedford General Hospital

Introduction

The vast majority of children's fractures are treated successfully by closed methods. Those requiring operative intervention form but a small proportion of the whole. These fractures may be divided into two groups.

(*1*) Certain fractures which involve the epiphyseal (growth) plate, where exact reduction is essential.

(*2*) Fractures of the shaft or metaphysis of long bones where an acceptable reduction cannot be obtained or maintained by conservative measures. The methods of treatment employed in this group are similar to those used for comparable adult fractures and are not discussed in this chapter.

EPIPHYSEAL INJURY

Three types of epiphyseal injury occur which were classified into five groups by Salter and Harris (1963).

1a

Fracture-separation of the epiphysis

The whole epiphysis is displaced; the line of separation runs across the epiphyseal plate through the zone of hypertrophied cartilage cells. In many cases the fracture extends obliquely into the metaphysis so that a triangular-shaped piece of metaphysis is attached to the epiphyseal fragment. Less frequently there is a pure epiphyseal separation without involvement of the metaphysis. The majority of these injuries can be treated by closed manipulation but there are a few exceptions where open reduction is needed. These include some fractures of the proximal radial epiphysis and traumatic separation of the capital epiphysis of the femur.

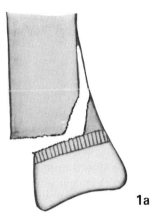

1a

1b

Transepiphyseal plate fractures

These form an important group of injuries and occur particularly at the elbow and ankle joints. The fracture line runs from the articular surface across the epiphyseal plate into the adjacent metaphysis. If this fragment is displaced then meticulous reduction is required for two reasons.

First, the articular surface is distorted and needs anatomical reduction.

Second, the break in continuity of the epiphyseal plate permits the formation of a bone bridge between the metaphysis and the epiphysis, causing a localized closure of the plate. Disturbance of growth will occur with progressive deformity of the bone, depending upon the age of the child. Clearly the younger the child the more severe will be the deformity.

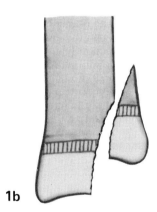

1b

1c

Crushing injuries of the epiphyseal plate

This type of injury is the least common. Often there is little radiographic evidence of injury to the epiphysis save for some buckling of the cortex at the metaphysis. It is only when disturbance of bone growth becomes apparent that the significance of the injury may be appreciated. Most commonly this type involves the ankle joint at the medial part of the tibial epiphyseal plate. It may cause a progressive varus deformity of the ankle with shortening. Less often the knee or wrist joints may be damaged by crush injuries of the epiphyseal plates.

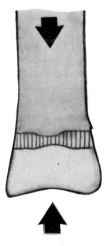

1c

INJURIES OF THE ELBOW JOINT

FRACTURES OF LATERAL CONDYLE OF THE HUMERUS

2

The fracture passes obliquely across the growth plate between the distal epiphysis of the humerus and the lateral side of the metaphysis. It produces a large epiphyseal fragment containing the whole of the capitulum, a portion of the adjacent trochlea, and a piece of the lateral cortex of the metaphysis.

In young children there is very little ossification of the articular surface of the humerus, so radiographs may show only a small metaphyseal fracture, and the slight shift of the ossific centre for the capitulum may not be noticed. Unless these appearances are interpreted correctly this fracture may be treated inadequately.

Open reduction and internal fixation of this fracture is indicated whenever the fragment is displaced by more than a few millimetres. Failure to do this may lead to non-union of the fragment, irregular growth of the distal end of the humerus and a progressive valgus deformity of the elbow. Firm fixation of the fragment is essential; soft tissue suture is inadequate.

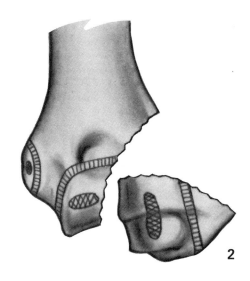

2

Position of patient

The child is placed in a supine position, the shoulder abducted and the arm supported on a side table with the elbow flexed at about 60°.

The operation must be performed in a bloodless field using a pneumatic cuff which is placed as high as possible on the upper arm so as not to encroach upon the operation area.

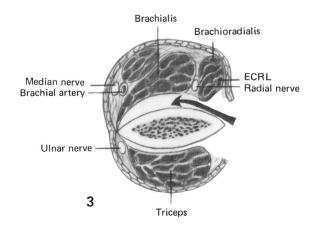

Brachialis

Brachioradialis

Median nerve
Brachial artery

ECRL
Radial nerve

Ulnar nerve

3

Triceps

Anatomical approach

3

This uses the lateral intermuscular septum attached to the lateral supracondylar ridge of the humerus. The radial nerve is protected by the extensor carpi radialis longus, the brachioradialis and brachialis muscles which are elevated from the anterior aspect of the humerus.

4

The incision

This runs along the lower two-thirds of the lateral supracondylar ridge across the lateral aspect of the elbow to terminate 1 cm distal to the head of the radius. It is deepened and the deep fascia divided down to the lateral supracondylar ridge cutting accurately down to bone. It is important not to allow the knife to stray to either side of the ridge.

The lower part of the origin of brachioradialis and extensor carpi radialis longus muscles can be detached from the supracondylar ridge by sharp dissection and are elevated anteriorly. Posteriorly the medial head of triceps is elevated by using a small rugine (Howarth's or Dewar's). By a combination of sharp dissection and gentle stripping with the rugine the muscle attachments are separated from the supracondylar ridge up to the fracture. The soft tissue attachments beyond this are disturbed as little as possible.

The elbow is now flexed to a right angle and the anterior surface of the metaphysis displayed by elevating the brachialis muscle across to the medial border. A MacDonald's dissector is placed around the medial border and the condylar fracture displayed by lifting the synovium forwards. Blood and blood clot within the joint should be mopped out until the articular surface is clearly seen.

The fragment is mobilized so that its fracture surface can be cleared of all clot and fibrin. It may be considerably rotated so that the articular surface faces laterally, and the fragment has to be turned into its correct location. After preparing the metaphyseal surface the fragment should be repositioned accurately and the whole articular surface inspected to ensure that the reduction is perfect. The position of the fragment is then secured with a light clamp.

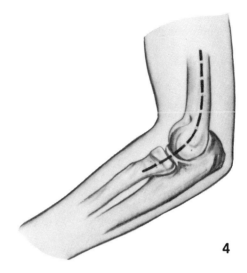

4

Wound closure

The deep fascia is closed with interrupted absorbable sutures and the skin with unabsorbable material. A well-padded plaster-of-Paris splint is applied to hold the elbow in flexion, with the forearm in neutral rotation and the wrist in moderate extension. If a complete plaster is applied this must be split before the child leaves the operating theatre. This is retained for 4 weeks; the plaster and stitches are then removed. Radiographs should be taken at this stage to confirm that the fracture is uniting. Cautious active movement may then be permitted within a sling for 2 weeks and progressive activity allowed thereafter.

The wires can be removed after 3 months but often they loosen and require removal before this time.

5

Fixation of the fragment

Unless the metaphyseal part of the fragment is large enough to accept a screw, the lateral condyle must be fixed with two Kirschner wires. The common extensor origin is split longitudinally so that the lateral epicondyle is exposed; a wire is introduced through the fragment across the fracture into the metaphysis. A second wire is then inserted in a different plane to stabilize the fragment. The wires are cut short so that they do not protrude through the skin. Radiographs are taken before closing the wound to confirm that the wires are placed correctly.

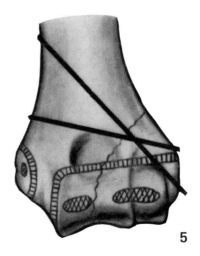

5

FRACTURES OF NECK OF RADIUS

Two varieties of fracture occur:

(*1*) Metaphyseal injuries.

(*2*) Fracture-separation of the proximal radial epiphysis.

The former may be greenstick or complete. In greenstick fractures there is a variable degree of tilt of the radial head. With complete fractures considerable displacement may occur; occasionally the upper end of the radial shaft may be subluxed anteriorly because of tearing of the annular ligament.

Epiphyseal displacements vary from a minor shift to total separation of the epiphysis. The majority of fractures of the neck of the radius may be treated conservatively: some need no reduction and many others can be reduced by closed methods.

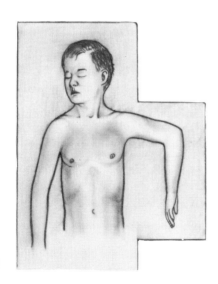

6

Indications for open reduction

(*1*) Failure to obtain a satisfactory position by closed methods. A persistent angulation of 30° or more in a child under 10 years of age, or 20° or more in a child over the age of 10 years should not be accepted.

(*2*) A widely displaced fracture.

(*3*) Fractures of the neck of the radius associated with subluxation of the upper end of the radial shaft.

Open reduction may have to be supplemented by internal fixation if the reduction is unstable. Although internal fixation of the radial head presents technical difficulties the fragment must be stabilized because the functional results of severe malunion are very poor.

Operative hazards

The posterior interosseous nerve is vulnerable during the exposure of the head and neck of the radius. To safeguard the nerve the forearm should be pronated during the dissection (Strachan and Ellis, 1971), the incision should not extend beyond the inferior margin of the annular ligament, and retraction of the soft tissues should be gentle at all times.

6

Position of patient

The patient is supine, the shoulder abducted so that the arm can be placed on a side table. The elbow is flexed to 90° supported on a small sandbag and the forearm is placed in pronation.

The operation is performed in a bloodless field by using a pneumatic cuff placed as high as possible around the upper arm.

7

The incision

This begins at the mid-point of the lateral supracondylar ridge and runs vertically to the tip of the lateral epicondyle. It then curves forward to run across the posterolateral aspect of the head of the radius and lateral aspect of the ulna (Boyd, 1971).

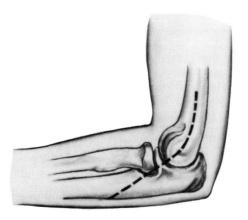

7

8

Exposure

The upper half of the incision is deepened by cutting down to the bone along the supracondylar ridge. The muscles are elevated from both aspects of the ridge by sharp dissection. The common extensor origin is elevated from the lateral epicondyle anteriorly and the origin of anconeus is reflected posteriorly; in this interval lie the lateral ligament and annular ligament. These structures are divided in line with the incision to expose the head and neck of the radius. MacDonald's dissectors are introduced around the neck of the radius and the soft tissues retracted gently. At the distal edge of the wound the upper fibres of supinator may be retracted gently with a hook for better exposure.

By rotating the forearm, hitherto in pronation, the extent of the fracture and deformity can be assessed.

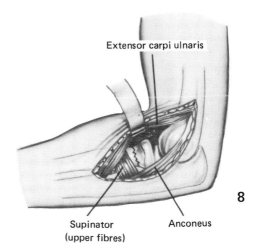

Extensor carpi ulnaris

Supinator (upper fibres)

Anconeus

8

Management of angulated fractures

The radius is rotated so that the maximum tilt of the radial head presents. Direct pressure over the margin of the head will correct the deformity. The stability of the reduction can be judged by rotating the forearm once more. If the reduction is stable no more need be done save for closure of the wound in layers, and the application of a plaster-of-Paris splint.

Management of unstable or severely displaced fractures

Where the radial head is completely unstable or when it has been separated from the shaft the corrected position cannot be maintained without internal fixation. Furthermore, occasionally the shaft of the radius is found to be subluxed anteriorly because the annular ligament has been torn. This is another indication for internal fixation.

Two methods are available which involve the insertion of Kirschner wires into the radius; each presents technical difficulties. It is recommended that the wires are inserted with the aid of a light-weight power drill.

9

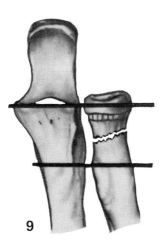

9

(*1*) The upper shaft of the radius is transfixed by a wire about 1 cm below the fracture. The annular ligament is incised in the long axis of the radius and the shaft is held in its correct position while the wire is driven into the ulna, thus stabilizing the distal fragment.

The radial head fragment is grasped firmly and a second wire is driven across this fragment transversely, avoiding the growth plate. The fragment is placed accurately in position onto the shaft making quite sure that it is not tilted. The wire is then driven into the radial notch of the ulna. The annular ligament is repaired with one or two catgut stitches.

10

(2) This method is useful in younger children, where the radial head fragment is small, and in fracture-separations of the epiphysis, where the first method might damage the growth plate.

A Kirschner wire is passed through the posterior aspect of the lower end of the humerus to emerge through the centre of the capitulum. The radial head fragment is held firmly by Allis' forceps in its correct position while the wire is driven through the fragment and down the medullary cavity of the radial shaft for 5 cm.

The most difficult part of this procedure is to ensure that the wire emerges at the centre of the capitulum. A towel clip can be used as a 'jig' to help guide the wire. One blade is placed with the point in the centre of the capitulum; the other blade grips the posterior aspect of the lateral condyle. The posterior blade is used as a guide for the point of entry of the wire which is inserted as close as possible to it. The wire is directed anteriorly through the capitulum, aiming for the anterior point of the towel clip, and should emerge centrally placed. The towel clip is removed and the wire is advanced into the radial head and then down the shaft.

It is advisable to obtain radiographs to ensure that the wires are correctly placed before closing the wound. The wires are then cut short so that the skin may be closed without them protruding. Great care must be taken during the wound closure to avoid moving the elbow.

A well-padded plaster cast should be applied. This must extend from the upper arm to the hand to prevent forearm rotation and to hold the elbow securely. Inadvertent movement of the elbow could bend or break the wires with disastrous results. The plaster should be split before the patient leaves the theatre.

Postoperative care

Plaster immobilization should be continued for 3—4 weeks. The plaster should then be removed but further radiographs must be taken to confirm that bony union is occurring. If wires were inserted they should be removed under anaesthesia. Active movements are now permitted but for the first week or two the constraint of an arm sling is advisable.

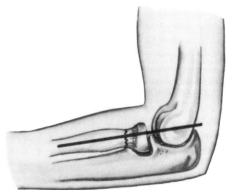

10

Complications

Malunion

This occurs if reduction of the fracture is incomplete or when the fracture redisplaces after open reduction. Persistence of severe displacement, particularly if the fragment is displaced as well as tilted, is likely to produce considerable impairment of function. Minor degrees of tilting of the head often correct with growth, particularly in young children.

Ischaemic necrosis of the radial head

This may occur when the radial head is completely displaced from the metaphysis. Early excision of the radial head must be avoided because the proximal end of the radius will fail to grow longitudinally and, as a result, progressive subluxation of the inferior radio-ulnar joint develops.

Late excision of the ischaemic radial head after the cessation of growth can be undertaken without the risk of growth disturbance and may even improve the range of forearm rotation.

FRACTURE-SEPARATION OF MEDIAL EPICONDYLE

The medial epicondylar apophysis develops from a centre of ossification which is separated from the articular epiphyses by a portion of metaphysis. It is extracapsular in position and unites with the metaphysis of the humerus.

It may be avulsed as a result of an abduction strain of the elbow or in association with a dislocation of the joint. The apophysis is usually displaced distally and such injuries are treated conservatively with good results.

With a severe abduction strain of the elbow the medial capsular ligament may be torn and the avulsed epicondyle drawn into the joint. If there is but a momentary subluxation then the bones regain their normal positions, leaving the epicondyle trapped within. Sometimes the epicondyle remains trapped after manipulative reduction of a dislocation.

Indication for operation

Failure to extricate the fragment from the joint by manipulation.

Operative hazards

The ulnar nerve may be damaged by the initial injury but it is also at risk during the operation because it is closely related to the medial epicondyle. It is important to find and protect the nerve at an early stage.

Position of patient

The patient is placed on his back but tilted towards the injured side. The shoulder is abducted and externally rotated so that the medial aspect of the arm is displayed. The limb is supported on a side table with the elbow flexed 60°–80°.

11

An alternative position is to place the child prone with the shoulder abducted about 60° and the forearm in neutral rotation (palm uppermost). The elbow is supported on a small sandbag.

The operation is performed in a bloodless field using a pneumatic cuff applied high around the upper arm.

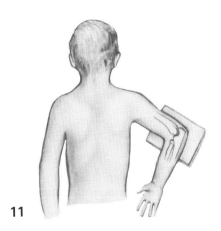

11

12

The incision

This commences at the junction of the middle and distal thirds of the upper arm and runs distally along the anterior border of the medial head of triceps following the line of the medial intermuscular septum. It continues around the medial aspect of the elbow onto the common flexor group of muscles for a short distance.

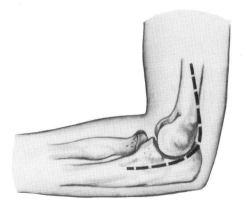

12

13

In the upper part of the wound the deep fascia is opened longitudinally along the intermuscular septum to display the ulnar nerve which lies just posterior to the septum. This is followed distally towards the elbow until it is close to the flexor origin. The nerve is carefully mobilized at this point so that it may be retracted gently away from the epicondylar groove.

The elbow is now extended; the flexor mass is grasped with forceps and the epicondyle is gently pulled out from the joint.

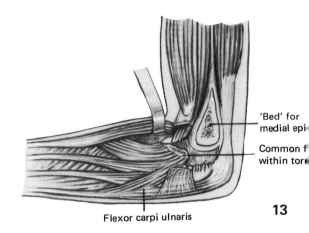

'Bed' for medial epi‹
Common f‹ within tor‹
Flexor carpi ulnaris
13

14 & 15

Replacement of medial epicondyle

It is important to ensure that the ulnar nerve is not caught up during this procedure and it should be retracted gently away from the epicondyle.

The elbow and wrist are flexed to relax the muscles; the raw area of bone is defined by retracting the brachialis, and the medial epicondyle is held in position with a light clamp. The fragment is transfixed by a Kirschner wire which is driven obliquely across the metaphysis towards the lateral cortex. The end of the wire is cut short so that it will not protrude through the skin, and the fixation may be re-inforced by suturing the tough fascia to the adjacent intermuscular septum.

In the older child the fragment is larger and may accept a screw. This provides much more effective fixation.

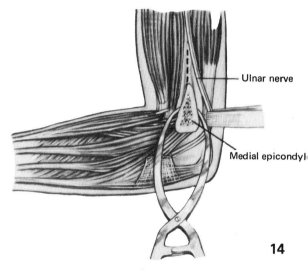

Ulnar nerve
Medial epicondyl‹
14

Wound closure

The deep fascia need not be closed and the skin is sutured taking care not to pick up the ulnar nerve in the stitches.

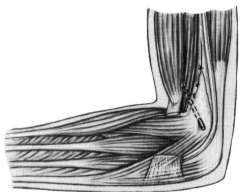

15

Postoperative care

A well-padded plaster cast is applied to hold the elbow flexed to 90° and the forearm and wrist in neutral position. The plaster is removed 4 weeks later and active movements are permitted. It is usual for the wire to become loose soon after activity is resumed, but it is a simple matter to remove it.

Usually the fragment heals by fibrous union but this does not affect the normal function of the limb.

Other indications for operation

Occasionally after conservative treatment of a displaced epicondyle the child complains of discomfort when the medial aspect of the elbow rests on a hard surface. This occurs if the fragment remains mobile and is lying very superficially. In these cases it is justifiable to excise the epicondyle from the flexor origin.

INJURIES OF THE ANKLE JOINT

TRANSEPIPHYSEAL PLATE FRACTURE OF THE DISTAL TIBIAL EPIPHYSIS

This is a shearing injury of the medial half of the tibial epiphysis. The fracture runs from the articular surface of the tibia across the epiphyseal plate into the adjacent metaphysis and through the medial cortex. Those cases with minimal displacement can be treated conservatively but where significant displacement has occurred then open reduction and internal fixation will be necessary.

16

Indications for operation

(*1*) Fractures where radiographs show an obvious 'step' in the articular surface.
(*2*) Fractures where there is a sufficient break in continuity of the epiphyseal plate for a bony bridge to be established between the epiphysis and metaphysis.

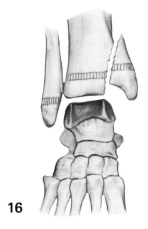

16

Operative hazards

The posterior tibial vessels, nerve and the tibialis posterior tendon are particularly liable to be damaged during the exposure of the medial malleolus. These structures must be carefully mobilized and protected during the operation.

17

Position of patient

The child is placed supine. The leg is positioned with the knee in about 45° of flexion so that the limb is externally rotated and the medial side of the ankle is uppermost. The outer side of the knee is supported by a firm pillow or sandbag. Operation must be performed in a bloodless field using a pneumatic cuff placed around the upper part of the thigh.

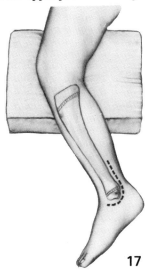

17

18

The incision

This is 'J' shaped: the vertical limb runs down behind the medial malleolus and then turns anteriorly across the ankle joint as far as the tibialis anterior tendon. The incision is carried down to the deep fascia and the flap reflected anteriorly to display the medial side of the ankle and the anterior aspect of the joint up to the tibialis anterior. Care must be taken to avoid injury to the long saphenous vein and nerve which lie superficial to the deep fascia close to the 'hinge' of the flap. The tibialis anterior tendon is mobilized and retracted laterally by incising the extensor retinaculum to the medial side of the tendon.

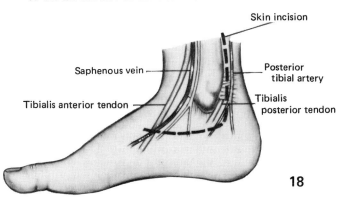

18

19

The structures directly posterior to the medial malleolus are now to be mobilized and retracted out of the way. The flexor retinaculum is divided at its malleolar attachment, exposing the tibialis posterior tendon and sheath. By using a small rugine the tendon and the other structures lying behind the medial malleolus can be elevated from the bone. A curved dissector can then be introduced between these structures and the malleolus.

To display the fracture completely the ankle joint must be opened anteriorly and medially. A vertical incision is made to the medial side of the tibialis anterior tendon from the tibial metaphysis to the joint. The capsule is opened anteriorly and the incision curves medially to the deltoid ligament. The articular surface of the tibia can be inspected by extending the foot. The whole malleolar fragment is now mobilized until it can be replaced in anatomical position and the articular surface can be seen to be restored.

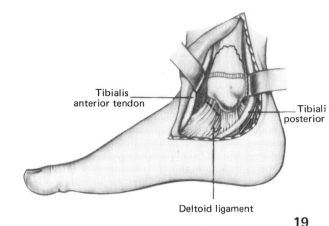

Tibialis anterior tendon

Tibialis posterior

Deltoid ligament

19

20

Fixation of the fragment

Two or three Kirschner wires are sufficient to hold the fragment securely; their precise placing will depend upon the size of the fragment and the extent of the metaphyseal portion.

The first wire can be inserted from near the tip of the malleolus obliquely upwards to cross the epiphyseal plate and traverse the metaphysis towards the lateral cortex. One or two more wires may be inserted in different planes to prevent the fragment from rotating.

The wires are cut short so that they will not project through the skin, but sufficient length is left outside the bone for ease of subsequent removal.

Wound closure

The capsular ligament is approximated with a few catgut stitches and the skin closed with interrupted sutures. A well-padded dressing is applied but there is no need for plaster splintage at this stage because the internal fixation is adequate.

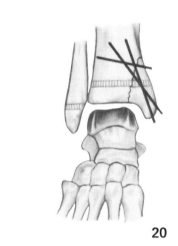

20

Postoperative care

The stitches are removed at 2 weeks, and a well-fitting below-knee plaster cast is applied. After 4 weeks this plaster is changed to a walking plaster.

When radiographs confirm sound union of the fragment then unprotected walking may be permitted. The wires can be removed as an out-patient procedure in a few months.

Complications

Despite the breach of the epiphyseal plate, if accurate re-alignment has been accomplished then growth continues. Only if there has been crushing of the epiphyseal plate will growth be seriously impaired.

FRACTURES OF THE HIP REGION

Fractures of the proximal end of the femur are relatively uncommon in children. They are usually associated with severe violence: road accidents or falls from a height. The injuries are classified into four groups.

(1) Traumatic separation of the capital epiphysis.
(2) Transcervical fractures.
(3) Basal fractures.
(4) Trochanteric fractures.

Undisplaced transcervical and basal fractures are treated conservatively, and most displaced trochanteric fractures can be reduced by closed methods and maintained in a plaster hip spica.

Indications for operation

(1) Displaced transcervical fractures.
(2) Traumatic separation of the capital epiphysis.

Various patterns of pins exist. The author prefers those designed by Adams where the distal portion is threaded in order to engage in the lateral cortex, and the base is triangular in section so that it may be gripped by a chuck.

Position of patient

The anaesthetized child is placed on an orthopaedic table with the lower limbs abducted and the foot of the sound limb strapped to the foot support. With the knee and hip flexed gentle traction is exerted upon the hip, and the limb is gently but firmly rotated internally. This foot is then attached to the footpiece to maintain the position while the reduction is checked by radiographs in two planes using either mobile machines or the image intensifier. If possible the amount of internal rotation should be adjusted so that the plane of the femoral neck is roughly horizontal in the lateral x-ray projection.

21

The principle of meticulous reduction and internal fixation applies just as much to the child as to the adult. The only difference is the method of internal fixation. Trauma to the epiphyseal plate must be kept to a minimum so that trifin nails should not be used. Instead several threaded pins are inserted along the neck into the epiphysis. They should be arranged so as to form a triangle within the epiphysis, taking care to avoid over-penetration.

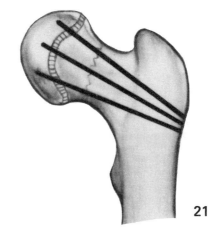

21

22 & 23

The incision

A vertical incision is made over the lateral aspect of the upper thigh from the prominence of the great trochanter distally for 10 cm. The incision is deepened down to the fascia lata which is incised vertically in the distal half of the wound. Proximally the fascia splits into two layers enclosing the tensor fascia muscle. The muscle fibres are split and separated and the whole layer held apart with retractors. The vastus lateralis and its fascia are now seen clothing the outer aspect of the femur.

The posterior border of this muscle is defined and separated and a bone lever inserted deep to the muscle and then lifted around the anterior aspect of the femur to hold the muscle belly forward. This displays the outer aspect of the upper femur covered by vastus intermedius, the fibres of which are split and cleaned from the bone with a periosteal elevator. Bone levers are then inserted around the femoral shaft.

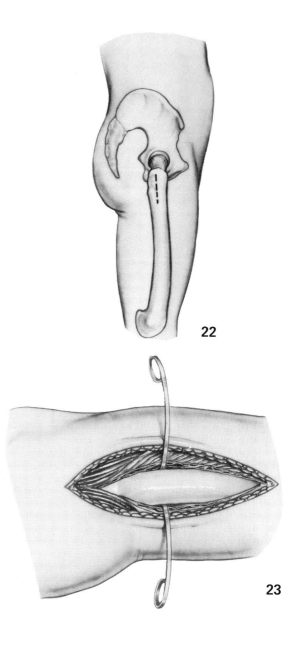

22

23

24

A small hole is made in the cortex with a bone awl 2–3 cm below the great trochanter, and a guide wire is introduced along the neck in a horizontal plane, directing the point towards the opposite antero-superior iliac spine. Check radiographs are taken or the image intensifier used to assess the position of the wire and to determine the length of pin needed. The wire is then withdrawn and the correct pin introduced along the same track. It is easiest to use a power drill in the early stages and change to a hand drill for the final adjustment of position. Check radiographs are taken at this stage.

Having introduced the first pin two more should be inserted in fairly close proximity to it, but varying the direction of the points in order to establish a 'spread' in the epiphysis. As the butt ends of the pins are fairly close together the Jacob's chuck may foul the pins already in position. An extension tube with a terminal box spanner which fits into the chuck can be used for final insertion of the pins. Radiographic control should be employed with each pin and a final assessment of the position made before wound closure. The wound is closed in two layers.

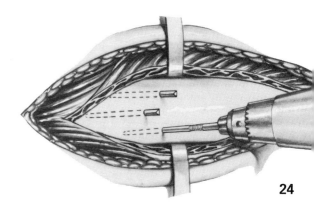

24

Postoperative care

Early active hip movements should be encouraged and the child can sit out of bed within a few days. 'Straight leg raising' against gravity should be avoided for several weeks.

The importance of avoiding premature weight-bearing must be stressed so that the parents and the child understand fully the reason for the restriction on activities. Union of transcervical fractures is often slow, and early weight-bearing may jeopardize healing. It is wise to insist upon the use of crutches for protected weight-bearing for 3—4 months before allowing sticks to be used.

Radiographs should be obtained at 6 weeks and 3 months and thereafter at intervals until positive radiographic evidence of bone union is seen. Removal of the pins should not be undertaken in less than 1 year from the injury.

Complications

Delayed union or non-union of the fracture occurs though it is difficult to estimate its frequency. Its occurrence is closely associated with imperfect reduction of the fracture or inadequate fixation. Intertrochanteric osteotomy may permit bony union to occur.

Avascular necrosis of the proximal fragment occurs in about 20 per cent of cases. In very young children substantial remodelling can occur.

Coxa vara deformity is frequent and is often associated with delay in union.

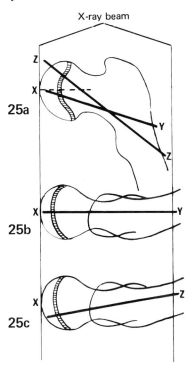

TRAUMATIC SEPARATION OF CAPITAL EPIPHYSIS

This injury is treated in the same manner as transcervical fractures, but two aspects merit particular attention.

First, the manipulative reduction should be performed as soon as possible and with the utmost gentleness.

Second, the epiphysis is much smaller than the transcervical fragment so that great care must be taken when inserting the pins to avoid damaging the joint surfaces and yet to obtain a sufficient grip of the fragment.

In this respect it is important to realize that the standard radiographs of the hips taken in two planes at right angles can give a false impression of the position of the points of the pins (Pollen, 1965).

25a,b &c

This paradox is explained in *Illustration 25* where *Illustration 25a* represents the proximal end of the femur with two pins, Y and Z, inserted. The vertical lines represent the direction of the x-ray beam producing the lateral radiographs and X marks the 'equator' of the femoral head where the x-ray beam meets the head at a tangent and casts a shadow.

Illustration 25b represents the lateral film showing pin Y directed towards the equator. The radiograph gives a true picture of the position.

Illustration 25c represents the lateral film of the femur with pin Z in position. Because this pin is directed to the upper and posterior quadrant of the femoral head it emerges through the bony head away from the equator. The shadow of the bony margin overlaps that of the pin and the film falsely indicates that the point is contained within the bone.

Similarly a false picture would be obtained in the anteroposterior projection.

This situation may arise whenever multiple pins are used, but the hazard is greatest where the epiphysis is to be secured. As a safeguard the points should not be placed closer than 5 mm from the bony margin.

Complications

Avascular necrosis of the epiphysis occurs frequently and may produce severe degenerative arthritic changes in the hip joint.

References

Adams, J. C. (1976). *Standard Orthopaedic Operations*. Churchill Livingstone: Edinburgh, London and New York

Boyd, H. B. (1971). In *Campbell's Operative Orthopaedics*. Volume I, page 121, 5th Edition. St. Louis: C. V. Mosby

Pollen, A. G. (1965). 'Fallacies in the interpretation of radiographs during nailing of the neck of the femur.' *Proc. R. Soc. Med.* **58,** 329

Salter, R. B. and Harris, R. W. (1963). 'Injuries involving the epiphyseal plate.' *J. Bone Jt Surg.* **45A,** 587

Strachan, J. C. H. and Ellis, B. W. (1971). 'Vulnerability of the posterior interosseous nerve during radial head resection.' *J. Bone Jt Surg.* **53B,** 320

[The illustrations for this Chapter on Fractures in Children were drawn by Mr. G. Lyth.]

Treatment of Delayed Union, Non-union and Mal-union of Fractures

E. L. Trickey, F.R.C.S.
Consultant Orthopaedic Surgeon, Royal National Orthopaedic Hospital, London

FRACTURE HEALING

Following the fracture of a bone the repair process starts immediately as the result of neuromuscular, hormonal and mechanical stimuli from the injured area. There is a general proliferation of mesenchymal cells which form osteocytes and osteoblasts and of tiny blood vessels. Fracture callus forms between and around the bone ends.

Immobilization is not essential for the union of all fractures. However, it is a principle of fracture treatment to employ enough to allow both vascularization of the site and the proper development of bone in the callus to bridge the fracture gap.

Internal (endosteal) callus forms between the bone ends, external (periosteal) callus around the fracture site. The amount of callus formed is dependent on certain factors. External callus is increased by movement so that around the bone ends of a mobile fracture there may be a large mass. If the blood supply to one or both fragments is poor external callus formation is small.

If a fracture is rigidly immobilized no external callus forms. Such rigidity is possible only with internal fixation. We must distinguish between two types of internal fixation. There is fixation which is rigid and fixation which simply apposes bone ends allowing a little movement, and the formation of external callus. After rigid fixation the development of actual bone strength is slow. Part of the strength is in the fixation material. The strength of external callus is missing.

DELAYED AND NON-UNION OF FRACTURES

The exact definition of delayed union is difficult as there is no fixed time for the union of a fracture. Union is delayed if progression to solid union is slow, judged by the mobility of the fracture and the appearance of the fracture line in the radiograph.

Non-union can be diagnosed when the fracture surfaces have become smooth and rounded or sclerosed after a reasonable period of treatment.

The most important causes of delayed and non-union are inadequate immobilization for an inadequate period of time and incorrect methods of conservative and operative treatment. In many cases of delayed union consolidation will take place if adequate conservative treatment is continued for long enough. However, each case must be considered individually and valuable time can be saved in some instances by surgery. In a case of established non-union there is no point in prolonged conservative treatment.

Surgical treatment

As the commonest cause of slow fracture healing is inadequate immobilization rigid internal fixation alone may effect union when there is evidence that the bone ends are vascularized. A large mass of external callus is adequate evidence. If no external callus has formed, internal fixation alone is not adequate and bone grafting is necessary. In practice bone grafting should be used in nearly all cases whether or not rigid fixation is employed. Methods of internal fixation will not be discussed in this chapter.

Bone grafting

Bone placed across or around a fracture acts as a scaffolding. It is absorbed and replaced by living bone. The more trabecular the graft the quicker is the replacement. Bone for grafting can be of cortical or cancellous types. It can be autogenous or homogenous prepared by one of a number of methods. There is no doubt that fresh autogenous bone is the best material and that cancellous bone is superior to cortical bone in nearly every situation. In the past, cortical bone has been used because the strength of the structure can be utilized by screw fixation to the recipient area. The disadvantages are that cortical bone can break and absorption and replacement of the graft by living bone is a slow progress.

A cancellous graft must be protected from an excess of movement until it is replaced. For delayed union when there is only a jog of movement plaster immobilization may be sufficient. However, for non-union and when there is a bone gap to be filled, cancellous grafting should be supplemented by adequate internal fixation using either a plate or an intramedullary device.

The best source of cancellous bone is the iliac crest. An alternative site is the greater trochanter of the femur.

MAL-UNION

When mal-union of a fracture is of such a degree that correction is necessary the exact treatment will vary according to the bone involved. Nevertheless, as a principle one can say that when the mal-union is near the end of a long bone a corrective osteotomy alone may suffice. Bony union through cancellous bone is rapid. However, if the site is in the cortical mid-shaft then a corrective osteotomy must be internally fixed and surrounded by a cancellous bone graft.

THE OPERATION

OBTAINING ILIAC BONE FOR GRAFTING

1a & b

Position of patient

This will be determined by the position required for the operation of bone grafting. If the patient is supine the iliac crest is made more prominent by placing a sandbag under the donor side buttock to rotate the pelvis.

Bone can be taken from any part of the crest and blade of the ilium and from the posterior superior iliac crest where bone is particularly plentiful. However, the sacro-iliac joint must not be opened. If necessary bone can be taken from each iliac crest at the same operation.

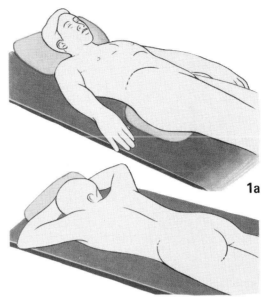

1a

1b

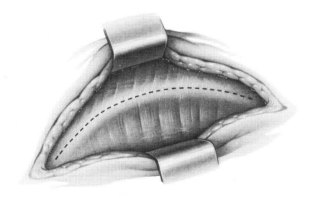

2

2

The incision

This is along the line of the iliac crest. The length is dependent on how much bone is required. After division of skin and subcutaneous tissues the exact position of the lateral edge of the crest is located. At this point the abdominal muscles above are delineated from the gluteal muscles below and an incision should be made along this line using cutting diathermy. It is a vascular area.

Preparing the ilium

The next stage is dependent on the amount and the type of bone required.

For iliac slivers

3a & b

These are required for the treatment of non-union of fractures of long bones. The gluteal muscles are separated from the blade of the ilium by subperiosteal dissection to the required depth. The blade of the ilium is cut with an osteotome along its length just distal to the crest. Both lateral and medial cortices are divided taking care to avoid deep penetration on the medial side. A length of the crest with attached abdominal muscles is now rotated upwards by a simple bone lever slid down the inner wall of the blade of the ilium under the periosteum.

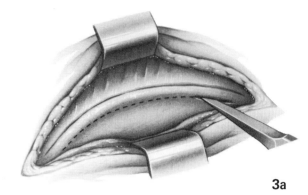

3a

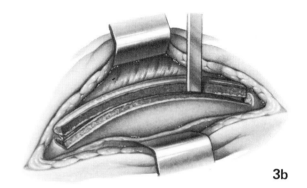

3b

3c

An osteotome is used to shave off slivers from the exposed bone. They should be 5 mm wider than the widest part of the ilium and may be straight or curved. The slivers consist of both cortices of bone with intervening cancellous bone and should be cut as thin as possible — up to 7·5 cm long. They are placed in normal saline until they are used.

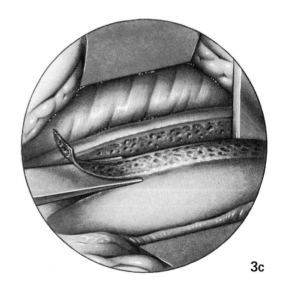

3c

4a & b

For iliac chips

When bone is needed to fill a cavity or when bone of a special shape is required to cover a space, iliac bone can be taken from the lateral cortex without disturbing the crest. The gluteal muscles are separated from the lateral blade. Bone is taken consisting of lateral cortex and underlying cancellous bone alone, either to be used as a block or to be cut up into chips or slivers. A gouge is used to remove as much of the exposed cancellous bone as is required.

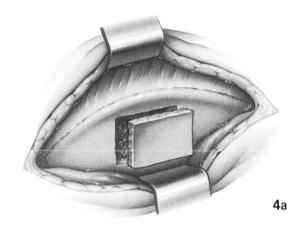

4a

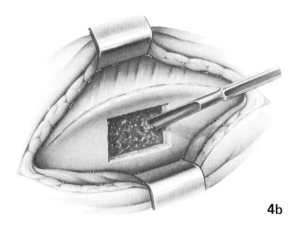

4b

5

Closure of wound

This is a vascular area and care should be taken with haemostasis. Bone wax may be needed to control persistent oozing from a cancellous surface. The wound should be drained for 24–48 hr. Sharp prominences of ilium which would project under the skin are nibbled off. The gluteal muscles are sutured back to the iliac crest and abdominal muscles.

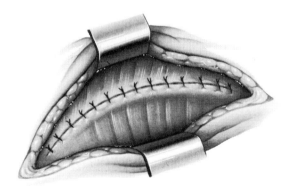

5

BONE GRAFTING FOR UNUNITED FRACTURE

6

The incision

A tourniquet is used if possible. The skin incision must be varied according to local disease. The most direct route to bone should be used and the incision should be straight but variations are needed with reference to previous scars. Following a successful skin grafting operation, bone grafting is delayed until 3 months after complete healing of the skin wound. A longitudinal incision is made through the periosteum of each fragment elevated. If the periosteum is adherent to bone, as is likely near the fracture site, a thin osteoperiosteal flap is elevated with an osteotome. The dissection must be right on bone. The periosteum should be separated circumferentially. If the periosteum is replaced by fibrous tissue, as is likely when there is a bone gap due to bone loss, this fibrous tissue should be excised back to living muscle to speed the vascularization of the graft.

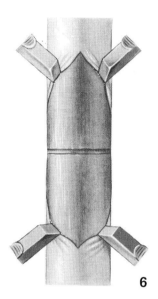

6

Treatment of ununited fractures of long bones

A mobile fracture in good alignment need not be taken apart. If the fracture is very mobile it should be fixed with an adequate plate or intramedullary device. This is essential when there is a bone gap to be filled. If the mobile fracture is mal-united however, the fracture should be taken apart and straightened at the fracture site. The bone ends are cleared of fibrocartilaginous tissue and fixed with some internal device, prior to bone grafting. It is not necessary to excise the bone ends drastically. When there is a bone gap to be filled some shortening should be accepted and the bone ends should be approximated if possible to increase the success of bone grafting.

7a-d

Insertion of graft

The appearance of the cortical bone at the fracture site should be inspected. If it looks white and avascular it should be shaved back to more healthy bone in which even a few blood vessels are apparent. Large abnormal bony swellings should be removed so that the bone ends resemble their normal shape. Their removal allows space for the graft and easier skin closure. Circumferentially the healthy cortical bone of each fragment should be elevated in narrow strips with a narrow osteotome to increase the total surface area from which new bone can be formed. Bone slivers are laid longitudinally around the fracture site under the periosteum.

If there is a gap to be filled between the bone ends, slivers can still be used. However, the space may be filled more easily by cutting the slivers into chips and by packing in cancellous bone.

Closure of wound

It is advisable to suture some soft tissues around the graft as it helps to keep it in place. It may not be possible to use periosteum. Suction drainage is advisable. It is essential that the skin is closed without tension.

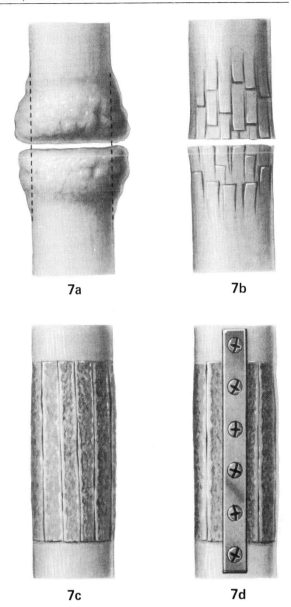

7a

7b

7c

7d

[*The illustrations for this Chapter on Treatment of Delayed Union, Non-union and Mal-union of Fractures were drawn by Mr. M. J. Courtney.*]

Spinal Injuries

Sir George M. Bedbrook, O.B.E., Hon.M.D.(W.A.), M.S.(Melb.), D.P.R.M., F.R.C.S., F.R.A.C.S.
Chairman, Department of Orthopaedic Surgery and Senior Spinal Surgeon,
Royal Perth (Rehabilitation) Hospital, Western Australia

APPLICATION OF SKULL CALIPER

Indications

(*1*) To assist in reduction of fractures, dislocations and fracture-dislocations of the cervical spine. The calipers are left in position for periods of up to 10 weeks and not less than 6 weeks.

(*2*) To maintain reduction obtained by closed manipulative reduction. The calipers remain in position for the same period as mentioned above.

(*3*) To assist postural nursing of all stable fractures and cervical spinal injuries (usually for short periods only).

Contra-indications

All stable injuries involving a fracture and even subluxation. These include compression and extension injuries. (Stability must be determined by flexion-extension lateral x-rays taken under sedation — if necessary.) The spine should be positioned by the surgeon.

Preparation of scalp

Adequate hair must be removed in all cases and the scalp thoroughly cleaned. All associated lacerations must be carefully cleaned and sutured, if necessary under local anaesthetic.

1

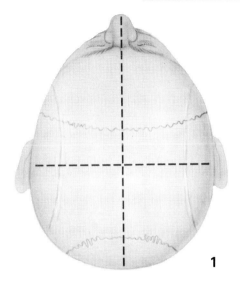

1

Towelling must be arranged so that the naso-occipital line is visible. The lines nasion to occiput and between the pinnae are then marked with Bonney's Blue or suitable marking ink.

2

Preparation for calipers

The calipers (Crutchfield, Bennet, Vinke) are opened to the maximum width and a suitable size selected so that the pins will be vertical to the calvarium and the points are either:

(*1*) in front of the coronal line if extension is to be assisted;

(*2*) on the coronal line if neutral traction is required;

(*3*) behind the coronal line if flexion is required.

The points should be marked clearly.

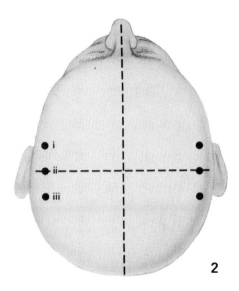

2

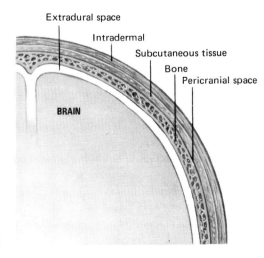

3

Anaesthesia

(*1*) Intradermal local anaesthesia with 2 per cent lignocaine, 1 ml.

(*2*) Subcutaneous local anaesthetic, 2 ml, bilateral over the marked spots.

(*3*) Five millilitres maximum each side, deep to the scalp in the pericranial space.

(*4*) Three to five minutes should elapse for adequate effect.

3

4

Instruments

No. 15 scalpel.
  Howarth dissector.
  Guarded twist drills with guard at 2, 3 and 4 mm
from distal end of 7/64 inch drill.
  Remember the caliper ends must *only* go through
the outer table of the skull — average depth being
4 mm.
  Hand drill.
  Select right size of head caliper.

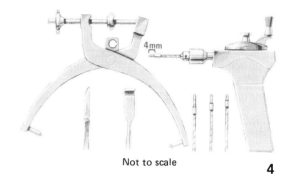

Not to scale

4

The incision

5

Compressing the marked spot on the first side (R or
L) with two fingers, a short incision is made in the
coronal plane usually 5 mm long, but never longer than
1 cm.

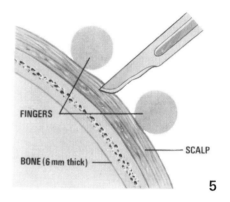

5

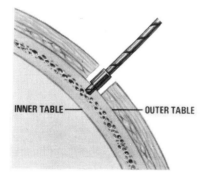

6

6

Bleeding is not usually excessive. A Howarth periosteal
resector is used to bare the bone. Then using a guarded
drill, a hole is drilled in the outer table only to a depth
of 4 mm (maximum 5 mm).

7

The drill is removed and using the open caliper point the hole is 'found' and the surgeon ascertains that it will locate well.

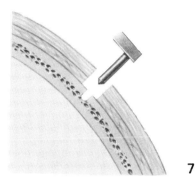

7

Second incision

With the caliper point in the first hole (R or L) the position of the second incision should be checked. The caliper is removed and a second incision is made. Drilling should be as for the first procedure with the assistant maintaining pressure over the scalp at the first incision if necessary to control any haemorrhage.

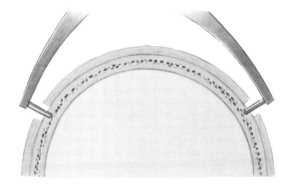

8

8

Locating the caliper

When the second hole is finished, the caliper is located first in one drill hole and then in the second. The caliper is tightened in a manner appropriate to the type used.

Around each pin anoint with either:

(*1*) sealed dressing with Friars Balsam or similar compound or;

(*2*) silver sulphadiazine cream changed daily as for burns.

Complications

(*1*) Penetration of inner table.

Remedy — re-insert properly.

(*2*) Infection — soft tissue cellulitis, osteomyelitis rare — incidence 1 in 500.

Remedy — treat with appropriate drug and prevent recurrence.

(*3*) Loosening of caliper.

Remedy — tighten with the finger daily.

POSTURAL REDUCTION, FRACTURE-DISLOCATIONS OF CERVICODORSAL AND LUMBODORSAL SPINE AND MAINTENANCE

Indications

All fractures and dislocations of the spine either with or without operative treatment.

Advantages

(*1*) Will effect total or partial reduction in all except 11 per cent of fracture-dislocations which have locked facets.
    (*2*) Allows muscle recovery.
    (*3*) Prevents further neuromuscular damage.
    (*4*) Encourages postural reflexes in extension.
    (*5*) Prevents flexion-contractures.

Duration

For the first 6–8 weeks as strictly as possible.

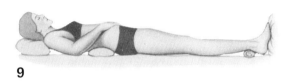

9

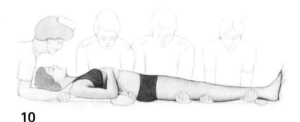

10

Method

9-12

On a regular hospital bed using pillows in the lordotic areas of the spine; in supine, prone or lateral position. Turning by special team every 2 hr.

On special beds such as the Stoke Mandeville Edgerton bed, where turning is carried out by automatic electrical devices with one attendant.

Using bed blocks of various heights made of blocked rubber or pillows.

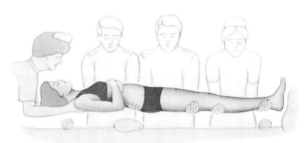

11

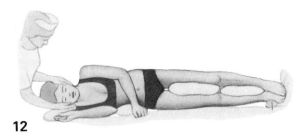

12

Special points

13 & 14

The level of sensory loss and level of fracture must be marked on the skin so that posturing can be accurate. When cervicodorsal fracture-dislocations are being postured a pillow is needed at the level of T1-T2 to achieve a good extension. At the lumbodorsal junction the pillow must not be too large at first, or else adynamic ileus will be aggravated. The height of pillows can be increased slowly until maximum is obtained.

All posture must be checked clinically and by x-ray in bed.

Whilst perfect reduction is always the goal, multiple fractures at two or more levels are the rule pathologically, so that the surgeon must judge the alignment and displacement, remembering that, only in cases with displacement on lateral x-rays greater than one half, is canal alignment grossly reduced.

Increasing accuracy with tomography including oblique and axial views has demonstrated the morbid anatomy as multifactorial in most flexion-rotation injuries.

Fracture-dislocations greater than half width on lateral plates can readily redisplace.

Contra-indications

There are no contra-indications.

This is the universal method needed in all cases. Rarely in lumbodorsal injuries (1–2 per cent), more commonly in cervicodorsal injuries (26 per cent), extension forces have caused displacement – usually minor. Reduction can be achieved by cautious introduction of flexion in the postural care management.

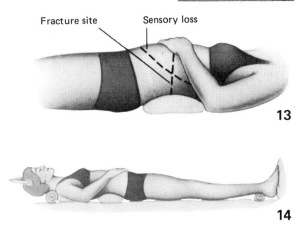

Fracture site   Sensory loss

13

14

REDUCTION OF CERVICAL FRACTURE-DISLOCATION WITH OR WITHOUT SPINAL CORD INJURY

Indication

Flexion-rotation dislocations of the cervical spine: (*1*) with single facet fracture-dislocation and (*2*) with bilateral facet fracture-dislocation.

Timing

As soon as possible after injury.

Methods

Slow 'manipulation' and reduction without general anaesthesia if over 24 hr.

Rapid instantaneous manipulation and reduction with general anaesthesia if under 24 hr.

Decision on method

Provided there is no contra-indication to general anaesthetic (such as pulmonary, cerebral or other injuries) all cervical fracture-dislocations with 'locked' facets, seen within 24 hr with or without spinal cord damage, should be treated by this method.

After 24 hr those without cord damage can be so treated, but with cord damage spinal cord oedema will cause the surgeon to select a method without general anaesthesia.

15

METHOD WITH GENERAL ANAESTHESIA

With manual traction applied by a halter, general anaesthesia is commenced including intubation and relaxant.

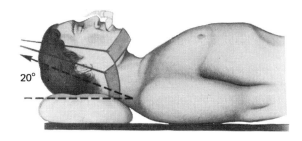

15

Bilateral dislocation

16

The head is flexed to 45°, applying manual traction to unlock, with pillow or sandbag under cervical spine.

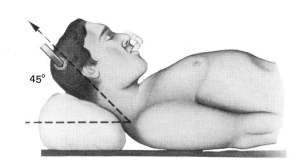

16

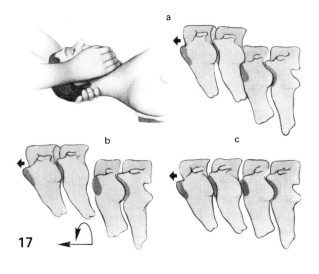

17 & 18

Maintaining traction, the head is slowly extended to completely unlock. A soft 'click' usually indicates reduction. The head should be extended 30°–40°.

A lateral x-ray film is taken to confirm reduction.

Crutchfield calipers are applied as described.

If reduction is not achieved the process is repeated once.

If reduction has still not been achieved, then one further attempt should be made by a more experienced operator or the slow reduction method should be progressed to (*see* below).

Head traction calipers are then applied as described with the head held in reduced position.

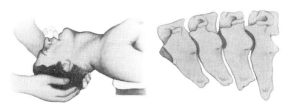

18

Unilateral dislocation (Walton manoeuvre)

19a & b

Head in flexed position.
  In coronal axis 45°.
  In sagittal axis 45°.
  To opposite side from facet dislocation with traction maintained.

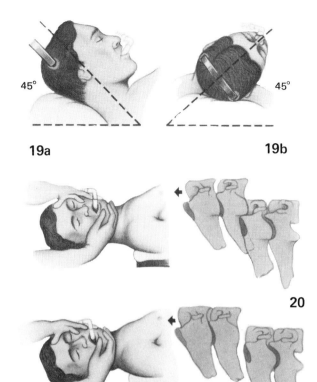

19a   **19b**

20

21

20 & 21

Maintaining traction, the head is rotated away from the side of dislocation around the intact side thus unlocking the dislocation.

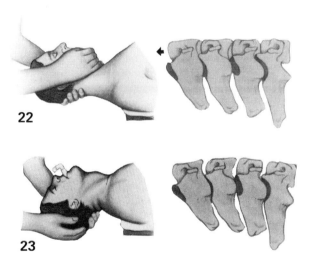

22

23

22 & 23

Then the head is rotated back to neutral as extension is increased. As this procedure is carried out, the head is then finally extended to maintain the reduction.

An x-ray is taken to check reduction.
The procedure is repeated if, after careful study of original plates to see that the sides are correctly identified, reduction has not been accomplished.

24

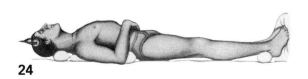

24

After reduction head calipers are applied and postural care commenced to maintain reduction.

REDUCTION OF CERVICAL FRACTURE-DISLOCATION

METHOD WITHOUT GENERAL ANAESTHESIA

Bilateral fracture-dislocation

25

Head calipers are positioned under local anaesthetic and using pillows traction is applied in flexion (30°–40°) with 15 lb (7 kg) weight.

26a-d

The x-ray is checked and if the fracture-dislocation is not distracted and unlocked the weights are increased by 5 lb (2 kg) every 30–45 min, the x-ray (lateral only) being checked each time. The patient is sedated until 'unlocking' occurs and flexion is adjusted as necessary.

27

Then maintaining the traction, a pillow is inserted under cervicodorsal area and the head lowered into the extended position. Unlocking is checked by x-ray.

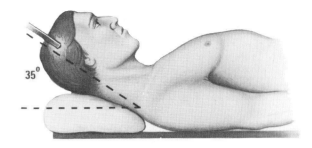

25

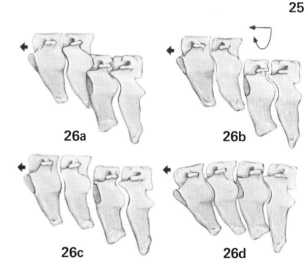

26a **26b**

26c **26d**

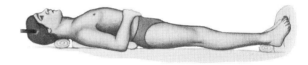

27

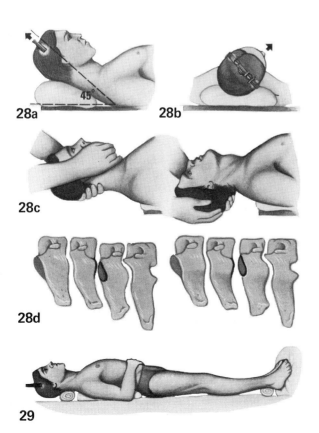

28a **28b**

28c

28d

29

Unilateral dislocation

Method

28a-d

Traction is applied slowly in two planes — coronal and sagittal. The traction is increased on both axes as for bilateral dislocation. Unlocking is checked by x-ray. The head is brought to neutral and then extended.

29

The reduction is maintained very carefully with posture and traction. Sufficient extension is maintained for 6–8 weeks.

CLOSED REDUCTION OF FRACTURE-DISLOCATION OF LUMBODORSAL SPINE WITH LOCKED FACETS WITH AND WITHOUT PARAPLEGIA

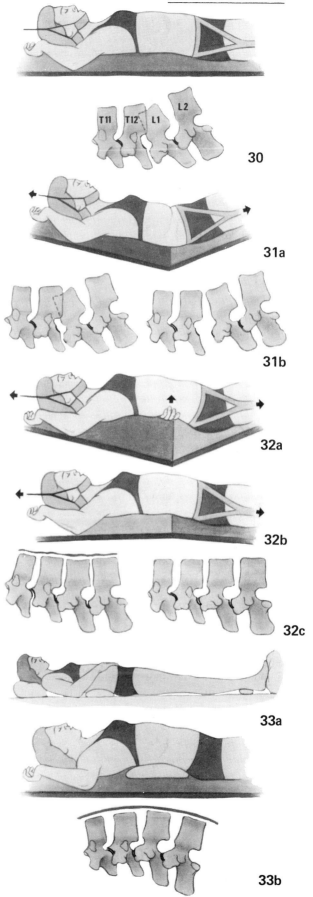

Indications

(*1*) When postural reduction fails.
(*2*) When open reduction is contra-indicated by:
   (*a*) infection;
   (*b*) multiple injuries;
   (*c*) other complications such as pulmonary; or
   (*d*) psychological or religious reasons.
(*3*) Before open reduction.

Method

Reduction under general anaesthesia

30

The patient is placed supine with relaxation, ensuring that the fracture site is at the break in the table so that the spine can be flexed or extended.

31a & b

Traction is applied manually or via harness to the head or thorax and pelvis to distract the fracture in the flexed position by 'breaking' table.

32a, b & c

With traction continuously applied the operator exerts a forward thrust to the prominent spinous process, thus lifting (patient supine) the lumbodorsal spine into lordosis. The lumbar column below the fracture-dislocation can usually be felt to move forward and be locked by the anterior longitudinal ligament.

33a & b

Traction and extension are maintained. The table is reversed and a gall-bladder rest is raised under a pillow to give hyperextension, thus 'fixing' the intact anterior longitudinal ligament. Traction is released but postural reduction is maintained.

The x-ray is checked. The above process is repeated if necessary, then the patient is allowed to recover from relaxant anaesthesia so that the muscle tone assists.

The patient is taken off the operating table by the sliding method onto a rigid surface to hold reduction. The rigid surface is removed in the ward when the patient is fully conscious.

Postural reduction is maintained.

OPEN REDUCTION OF FRACTURE-DISLOCATION OF LUMBODORSAL SPINE WITH OR WITHOUT PARAPLEGIA

Indications

(*1*) Failed conservative method.

(*2*) Locked facets.

(*3*) Gross dislocation (in presence or absence of paraplegia).

(*4*) Central nervous system deterioration.

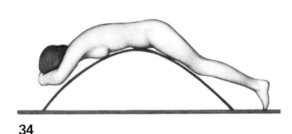

34

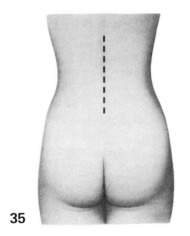

35

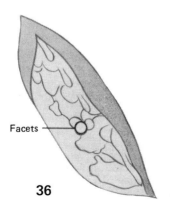

Facets

36

This procedure may include laminotomy but is *not* a laminectomy, for which there are only rare indications, e.g. when an intraneural canal space-occupying lesion is present either:

(*5*) bony — laminal or vertebral; or

(*6*) disc with bony injury — rare; or

(*7*) tumour and, rarely, localized haemorrhage.

Contra-indications

(*1*) Multiple injuries.

(*2*) Infection of skin.

(*3*) Other, e.g. chest injuries.

This procedure does *not* increase the chance of central nervous system improvement.

34

Procedure

Maintaining partial postural reduction, the patient is taken to the operating theatre and anaesthetized with a general anaesthetic.

The patient is turned with a 'log roll' by staff and placed carefully on a suitable frame to prevent abdominal compression. This will usually flex the spine at the fracture site, but will not reproduce the original deformity at the time of the accident.

35

The incision

A mid-line incision is made centred over the site of the fracture-dislocation, extending two or three segments above and below the fracture site. The fascia is incised to the spinous processes, which are then carefully cleared by cutting and coagulation diathermy; the laminae are cleared.

It is usual for the erector spinae muscles to have been stripped and lacerated by the accident.

Retractors are inserted.

36

Clearing the laminae

Carefully the two laminae above and below are cleared, making certain the posterior primary rami above and below are *not* damaged, or the erector spinae will be further denervated.

37 & 38

Reduction of dislocation

Using intact spinous processes and suitable bone-holding forceps, the dislocation is reduced first by caudocephalic traction and then suitably lifting the upper over the lower. If this is not possible, laminotomy and facet removal will help, using a distraction device with great care.

Splintage

The spine should be allowed to extend by removing the frame, after which some type of metal fixation or splintage may be employed.

39a & b

Instruments

In selecting instruments for this procedure one should consider the less bulky ones that do not damage muscle or nerve, and hold the laminae together.

The following instruments are suitable:

(*1*) Knodt's clamps.

(*2*) Harrington compression and/or extension rods.

Application of clamps by the Harrington technique should be carried out only by experienced surgeons using equipment for scoliosis. *This is no operation for the 'occasional' surgeon.*

After fixation is tested the wound is closed.

40

Posture

Still in a prone position, the patient should be log-turned onto a trolley with a pillow to help maintain postural extension. The clamps are *not* to be regarded as a quite rigid method of internal splintage.

Postoperative care

Posture is maintained and erector spinae exercises introduced early. Depending on the degree of sensation and available materials, after 2 weeks a cast should be used to help fixation. The cast is made on a mould taken in two halves by the orthotist, and can be made of plaster-of-Paris, Orthocast or polythene lined with Plastazote. It is often desirable to remove the internal fixation device after one year when spinal fusion has occurred.

Addition

Articular facet fusion may be carried out, but *not* laminal fusion as this can induce canal stenosis.

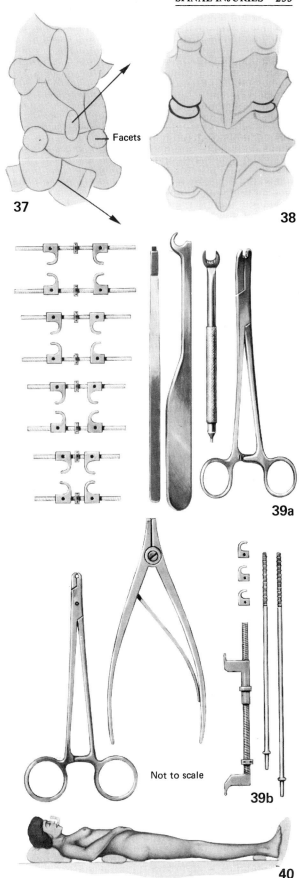

Facets

37
38
39a
39b
Not to scale
40

SPINAL FUSION OF GALLE TYPE

Indications

(*1*) Ununited fracture of the dens.
   (*2*) Subluxations of the atlanto-axial joint.

Method

State 1

41 & 42

(*1*) A mid-line incision from the occiput to C5.
   (*2*) Incised skin and deep fascia are tough and need sharp dissection.
   (*3*) The incision is made in the mid-line between the trapezii and the right and left splenius capitus to expose the spinous processes.
   (*4*) Muscle is dissected off the spinous processes with a sharp cutting and coagulating diathermy.

43

The laminae of C1, C2, C3 and the occiput are cleared by subperiosteal dissection.
   (*1*) Using a Cobb elevator sharp dissection is carried laterally.
   (*2*) The surgeon should watch for venous bleeding laterally.
   The muscle masses are retracted:
   (*1*) using Gelpys' retractors first; and
   (*2*) as dissection proceeds, a laminectomy retractor.

   The arch of the atlas is exposed.
   (*1*) With great care subperiosteal dissection is carried laterally.
   (*2*) The vertebral artery at the junction of the lateral one-third and medial two-thirds should be carefully avoided.
   (*3*) Wide lateral dissection of the laminae of C1, C2 and C3 will thus be obtained.
   (*4*) The venous channels are sealed off with cautery, gauze swabs or felt squares.
   (*5*) Decortication of the laminae can be effected by using the Capener chisels and nibblers.
   The graft is removed from the ilium and cut like an inverted 'U' to fit the laminae of C1 and spinous processes of C2.

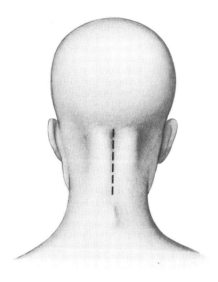

41

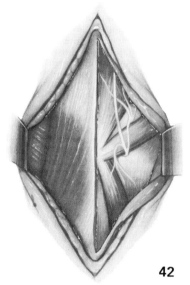

42

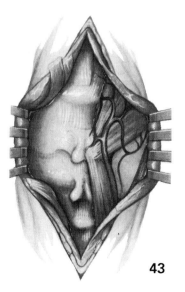

43

44

A long incision is made vertical to and deepening to the iliac crest.

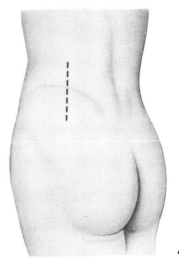

44

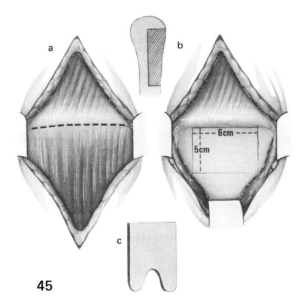

45

45 a, b & c

Then the gluteal muscles are cleared from the iliac wing by subperiosteal dissection.

Using adequate retraction, a quadrilateral area of about 5 cm in diameter is marked out and then the outer table only is removed, using sharp chisel dissection. This gives a graft of about 1 cm thick, curved in the line that will take the cervical spine and can then be cut into the inverted 'U'.

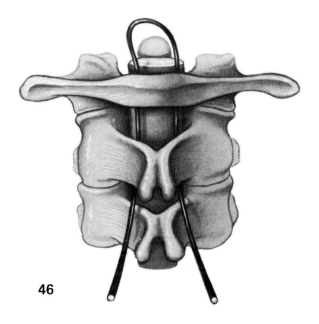

46

46

Using suitable curved dissectors between the dura and laminae a strong wire loop is passed (using McCormack dissectors), as shown, under the arch of C1 and C2.

47

The graft is placed, cancellous surface down, into the laminae after a cancellous bed has been prepared and laid.

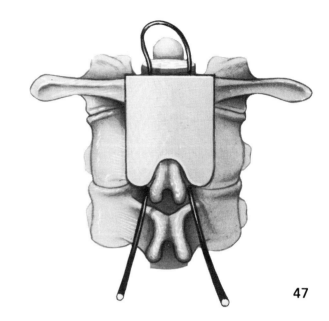

47

48

The wires are tightened to fix the graft securely in position.

The wound is closed in layers sewing the splenius muscles together, the trapezius muscles together, the subcutaneous fascia and the skin using drainage.

Postoperative care

The patient is sat up in bed as soon after the operation as possible. Traction is discontinued if used prior to operation and a polythene collar is applied about 4–5 days postoperatively, after an immediate soft collar used for support.

Time of fusion

Fusion usually takes about 3 months.

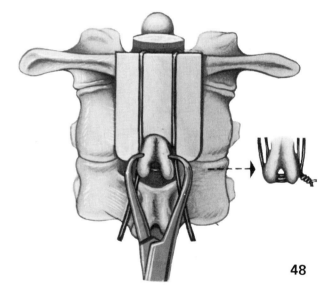

48

SPINAL FUSION IN TREATMENT OF SPINAL FRACTURES

Indications

(*1*) To treat non-union at all levels.

(*2*) To stabilize the spine in fractures of the cervico-dorsal area proven to be unstable, 6—8 weeks after the accident. These are usually of the flexion-rotation type.

(*3*) To fuse and stabilize after extensive laminectomies. Such an indication is very small, with the proven lack of usefulness of laminectomy in the management of spinal fractures with paraplegia.

(*4*) To correct spinal deformity.

METHOD

Anterior approach

Cervical approach

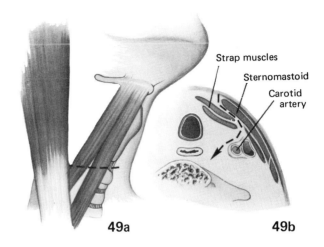

49a   **49b**

49a & b

A transverse incision is made at the level of the cricoid or above and below this level, depending on the vertebrae to be approached, with incision through the platysma down to the anterior border of the sternomastoid — then along this anterior border and between the strap muscles and carotid sheath onto the prevertebral fascia.

50

The prevertebral fascia is thus exposed. The disc spaces of C4-5, C5-6, C6-7 and even C7-T1 are exposed.

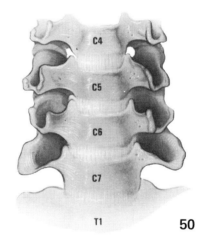

50

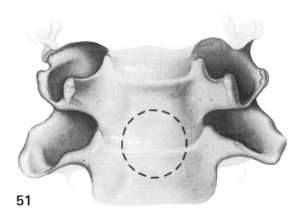

51

51

Identification with lateral x-ray is important. After exposing the disc space required it can then be prepared by diathermy of a circle approximately 1·5 cm in the mid-line to prevent excessive bleeding.

52 & 53

A serrated dowel drill is then used to cut a circular hole of suitable depth to leave the posterior cortex intact. A drill is then inserted inside the dowel cylinder, and disc and bone are removed.

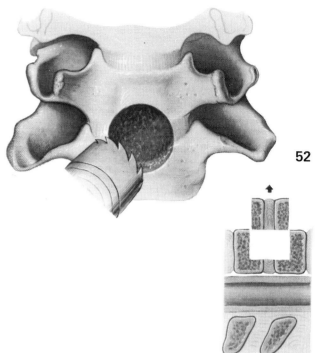

52

53

54

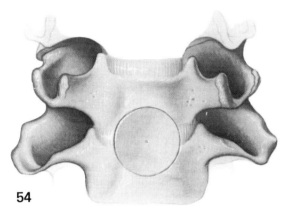

54

The cylindrical hole is cleared carefully and then, with the anaesthetist effectively inducing traction, a dowel is inserted firmly to give a tight fit.

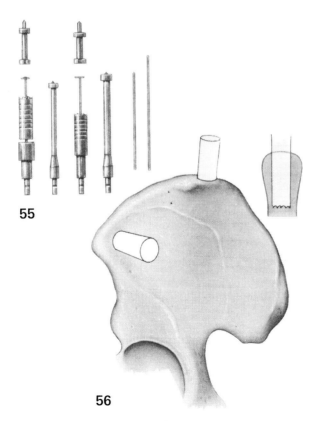

55

56

Taking of dowel graft

55 & 56

Using the dowel set illustrated, dowels are cut from the iliac crest behind the anterosuperior iliac spine.

57

If an iliac fibula strut is to be used to bridge two or three discs, a trench is fashioned with chisels.

The graft is fractionally longer than the trench or is fashioned with pegs or angles to lock. By maintaining traction as the graft is inserted, a tight fit is achieved.

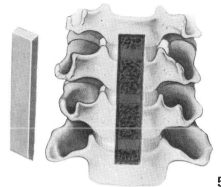

57

58

Thoracic approach

This usually entails a thoracotomy using the usual techniques — removing a rib, opening the thorax and finding the area concerned.

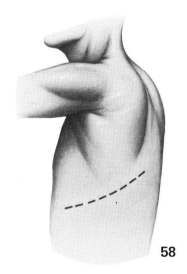

58

Lumbar approach

A lumbar incision as for a nephrectomy is used, exposing the retroperitoneal areas by sweeping the peritoneal structures towards the medial side, making certain that the ureter is swept forwards. Then the disc spaces of L2-3, L3-4, and L4-5 can be exposed. At the thoracolumbar junction, a much more extensive incision is used along the tenth or eleventh rib, extending down to the extraperitoneal space once again and dividing the diaphragm.

The incisions and surgical approaches are usual for gastric or splenic conditions. Having exposed the disc space, the surgeon can then select either a dowel or a wedge technique for spinal fusion.

ANTERIOR DECOMPRESSION

Before the use of bone grafting, anterior decompression may be required.

Indications

Traumatic paraplegia which has plateaued in its recovery.
    Pathological fractures.
    Spinal stenosis.

Method

Anterior decompression is undertaken with the following steps.

59

(*1*) The transverse process and the rib head are identified, the latter being removed if this is necessary.
    (*2*) The vertebral body is then cleared and the segmental vessels are divided at about the mid-vertebral level.

60 & 61

(*3*) The nerve root is retracted but is then used as a guide to follow into the neural canal. The pedicle may be removed and the dura is thus exposed from the lateral side.
    (*4*) The vertebral body is then excised using chisel cuts, maintaining the posterior cortex and the posterior longitudinal ligament.
    (*5*) After the vertebral body has been removed the vertebral cortex and posterior longitudinal ligament remains intact. It is then possible to remove the bone at the apex of the curve, opening the extradural space through the posterior longitudinal ligament.

62

The surgeon continues cephalad or caudad until the whole of the hump has been removed. It is important to move right across the mid-line to the opposite side and to ensure that all of the vertebral body is thus excised. The cord will move forward.
    (*6*) Then grafts of fibula and/or ribs are placed into the quadrilateral socket so formed. The grafts must fit firmly.

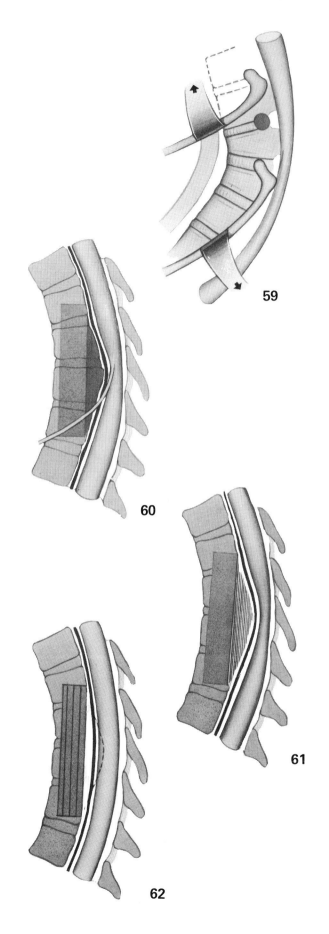

59

60

61

62

POSTERIOR FUSION

This is usually done to re-inforce an anterior approach, which has already been described. Instrumentation, such as the Harrington rod and Knodt clamps, may be used to fix the fractures (*see* page 233).

Method

After laminectomy

When a laminectomy has already been performed, the surgeon must carry out a posterolateral fusion on both sides. A mid-line incision is usually best with the muscles retracted laterally, making certain that the dura is not entered. The transverse processes, the articular column and the heads of the ribs in the thoracic and/or lumbar areas can then be exposed.

Bone graft is then placed *in situ,* using matchstick grafts after an adequate bed has been prepared.

Laminectomy not performed

If a laminectomy has not been performed, the laminae are cleared in the usual manner. They are exposed adequately right out to the transverse processes. The laminae are decorticated and the articular facets are fused in the same way as for scoliosis. Then with or without internal fixation, a bone graft is placed on to the raw bed of the laminae.

Nursing

Techniques differ depending on the area involved. Usually after careful 'log rolling' nursing for 10 days, an exoskeleton of plaster-of-Paris or polythene can be provided which is maintained for 3 months or until fusion occurs.

[*The illustrations for this Chapter on Spinal Injuries were drawn by Mr. M. J. Courtney.*]

Use of Hyperbaric Oxygen

R. H. Maudsley, F.R.C.S.(Eng.)
Consultant Accident and Orthopaedic Surgeon, King Edward VII Hospital, Windsor,
Maidenhead General Hospital, Wexham Park Hospital, Slough
and Heatherwood Hospital, Ascot

Under increased pressure more oxygen is made available in the plasma to the tissues. When hypoxia exists due to injury or disease the oxygen level in the plasma can be raised in a hyperbaric chamber.

This may be of advantage in ischaemia in maintaining normal metabolism until collaterals open up, and in anaerobic infections.

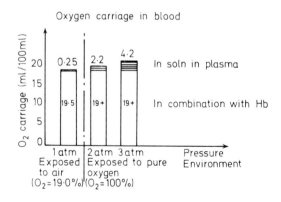

A pressure chamber is required to administer hyperbaric oxygen. There are two current types as follows.

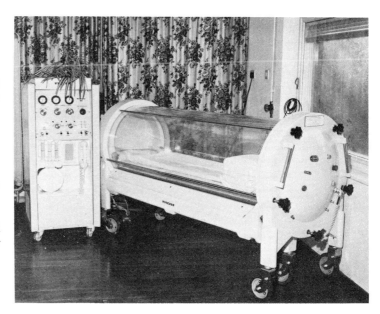

Large chamber

Patient and staff can enter and procedures can be carried out within the chamber. Compression is by air but oxygen is supplied by mask to the patient.

Small chamber (see illustration)

Only the patient enters and is compressed in 100 per cent oxygen.

The large chamber requires a team to manage it but the small chamber can be managed by a nurse or technician with some special training.

Availability

To use this facility it is either necessary to have it installed in the hospital or know where the facility exists, since time is of the essence.

The accompanying map shows centres in the United Kingdom.

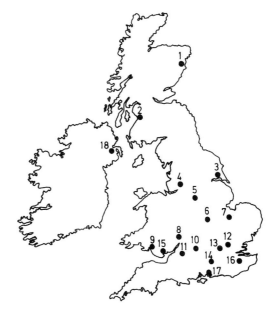

1 = Aberdeen; 2 = Glasgow; 3 = Hull; 4 = Manchester; 5 = Derby; 6 = Northampton; 7 = Peterborough; 8 = Monmouth; 9 = Swansea; 10 = Swindon; 11 = Bristol; 12 = London; 13 = Ascot; 14 = Winchester; 15 = Cardiff; 16 = Maidstone; 17 = Portsmouth; 18 = Belfast

Hazards

Great care must be exercised to prevent the following.

Risk of fire. This is minimized by avoiding:
(*1*) static build-up (through maintenance of cleanliness of chamber; removal of grease on hair, dressings etc.; not using artificial fibres in gowns etc.);
(*2*) spark – electrical contacts;
(*3*) smoking.

Oxygen toxicity. In the small chamber 2 atm (200 kPa) for 2 hr is standard and unlikely to produce toxicity when repeated with intervals.

Baratrauma. This is unlikely with 100 per cent oxygen in the small chamber.

Preparation of patient

Careful and sympathetic explanation to patient.
Clothes removed and cotton gown applied.
Dressings changed to dry dressings.
Grease removed from hair.

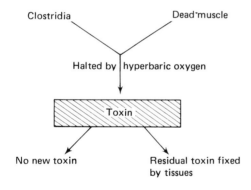

Regimen

The 2-hourly compression is generally accepted as ideal, with a gap of 2–6 hr before the next compression, and this is continued for several days according to the response and then tailed off gradually.

Adjustments to this regimen may be necessary if the unit is being used for other patients. During compression, which builds up to 2–2·25 atm (200–225 kPa) in 15 min, the attendant carefully explains what is happening, and stopping due to claustrophobia is rare. Decompression takes place after 1 hr 45 min, over a period of 15 min, though rapid decompression can be achieved in emergency. Myringotomy is not necessary when 100% oxygen is used but patients with colds should have a respiratory astringent available.

Use in gas gangrene

As soon as the patient is received in the unit a rapid examination is made, blood taken for investigation, a diagram of colour changes made and photographs taken before treatment is commenced. Emergency surgery is not normally necessary but if the swelling and tension are gross, surgical decompression can be performed between treatments. After a few days, evacuation of muscle and debris, slough etc. will be required.

Only if the limb has severe residual damage is amputation necessary as a late elective procedure.

In considering the use in acute and chronic conditions it should be remembered that hyperbaric oxygen is a supplementary treatment and not an alternative one to normal management.

Acute Infections of Bone and Joints

N. J. Blockey, M.Ch.(Orth.), F.R.C.S.(Eng.), F.R.C.S.(Glas.)
Consultant Orthopaedic Surgeon, Royal Hospital for Sick Children, Glasgow
and Western Infirmary, Glasgow

ACUTE OSTEOMYELITIS

Pyogenic bacteria reach the bone by haematogenous spread from an infection elsewhere — a boil, pustule or infected wound are common. They multiply in the vascular metaphysis and destroy bone. If untreated an abscess forms — the periosteum is lifted from the cortex causing sequestrum formation. Sinuses may then develop as the extracortical abscess enlarges. The epiphyseal growth plate and the adjacent joint may be invaded and further metastatic spread may occur. These serious complications can be avoided by correct early management.

Bacteriology

In Britain now:

Staphylococcus aureus	86—90 per cent (90% resistant to benzyl penicillin)
Streptococcus pyogenes	4— 7 per cent
H. influenzae	2— 4 per cent
Salmonella, E. coli, B. proteus etc.	1— 2 per cent

Over the past 15 years there has been a marked increase in penicillin-resistant staphylococci and a slight increase in *H. influenzae* infections.

1

Pathology

The commonest sites are the lower end of the femur, the upper end of the tibia, the upper end of the humerus and the lower end of the radius. In every metaphysis of a child there is a vascular honeycomb of bone with a thin cortex. Staphylococci arrive by haematogenous spread to this vascular area, organisms digest medullary bone, pierce the cortex and finally raise the periosteum. In children the old concept of pus entering the medullary cavity and building up pressure is not valid. Coronal sections of the lower femur of a 4 year old show no such cavity.

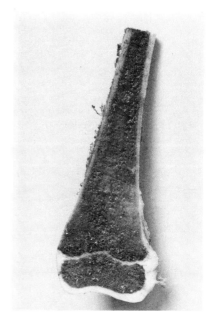

1

2

Diagnosis

The patient, often a child, develops pain of sudden onset in the metaphyseal region of a limb bone. In 40 per cent there is a reliable history of previous minor trauma. This pain worsens leading to loss of function and the adoption of the position of rest in the adjacent joint. Swelling develops and the underlying skin becomes red and looks stretched and tight. The child has a pyrexia and becomes ill. Tenderness is very marked and is maximal over the metaphysis, not over the joint as in acute rheumatism or traumatic joint effusions. The affected area becomes indurated and if untreated an area of fluctuation develops in this area of induration and discoloration. Toxicity increases, swelling spreads to the whole segment of the limb and pain becomes extreme. Rigors and spikes of hyperpyrexia indicate septicaemic spread. If the clinical signs are as described and illustrated the diagnosis of osteomyelitis is certain. The site, however, is uncertain at this early stage — another reason for not operating at once. Effective antibiotics should be given immediately.

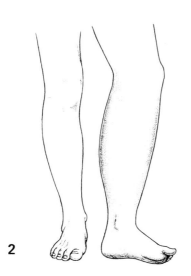

2

3

The widely indurated area will, in a few days, diminish as localization occurs under antibiotic treatment.

The presence of fluctuation in this smaller indurated area indicates the correct site for surgical drainage.

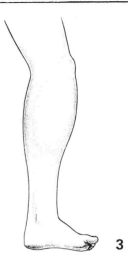

3

Investigations

After admission to an orthopaedic ward blood is withdrawn for white cell count, for erythrocyte sedimentation rate (E.S.R.) and for culture of organism. A 4 hourly temperature chart is kept and radiographs are taken.

Likely results in acute disease

Temperature raised above 39° C.

Erythrocyte sedimentation rate raised above 20 mm in first hour.

White cell count raised.

X-ray — no bony change for first 7 days.

Blood culture — two-thirds will be positive.

Management

The affected limb is placed at rest in a removable splint. The infected area is palpated every day to detect fluctuation, which is the indication for operation.

Antibiotics

Drugs, chosen on a best-guess basis, are given by intravenous or intramuscular route to ensure a high bactericidal tissue concentration for the first 48 hr (flucloxacillin, 1g, 6 hourly by intramuscular injection for 48 hr is suitable in most cases). The best results have in the author's experience been achieved using Fucidin and erythromycin 30 mg/kg each day for 21 days in four divided oral doses after the first 2 days of parenteral antibiotic therapy.

SURGICAL TREATMENT

4

Operation plays no part in the early management. 'Decompressing' the infected metaphysis conveys no benefit. *When pus is clinically detectable* operations should be performed forthwith. This may be present on admission in neglected cases, may never arise in treated cases or may be diagnosed 3–7 days after starting treatment.

Operation is performed if and when the widespread area of induration contains a softer central area of fluctuation.

5

The incision

A tourniquet is applied. A linear incision is made over the area of fluctuation. Skin, subcutaneous tissue and periosteum are cut in the same line; pus will well up into the wound.

6

The periosteum will have been lifted off the cortex by the abscess and no further stripping is necessary. The pus is mopped out of the space between periosteum and cortex and sent for culture. The cortex itself is drilled with a $^7/_{64}$ inch hand drill to enter the medulla. In an adult a gutter is cut so that the medullary contents can be seen. Any further pus is mopped out; all necrotic bone and tissue are removed with spoon or gouge until the walls of the cavity so created are of a healthy pink bone.

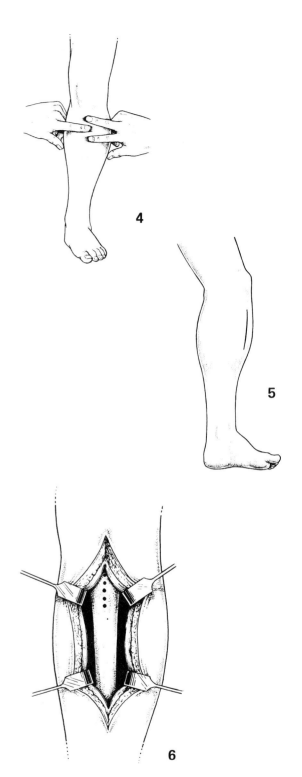

The whole cavity, medulla and subperiosteal space are now liberally washed out with 2 g cloxacillin in 20 ml sterile water. The periosteum and skin are then closed as one layer using strong braided silk and the limb is returned to its splint.

The pus is sent for culture. Antibiotics are continued for 21 days in all cases and for 6 weeks in cases slow to settle. They are changed only if original blood culture or postoperative pus culture reveals an unexpected organism.

At 21 days the E.S.R. is repeated. Repeat radiographs are taken and thorough clinical examination is made. Any cavity remaining in the bone at this time thought, by clinical signs and high E.S.R., to contain infection should be opened using the same technique described.

SEPTIC ARTHRITIS OF JOINTS

Pyogenic organisms can enter joints either by haematological spread to synovial tissues or by direct spread from an osteomyelitic focus.

Bacteriology

Similar to acute osteomyelitis except that in the age group 6 months to 2 years *H. influenzae* infections exceed the otherwise commoner *Staphylococcus aureus*.

7

Diagnosis

A warm swelling of the synovial cavity not obviously due to trauma should suggest this diagnosis. The cardinal signs are distension of the joint and pseudo-paralysis. In infants where infection of deep joints makes palpation difficult these signs may have to suffice. Thus the leg will be held flexed, the buttock regions will look full and tight, and the hip will have no active movement.

In older patients pain, pyrexia, heat, joint tenderness and assumption of the position of rest with very severe pain on attempting movement from that position will be diagnostic.

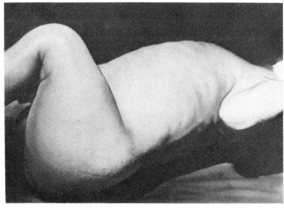

7

Investigations

As for acute osteomyelitis but in infants septic arthritis is usually secondary to bone infection and thus radiographs often show metaphyseal destruction.

Management

After clinical diagnosis and investigations the affected joint should be aspirated to confirm the diagnosis, relieve pain and prevent further articular cartilage damage. Effective antibiotics should be given by the intravenous, intramuscular or oral route, as for osteomyelitis.

Here lies the difference between the two conditions. In acute osteomyelitis antibiotics should always be given before surgery, in septic arthritis antibiotics should always be given after aspiration.

TECHNIQUE OF ASPIRATION

General anaesthesia is used in a baby or child in severe pain although local anaesthetic may be used for adults. Strict aseptic precautions are taken.

8

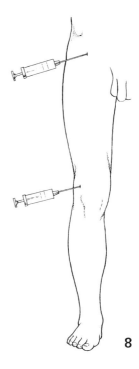

8

In most joints the needle is introduced into the area of greatest capsular distension. An 18-gauge 8 cm aspiration needle is used. (If aspirate is thick or fibrinous one can introduce a bigger needle, i.e. up to 14-gauge, but this or a bigger size may give a synovial leak after withdrawal which is undesirable.) A spinal 18-gauge needle with stilette may be used. A trocar and cannula is not advised. For the hip in a large child or adult the needle is inserted 2 cm medial to a spot 3 cm below the anterosuperior iliac spine; the needle is inclined posteromedially and one expects to feel it enter the capsule. A 10 ml syringe is attached and aspiration is begun. If this fails, one should aim to place the needle tip in the femoral head, checking this position by gently rotating the thigh, then gradually withdraw the needle, aspirating throughout.

In the knee, the needle is inserted 1 cm beyond the upper outer corner of the patella; pointing medially again, one feels the suprapatellar pouch being entered. Aspiration with pressure on the medial side of the joint is carried out in order to empty the synovial cavity.

The contents of the syringe are examined. Then the specimen so obtained is divided into two parts, injecting part into sterile broth culture for aerobic incubation and another part, again under strict aseptic conditions, into a second bottle of broth for anaerobic incubation.

The value of injecting drugs into the synovial cavity is not established. Penicillin and cloxacillin in solution are certainly harmless. The others cannot be so described. Many antibiotics given orally or parenterally produce bactericidal concentrations in synovial fluid.

These include cloxacillin, erythromycin, lincomycin, cephaloridine and Fucidin.

In septic arthritis of the infant hip aspiration must often be followed by open drainage of the joint. This is performed through a posterior muscle-splitting incision to evacuate the abscess entirely.

Systemic antibiotics should be continued for 21 days. Repeated aspirations may be necessary if the joint becomes hot and distended again. Open drainage of joints other than the hip are almost never necessary.

[The illustrations for this Chapter on Acute Infections of Bone and Joints were redrawn by Mr. J. M. P. Booth from originals by Mr. R. Callander.]

Chronic Infections of Bone and Joints

N. J. Blockey, M.Ch.(Orth.), F.R.C.S.(Eng.), F.R.C.S.(Glas.)
Consultant Orthopaedic Surgeon, Royal Hospital for Sick Children, Glasgow
and Western Infirmary, Glasgow

BRODIE'S ABSCESS

This abscess is a central metaphyseal collection of pus surrounded by a dense thickened wall of ivory-hard cortical bone. Because of low virulence of the causative staphylococci symptoms of aching pain and signs of heat, swelling and tenderness can persist for many months or years. A few such abscesses present in an area previously affected by the acute disease.

TREATMENT

The lesion is localized by palpation and radiographs. Tomograms are useful to determine the size and depth of the cavity.

Antistaphylococcal antibiotics are commenced before operation.

A tourniquet is applied.

1&2

The skin and periosteum are incised in the same line and the incision is continued down to the bone.

A window on the thickened cortex is mapped out using a $^7/_{64}$ inch drill bit. Escape of pus confirms the correct site.

The holes so made are joined up with a ½ inch (13 mm) osteotome. The cortex may be $^1/_4$ inch (6 mm) thick.

The trap-door of cortex is lifted off and discarded. The cavity is evacuated with gauze and swab and the contents sent for culture.

One gram of cloxacillin powder is placed into the dried clean cavity.

The periosteum fat and skin are closed as one layer.

Cloxacillin, 5 g/day, is continued for 21 days unless culture indicates otherwise.

The affected part is splinted until removal of sutures at 14 days.

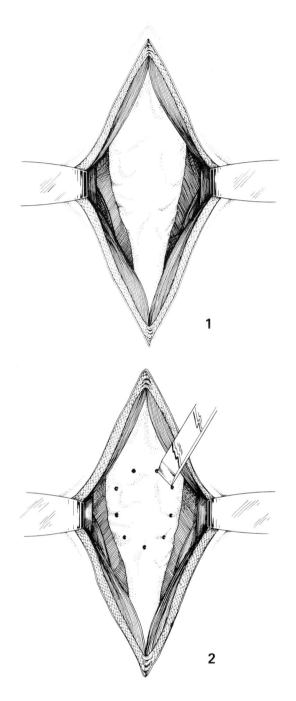

CHRONIC INFECTION WITH SINUSES

Cortical bone deprived of its blood supply by pus dies and becomes a sequestrum. Living periosteum builds an involucrum around the infection. This is incomplete at the most superficial part of the infection and pus escapes through sinuses onto the skin.

Sequestra must be removed. There is no urgency. Removal should not be performed until the involucrum restores continuity of the bone.

Chronic osteomyelitis is staphylococcal but there may be secondary invaders.

If sinus tracks become epitheliomatous or the patient has amyloidosis secondary to long-standing infection the treatment is amputation.

General care

Surgical treatment will only succeed if all infected tissue and all dead bone are removed. This major operation demands blood replacement and optimum conditions.

The patient is admitted 10 days before operation.

The affected limb is elevated and washed daily with 0·5 per cent chlorhexidine solution.

Check Hb% and transfuse if necessary.

Flucloxacillin, 500 mg 6 hourly, is commenced.

THE OPERATION

3&4

An elliptical incision is used to excise adherent skin with sinuses and their tracks.

The thickened periosteum is incised in the line of the skin incision and scraped off the thickened cortex ½ inch (13 mm) on each side.

Drill holes are inserted over a wide area keeping away from the sinus tracks.

White bone is dead. Pink bone is living. All dead bone on this subcutaneous surface is removed by lifting a window of cortex with sinuses and adherent skin still attached.

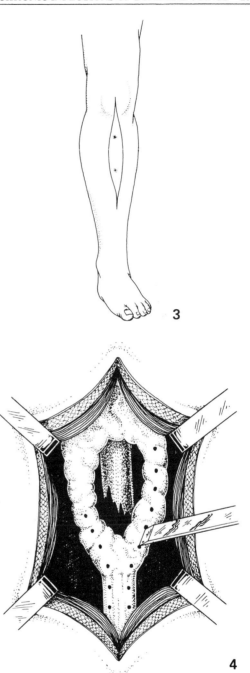

3

4

5

This trapdoor of dead cortex is discarded.

With Volkmann spoon, gauge and osteotome, the entire contents of the infected cavity are scraped out.

Every strand of granulation tissue is followed. Every cloaca is opened up and every sequestrum removed until living pink bleeding bone lines the cavity.

Penetration of the living involucrum should be avoided and the periosteum, which is adherent, should not be separated.

Avoid any overhanging edge.

When all infected material is removed cloxacillin powder is inserted.

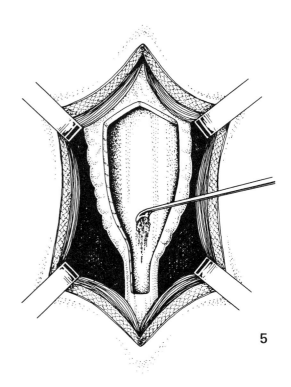

5

Primary closure with tension sutures through skin and periosteum is attempted.

In some sites it is possible to allow living muscle to fall into the dead space.

The limb is returned to splintage and elevation.

Antibiotics are continued for 6 weeks.

Heavy staining of the plaster is to be expected.

Blood lost is replaced.

The wound is examined at 2 weeks and the now uninfected bone is covered with split-skin grafts.

Relaxing skin incisions, wound irrigation through plastic tubes and the insertion of sterile gauze packs are not advised except in special circumstances.

[*The illustrations for this Chapter on Chronic Infections of Bone and Joints were redrawn by Mr. J. M. P. Booth from originals by Mr. R. Callander.*]

Surgical Management of Patients with Haemophilia

R. B. Duthie, M.A., Ch.M., F.R.C.S.
Nuffield Professor of Orthopaedic Surgery,
Nuffield Department of Orthopaedic Surgery, University of Oxford

and

John Tricker, M.B., B.S., F.R.C.S.
Lecturer, Nuffield Department of Orthopaedic Surgery,
University of Oxford

INTRODUCTION

The haemophilias are a group of genetically transmitted bleeding disorders which affect males. Approximately 30 per cent of haemophiliacs present as spontaneous mutants. The disorder is classified as follows.

Haemophilia A

This is the classic form of haemophilia and is due to the absence of active circulating Factor VIII (antihaemophiliac globulin). The defect is present on the gene on the X-chromosome which affects the reticuloendothelial system and causes an aberrant type of Factor VIII glycoprotein to be formed which lacks the normal clotting activity.

Haemophilia B

This is otherwise known as 'Christmas disease' and is due to a deficiency of active Factor IX. It is also transmitted by a sex-linked recessive gene and is six to eight times less common than Haemophilia A. The clinical manifestations, however, are identical as are the management details.

Antibodies

Antibodies are thought to arise in response to infusion and occur in 5–10 per cent of patients with haemophilia. Patients with Factor VIII antibodies are no more susceptible to haemorrhage than any other haemophiliac, but if bleeding occurs, it is difficult to control as transfused Factor VIII is rapidly inactivated. In the presence of Factor VIII antibodies, elective surgery is absolutely contra-indicated and treatment is directed towards analgesia and immobilization. The development of antibodies is a theoretical risk when massive infusions of Factor VIII are administered during surgery.

CLINICAL MANIFESTATIONS

Haemophilia presents with repeated bleeding episodes, the severity of which correlates with the level of Factor VIII in the blood (*see Table 1*). The incidence and site of haemorrhages are shown in *Table 2* which summarizes 12 years of experience (1966–1977) in the management of haemophilia in Oxford.

Table 1

Blood level of Factors VIII and IX	Haemorrhagic manifestations
50–100	None.
25–50	Tendency to bleed after major injury.
5–25	Severe bleeding after surgical operations or minor injury.
1–5	Severe bleeding after minor injury occasional spontaneous bleeding.
0	Severe haemophilia with spontaneous bleeding into muscles and joints.

After Biggs, R. (1976)

Table 2

Incidence 1966 – 1977

Haemarthroses		Muscle haematoma	
Knee	336	Iliopsoas	56
Elbow	190	Arm/forearm	33
Ankle	107	Thigh	30
Shoulder	25	Calf	41
Wrist	20	Shoulder	6
Hip	19	Buttock	6
Hand	18	Miscellaneous	4
Pseudotumour	6	Peripheral nerve lesions	
		Femoral	34
Fractures		Sciatic	3
Femur	11	Anterior tibial	2
Tibia	4	Posterior tibial	3
Olecranon	2	Median	3
Humerus	1	Ulnar	5
Clavicle	1	Others	3
Radius/ulna	3		
Axis	1		
Dislocations	2		

Haemarthrosis

This accounts for the majority of the emergency admissions to the haemophilia unit. The high incidence of haemarthrosis into the knee, elbow and ankle is attributed to the very large amount of synovium in these joints, which may be trapped within the articulation. In addition, di-arthrodial joints are unable to withstand minor rotatory and angulatory strains. Repeated haemarthroses result in synovial thickening, intra-articular fibrosis and cartilage destruction, leading to joint stiffness. Secondary arthrotic changes occur in adjacent bone and perarticular tissues. The joints involved are those which commonly suffer acute haemarthroses (Bentley and Duthie, 1975).

Muscle haematomas

Unlike haemarthroses muscle bleeds are usually self-limiting owing to the confinement of fascial sheaths. The injured muscle heals by fibrosis and contracture and the original site of haemorrhage is obliterated. Cysts and joint contractures occur commonly. Muscle haematomas are associated with nerve compression and compartment syndromes with consequent limb ischaemia and paresis.

Haemophilic cysts and pseudotumours

These are uncommon and are either within a fascial envelope of muscle or extend to the periosteum with consequent cortical bone thinning. Very occasionally they may arise from intra-osseous haemorrhage.

PREPARATION FOR SURGERY

Circulating levels of Factor VIII are confirmed and the blood is screened for the absence of Factor antibodies.

Hepatitis

All haemophiliacs are potential carriers of the hepatitis B antigen and the serum should be screened for its presence prior to surgery. The presence of hepatitis antigen does not rule out elective surgery as long as special precautions are taken to prevent risk to the operating team (Houghton and Duthie, 1978).

PRINCIPLES OF COAGULATION CONTROL
(Biggs, 1976)

Haemorrhage both during and following surgery is controlled by replacing the missing clotting Factor in the patient's blood to an adequate level in order to maintain haemostasis until the wound is completely healed. The total amount of Factor that is required for the operative and postoperative period is estimated, obtained and banked prior to surgery. The relative merits of various therapeutic materials are listed in *Table 3*. Usage depends upon:

(*1*) type of material;
(*2*) potency of material;
(*3*) volume of dose;
(*4*) the patient's plasma volume.

There is much variation in patient response to Factor VIII infusion. Despite these variations the following formula serves as a rough guide to dosage:

$$\frac{\text{Patient's weight (kg)} \times \text{desired rise in Factor VIII (\%)}}{\text{Total units of Factor VIII in the dose}} = K$$

where K is a constant for any given type of therapeutic material (plasma K = 2, cryoprecipitate or human AHG K = 1·05, animal AHG K = 1·0). A unit of Factor VIII is defined as the Factor VIII activity contained in 1 ml of fresh citrated normal plasma.

Effective antihaemophilic therapy must be continued until the wound has completely healed. Any subsequent interference with the wound (removal of sutures and dressings, or mobilization of a limb following joint surgery) must be accompanied by Factor replacement – in practice, lyophilized human AHG or cryoprecipitate is generally used. The biological half-life of Factor VIII in the patient is approximately 12 hr, so repeated infusions of Factor VIII must be carried out 12 hourly and evaluation of serum levels assessed following each infusion, as in individual cases theoretical Factor VIII levels may not be achieved.

The Factor VIII serum level must be maintained above 40 per cent. This means that each dose of Factor VIII must raise the serum level to over 80 per cent of normal (Rizza, 1976). The first dose is administered 1 hr pre-operatively with premedication.

Epsilon aminocaproic acid (Epsicapron, EACA)

This is used to decrease the amount of bleeding following surgery (Tavenner, 1968). It acts by promoting clot stabilization, by inhibiting plasminogen activation, by preventing clot lysis and reducing postoperative requirement of AHG. The dose of Epsicapron is 0·01 g/kg 6 hourly and it is given until wound healing is well advanced, which is usually 2–3 weeks after surgery.

Factor IX concentrate

Plasma, cryoprecipitate, and AHG concentrate contain only small amounts of Factor IX and are therefore of little value in the treatment of haemophilia B. For major surgery to be carried out on a patient with Christmas disease, the Factor IX level must be kept above 25 per cent and this can only be achieved by the transfusion of protein concentrate, rich in Factor IX which has a biological half-life of 18 hr.

Table 3

Therapeutic materials available for the treatment of haemophilia

Source of Factor VIII	% Level of Factor VIII which may be achieved in patient's blood	Advantages	Disadvantages
Fresh whole blood	4 – 6	No preparation needed.	Insufficient quantity of Factor VIII. Factor VIII unstable in stored blood.
Fresh-frozen plasma	15 – 20	Cheap.	May overload circulation. One hour to administer. Serum hepatitis in pooled plasma.
Cryoprecipitate	60 – 80	One donor only: little risk of hepatitis.	Cannot be assayed until the time of transfusion. Stored below – 20°C.
Lyophilized human AHG	60 – 80	Units of Factor VIII known.	Hepatitis risk.
Lyophilized animal AHG	150	Very potent source of Factor VIII.	Antigenic.

PRINCIPLES OF SURGICAL TECHNIQUE (Duthie *et al.*, 1972)

Standard surgical approaches and techniques are used wherever possible and a pneumatic tourniquet is used to obtain a bloodless field. Local haemostasis is achieved using diathermy coagulation and electro-cautery for tissue dissection. Exposure is kept to the minimum required to perform the procedure and there is minimal stripping of tissue planes, as this will predispose to pocketing of haematoma in the recovery phase. The wounds are closed by coaptation of tissue planes by continuous haemostatic polyglycolic acid (Dexon) sutures. Also, they are not drained, but a firm compression bandage is applied and immobilization achieved with a plaster-of-Paris splint. Splintage secures immobilization of the operated area and discourages the formation of a haematoma. Percutaneous and external fixation devices are not used in order to avoid the complication of pin-track bleeding and infection. In general, definitive operations with predictable good results are preferred to multiple or staged procedures.

Implant surgery is carried out in a laminar flow operating theatre and prophylactic antibiotics are administered immediately pre-operatively and until the wound has healed and the sutures have been removed.

Postoperative care

The operated part is immobilized in a compression bandage and plaster-of-Paris, until the skin and soft tissues have healed. Isometric exercises are encouraged as soon as the patient is comfortable. The wound is inspected and the sutures removed under Factor VIII cover, which is maintained during early mobilization to prevent secondary haemorrhage. Limb rehabilitation is commenced in the hydrotherapy pool and then with appropriate walking aids on land. Postoperative rehabilitation and physiotherapy is always carried out in hospital until the patient is fully independent.

THE OPERATIONS

THE HIP

TOTAL HIP REPLACEMENT (Duthie, 1975)

Indications

Chronic hip arthropathy in the young or middle aged adult is becoming an increasing problem. Clinically, there is increasing hip pain with rest and night pain and all hip movements are restricted. Radiologically there are marked changes of chronic haemophilic arthropathy with secondary degenerative changes.

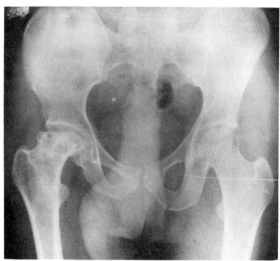

1

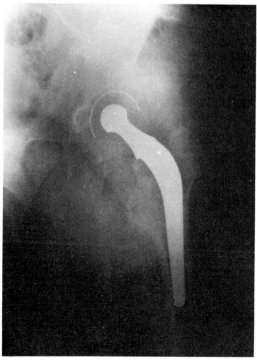

2

Procedures (see Chapter on 'Total Prosthetic Replacement of the Hip' in Orthopaedics Part II)

A standard approach and technique is used following the general principles of meticulous haemostasis and the use of electrocautery for tissue dissection employing a metal-on-polythene prosthesis. To reduce haemorrhage the greater trochanter is not removed.

Coagulation control

Haemostasis is maintained following the principles of coagulation control outlined above. The dose of Factor VIII required is calculated from the patient's weight and the initial level of serum Factor VIII. Factor replacement is given by intravenous infusion using a 21-gauge needle. A separate venepuncture is required for each dose.

Postoperative care

The hip is immobilized in a plaster-of-Paris hip spica incorporating the ankle joint, applied over a compression bandage. This immobilization is maintained for 3 weeks; it reduces the amount of haematoma formation and allows primary healing of soft tissues and thus reduces the Factor VIII requirement. Following removal of the cast and sutures at 3 weeks under Factor cover, mobilization is commenced in the hydrotherapy pool and the patient graduates to walking with elbow crutches.

Case history

A 32-year-old haemophiliac with 1 per cent of circulating Factor VIII and no antibodies to AHG had suffered multiple bleeds into both knees and had pain and stiffness of both these joints, but for the last 18 months he had had increasing pain in the right hip associated with giving way of that joint.

1&2

Examination of the right hip showed a marked antalgic gait, a range of movement from 10° of fixed flexion deformity with flexion of 70° with pain. Adduction was fixed at 10° and rotation was limited to 10° and was painful. Radiographs showed superior segment joint space narrowing with subchondral sclerosis and a small marginal osteophyte.

A standard total hip replacement was performed with full AHG cover, with the initial dose being given 1 hr prior to surgery.

3 & 4

Postoperatively the limb was enclosed in a full length hip spica for 3 weeks. After removal of the spica the sutures were removed and mobilization was started in the hydrotherapy pool. Mobilization continued initially with elbow crutches and he was discharged 5 weeks following surgery with a well healed wound and a range of movement of the right hip of flexion from 0° to 90°, abduction 20°, adduction 10° and a combined rotation of 20°. All these movements were pain-free. The Factor VIII requirement and serum levels achieved are shown in *Illustration 4.*

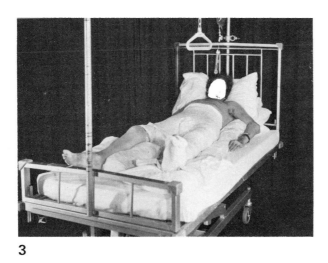

3

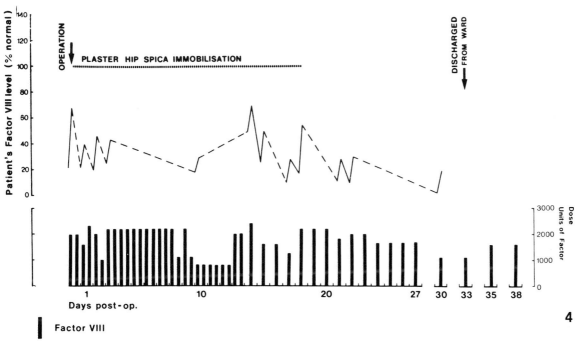

4

THE KNEE

SYNOVECTOMY (Storti *et al.*, 1969)

Indications

A history of recurrent episodes of haemarthroses with the clinical features of considerable synovial thickening. Failure of conservative management by repeated compression bandaging and adequate Factor infusion with strict bed rest for at least a 3 week period is the main indication. Minimal fixed flexion deformity and a range of flexion to at least 90° are prerequisites for synovectomy. Ideally, there should be only moderate radiographic changes of haemophilic arthropathy and there should be a persistent chronic thickened synovitic swelling despite conservative treatment.

Procedure

An anterior two-thirds synovectomy is performed using a medial parapatellar incision (*see* Chapter on 'Synovectomy of the Knee', in *Orthopaedics Part II*). Meticulous haemostasis is maintained throughout.

Postoperative care

Coagulation control is maintained following the principles outlined above. Following the operation, the limb is immobilized in a Robert Jones compression bandage with a plaster-of-Paris backslab until wound healing is complete. Isometric quadriceps exercises are commenced in the compression bandage. At 2 weeks the sutures are removed and physiotherapy started with Factor VIII cover. By 4 weeks, 90° of flexion should have been regained and weight-bearing is then permitted.

Case history

A 24-year-old accountant with 0 per cent circulating Factor VIII and no antibodies to AHG had had many haemorrhages in his elbows, ankles and left knee. In the 6 months prior to operation he had suffered recurrent haemorrhages into the left knee with an average of three haemarthroses a week.

5 & 6

Examination of the left knee showed considerable synovial thickening and a range of movements of 15°–100°. Radiographs showed mild haemophilic arthropathy.

Anterior two-thirds synovectomy of the left knee was carried out following an initial infusion of Factor VIII concentrate. Postoperatively a Robert Jones compression bandage with a plaster-of-Paris backslab was applied.

The wound healed by primary intention. There was a minor haemorrhage into the joint at 3 weeks; this settled rapidly. He was allowed to weight-bear at 4 weeks after the operation, at which stage he had regained 90° of flexion in the joint. Following the operation he had had several extra-articular haemorrhages which had required treatment, but these were localized around the infrapatellar regions and were painful. There had not been generalized swelling within the knee joint itself.

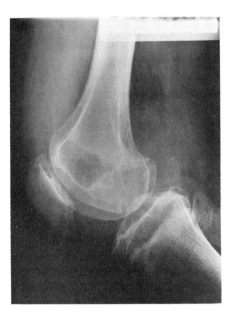

5

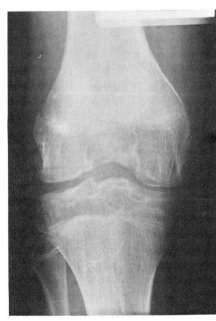

6

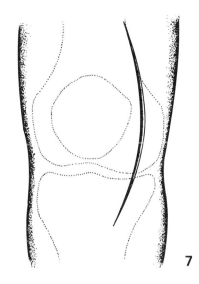

7

ARTHRODESIS (Houghton and Dickson, 1978)

Indications

The main indication for arthrodesis of the knee is pain. This may be associated with fixed contractures, gross deformity, instability and recurrent haemarthroses, which are functionally disabling.

7, 8 & 9

Procedure

A medial parapatellar incision is made and the under-surface of the patella is excised. The condylar surfaces of the femur are removed up to the level of the inter-condylar notch, and the surface of the tibia is excised just below the subchondral bone layer. Fixation is achieved with crossed compression screws. The knee should be arthrodesed in from 10° to 30° of flexion, depending on co-existent knee or ankle deformity.

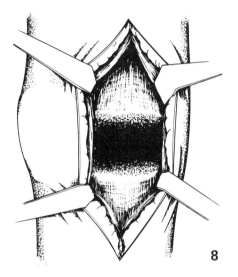

8

Postoperative care

The arthrodesis is protected by external splintage until bandage and a long leg plaster-of-Paris cast. At 2 weeks the sutures are removed and the cast is changed with Factor replacement to raise the serum level of Factor VIII to 80–100 per cent during the procedure. Isometric quadriceps exercises are started in the cast and the patient is mobilized without weight-bearing. The arthrodesis is protected by external splintage until there is radiological union at the site of the arthrodesis.

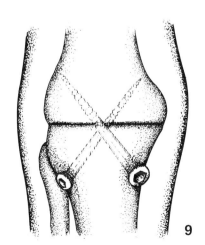

9

Case history

10 & 11

A 16-year-old schoolboy was a severe haemophiliac with 0 per cent Factor VIII and no antibodies to AHG. He had had recurrent bleeding into the left knee, right knee and elbow. On examination, he had a painful left knee, which was fixed at 60° of flexion, with posterior subluxation of the tibia on the femur.

Immediately prior to operation, an infusion of Factor VIII concentrate was given and an arthrodesis of the left knee was carried out with wedges cut in the tibia and femur to counteract the flexion deformity. Fixation was obtained using crossed screws and a plaster-of-Paris cast was applied.

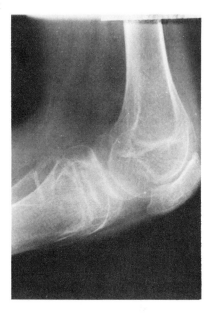

10

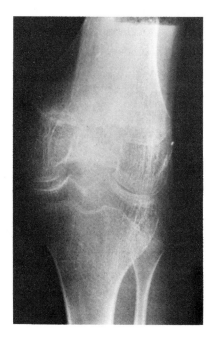

11

12, 13 & 14

The wound healed by primary intention and in 12 weeks the arthrodesis was soundly healed in the improved position of 20° of flexion. The result of the operation was that the patient had increased function in that limb and no pain from the knee. The Factor requirement and serum level achieved are shown in *Illustration 14*.

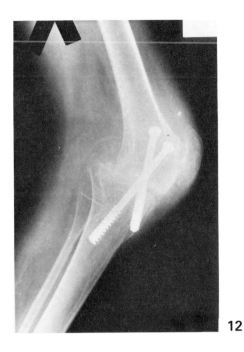

12

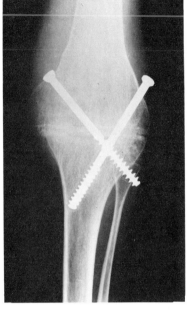

13

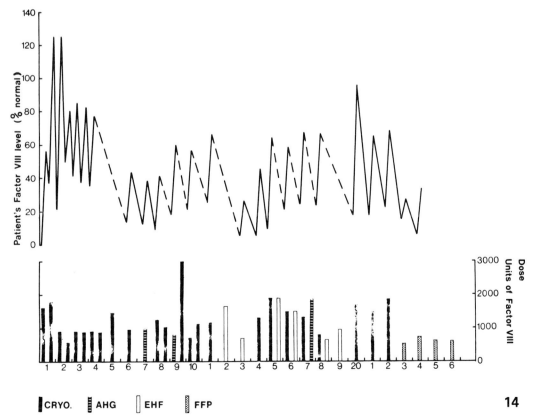

CRYO.   AHG   EHF   FFP

14

15

REVERSED DYNAMIC SLINGS
(Stein and Dickson, 1975)

Indications

Fixed flexion deformity of the knee (or elbow) secondary to intra-articular fibrous and capsular adhesions. The main features of the apparatus are shown. The affected limb is placed in a Thomas splint and supported in a knee flexion piece. Force *a* is converted to a downward pressure on the lower end of the femur via a canvas sling passed around the Thomas splint. Longitudinal skin traction is applied to the leg (Force *b*). Over a period of 10–14 days the knee flexion piece is approximated to the Thomas splint, thus straightening the leg.

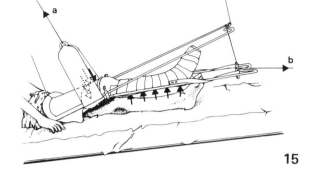

15

Factor VIII replacement is only occasionally required during this treatment if there is haemorrhage into the knee joint. This method has now superseded serial plasters in the treatment of knee flexion contractures and is equally successful in fixed flexion contracture of the elbow.

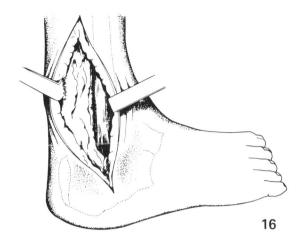

16

THE ANKLE

ARTHRODESIS (Houghton and Dickson, 1978)

Indications

The main indication for arthrodesis of the ankle is pain. This may be associated with fixed equinus deformity.

16, 17 & 18

A lateral incision is made and is deepened down to the fibula. The fibula is divided 8 cm from the tip of the malleolus and removed, and the cortex and articular cartilage are removed from the medial surface of this bone block. The ankle joint surfaces are excised horizontally and the bone block is fixed across the decorticated lateral surfaces as an onlay graft using screws. Accurate haemostasis is maintained throughout surgery.

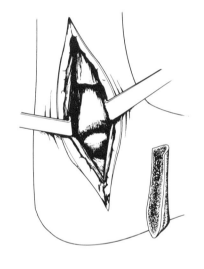

17

Postoperative care

The arthrodesis is immobilized with a compression bandage and a plaster-of-Paris cast in order to decrease haematoma formation and promote soft tissue healing. The sutures are removed at 2 weeks and a further cast is applied until the arthrodesis is fused. The time to radiological union is approximately 4 months and weight-bearing is then started. Factor VIII replacement is maintained following the principles outlined above.

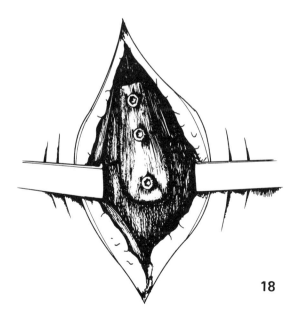

18

Case history

Five years prior to operation a 25-year-old tailor with 0 per cent Factor VIII and no antibodies to AHG sustained a left sciatic nerve palsy following haemorrhage into his left buttock. He had also suffered recurrent bleeds into his left calf.

19-23

On examination he had a severe equinocavus deformity of the left foot with a contracted tendo Achillis.

Operation was preceded by an initial infusion of Factor VIII concentrate. The equinus deformity of the ankle was corrected by the removal of an anterior wedge of the talus and tibia and the ankle was held in the correct position using the lower end of the fibula as a strut graft which was held with screws to the lower end of the tibia and to the talus. An Achilles tendon lengthening and a posterior capsulotomy of the left ankle joint was performed at the same time.

Postoperatively the limb was placed in a plaster-of-Paris cast and at 4 months this was removed and he was fitted with a below-knee caliper. At 8 months after surgery the caliper was discarded and it was noted that he had a marked improvement in the foot position and gait. The Factor VIII administered and levels achieved are shown. Factor VIII infused was kept to a minimum by the administration of EACA.

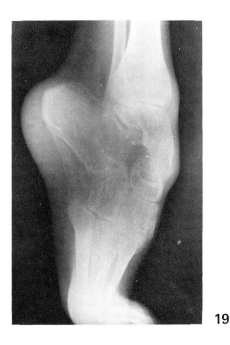

19

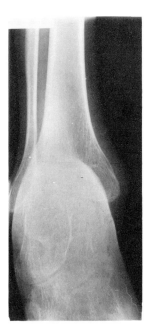

20

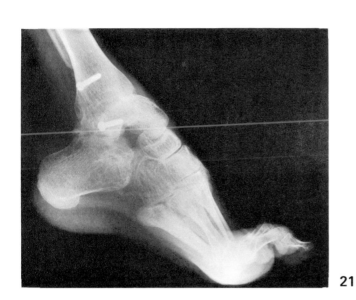

21

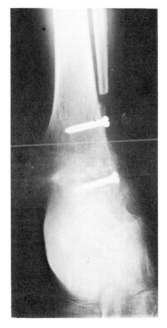

22

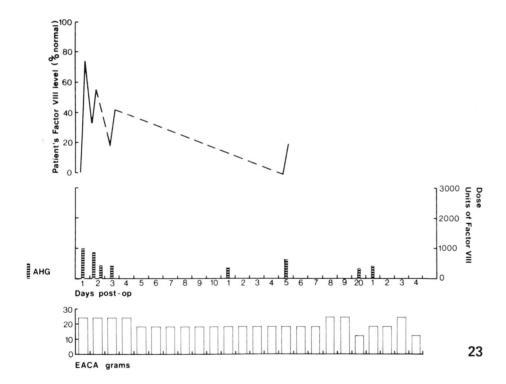

23

MANAGEMENT OF FRACTURES IN HAEMOPHILIA

Fractures are uncommon in patients with haemophilia. The important principles in the management of such fractures are as follows.

Coagulation control

The serum level of Factor VIII must be raised to 30–40 per cent of normal by intravenous infusion of AHG. This level of Factor VIII must be maintained for 3–4 days in a minor undisplaced closed fracture, but should be continued for 2–3 weeks in a more major fracture with displacement or in an open fracture. If surgical treatment is required or if the fracture is complicated, the Factor VIII level should be raised to 80–100 per cent in a similar manner to that for a surgical procedure. With adequate serum levels of Factor VIII there is less haematoma formation with less soft tissue destruction and the fracture can be expected to unite and consolidate in the usual way.

Fracture treatment

The best method of immobilization of the fracture is that which adequately holds the reduction and has the least chance of initiating further bleeding.

All children's fractures and stable fractures in the adult can be treated conservatively using plaster-of-Paris splintage.

Unstable fractures and intra-articular fractures, where there is incongruity of joint surfaces, are best treated by internal fixation.

Skeletal traction using percutaneous pins and wires are avoided as they may result in further bleeding or infection.

Secondary manipulations and operations should be avoided, but if they are required adequate Factor VIII replacement with AHG should be given both before and after the procedure. Factor VII replacement is also needed when removing sutures, renewing or changing the plaster cast and during the early phase of mobilization.

MANAGEMENT OF HAEMOPHILIC CYSTS AND PSEUDOTUMOURS

Haemophilic cysts and pseudotumours are rare. The initial treatment is conservative using the following principles:

(1) Immobilization of the affected part to reduce haematoma formation and to potentiate healing.

(2) Adequate Factor VIII replacement to achieve a serum level of 30 – 40 per cent of normal. This method of conservative management is continued until there is little pain and until the swelling is noted to subside. Radiographs should also show that resolution of the cyst is taking place.

Mobilization is then commenced initially with Factor replacement.

Surgical excision of the cyst is a major procedure and is only indicated if the lesion progresses despite adequate surgical treatment, and if the complications of skin ulceration, infection or haemorrhage occur. Amputation is then the only method of treatment if the cyst lies in an extremity.

COMPLICATIONS OF SURGERY IN HAEMOPHILIA (Houghton and Duthie, 1978)

The complications that have been encountered are summarized in *Table 4*. The commonest complication is haemorrhage often associated with secondary infection. Rarely antibodies develop in the postoperative period when high levels of antigenic Factor VIII are administered. This serious complication renders effective treatment difficult and rigid immobilization and compression, together with animal AHG, offer the best prospect of arrest of haemorrhage.

Table 4

Complication of surgery

Operation	Complication	Cause	Management
Knee arthrodesis	Delayed union 7 months.	– –	Prolonged immobilization.
Knee arthrodesis	Delayed union 11 months.	– –	
Knee arthrodesis	Delayed union 12 months.	– –	
Knee arthrodesis	Haematoma.	Poor coagulation control (1968).	Aspiration under Factor VIII cover.
Knee arthrodesis	Wound infection.	Secondary to haematoma.	Antibiotics; Factor VIII replacement.
Ankle arthrodesis	Haematoma.	Inadequate compression bandage.	Compression bandage and Factor VIII replacement.
Ankle arthrodesis	Haematoma and wound dehiscence.	Poor coagulation control (1967).	Factor replacement and daily dressings for 4 months.
Total hip replacement	Died.	Intra-operative collapse; cardiac arrest.	–
Total hip replacement	Dislocation fifth day.	Inadequate hip spica.	Conversion to full hip spica.
Femoral plate for fracture (at other hospital).	Infection and antibody development.	Poor coagulation control with haematoma.	Multiple debridement under Factor VIII cover; died 18 months post fracture.
Excision pelvic pseudocyst.	Died.	Uncontrollable haemorrhage day 3 prior to operation.	Re-exploration failed to stop bleeding from aberrant arteriovenous blood vessels.

CONCLUSIONS

Many other orthopaedic operations have been reported as having been performed on patients with haemophilia. Standard surgical approaches and techniques are used, but great care is taken to maintain haemostasis both operatively, by attention to detail, and by adequate Factor replacement both during the surgical procedure and during the postoperative period.

However, the best results of orthopaedic surgery in haemophiliacs are achieved in centres where there has grown up over the years an expertise, and where there is a greater experience of both the surgical and haematological complications and their treatment. It is recommended that elective surgery should only be carried out in such centres.

Acknowledgement

We would like to acknowledge the Physicians of the Oxford Haemophilia Centre – Drs Charles Rizza and James Matthews – for their assistance in the management of patients with haemophilia.

References

Bentley, G. and Duthie, R. B. (1975). 'Orthopaedic management of the haemophilias.' In *Recent Advances in Orthopaedics.* Edinburgh: Churchill Livingstone

Biggs, R. (Ed.) (1976). *Human Blood Coagulation, Haemostasis and Thrombosis,* 2nd Edition. Oxford: Blackwell

Duthie, R. B. (1975). 'Reconstructive surgery in haemophilia.' *Ann. N. Y. Acad. Sci.* **240,** 295

Duthie, R. B., Matthews, J., Rizza, C. R. and Steel, W. S. (1972). *The Management of Musculor-skeletal Problems in the Haemophilias. and Thrombosis,* 2nd Edition, Edited by R. Biggs, pages 365–398. Oxford: Blackwell

Houghton, G. R. and Dickson, R. A. (1979). 'Lower limb arthrodeses in haemophilia.' *J. Bone Jt Surg.* **60B,** 143

Houghton, G. R. and Duthie, R. B. (1978). 'Orthopaedic problems in haemophilia.' *Clin. Orth.* (In Press)

Rizza, C. R. (1976). 'The management of patients with coagulation factor deficiencies.' In *Human Blood Coagulation, Haemostasis and Thrombosis,* 2nd Edition, Edited by R. Biggs, pages 365–398. Oxford: Blackwell

Stein, H. and Dickson, R. A. (1975). 'Reversed dynamic slings for knee flexion contractures in the haemophiliac.' *J. Bone Jt Surg.* **57A,** 282

Storti, E., Traldi, A., Tosatti, E. and Davoli, P. G. (1969). 'Synovectomy, a new approach to haemophilic arthropathy.' *Acta haemat.* **41,** 193

Tavenner, R. W. (1968). 'Epsilon-aminocaproic acid in the treatment of haemophilia and Christmas disease, with special reference to the extraction of teeth.' *Br. dent. J.* **124,** 19

[*The illustrations for this Chapter on Surgical Management of Patients with Haemophilia were drawn by Mr. G. Bartlett.*]

Amputation Surgery

J. C. Angel, F.R.C.S.
Consultant Orthopaedic Surgeon, Royal National Orthopaedic Hospital,
Stanmore, Middlesex

INTRODUCTION

Amputation, one of the oldest procedures in surgery, was once employed only as a desperate and often unsuccessful bid to save life. Nowadays it is used not simply for that purpose, but to create a stump that, when fitted with a prosthesis, restores the function of the limb to the maximum possible degree.

INDICATIONS FOR AMPUTATION

During the year 1976, 4999 amputees were referred to the artificial limb fitting service in England (Chief Medical Officer, D.H.S.S., 1977). The causes of these amputations were as follows:

Vascular disease and diabetes mellitus	4087	81·7%
Injury	527	10·6%
Infection	77	1·5%
Tumour	256	5·1%
Neurogenic deformity	52	1·0%
Total	4999	99·9%

Seventy per cent of the patients were male and seventy-three per cent were over the age of 60 years. The upper extremity was involved in 250 cases (5 per cent).

Vascular disease

Atherosclerosis tends to affect the large and medium sized arteries leaving the distal vascular tree relatively intact. Thus gangrene of the toes in this condition indicates the presence of a much larger mass of disordered tissue. Demarcation of the gangrene is poor and local amputations are unlikely to succeed unless it is possible to relieve the proximal block by reconstructive arterial surgery. If there is no steep temperature gradient above the ankle the long posterior flap below-knee amputation is successful in the majority of cases (Burgess, 1969). Occasionally amputation is required for uncontrollable rest pain in the absence of gangrene.

In diabetes mellitus gangrene may be due to a proximal atheromatous block, pressure necrosis in the presence of peripheral neuropathy or small vessel block caused either by diabetic arteriopathy or arterial involvement in a septic process. These factors are usually found in combination rather than in isolation and even though the pedal pulses may be absent distal amputations are often justified. These include digital and ray resections and Syme's amputation.

The chronic debility associated with venous ulceration can sometimes be resolved only by ablation.

Injury

Amputation is required in trauma when conservative surgery does not offer a reasonable chance of restoring function. Where it may be acceptable to plan a prolonged course of reconstructive surgery and rehabilitation in a young person, the same may not apply in the elderly whose shorter life expectancy does not justify such a heavy investment of time and effort on the part of the patient.

In the case of burns and frostbite much potentially viable tissue can be saved by allowing time for a clear-cut line of demarcation to appear before amputating. Electrical burns often involve deep tissues to a far greater extent than indicated by the superficial wound, necessitating amputation at a higher level than at first anticipated.

Tumours

For those primary malignant tumours, the site and character of which does not allow them to be treated by local resection, amputation offers hope of a cure if a thorough search for metastases has been negative. The amputation may be justified even if distant metastases are known to be present or for secondary deposits if these tumours cause pain that cannot be relieved in any other way. It is very important that the amputation flaps should be clear of the neoplastic process in order to prevent the extremely difficult problem of stump recurrence.

Infection

Nowadays it is uncommon for acute infection to be the primary cause of an amputation. However, its presence not infrequently calls for a higher amputation than might otherwise have been the case and it is the reason for a number of revisions of amputations. The infection caused by gas-forming organisms has a particular capacity for rapid spread through the tissues. Of these *Clostridium welchii* is much the most virulent but certain gas-producing coliforms and streptococci are dangerous, particularly in diabetics. The level of amputation should be high enough to exclude surgical emphysema from the stump which should be left unsutured.

Chronic infection, usually in the form of osteomyelitis, may necessitate amputation because of chronic debility, associated deformity and functional loss or the development of malignant change. Except where malignant change has occurred, it is not essential to skirt the lesion by more than 1 or 2 cm as long as the amputation flaps have a good blood supply and are free from infected tissue. Attempting to cut away all oedematous tissue and secondary changes may result in unnecessary shortening of the stump.

Neurological disorders

Neurological disorders can lead to repeated skin breakdown and deformity. It may be possible to reduce the resulting functional deficit by amputation and prosthetic replacement. In paraplegics joint contractures of such severity that they cause problems in nursing may occur and the limb may sometimes be better amputated.

Congenital deformities

Some congenital deformities, particularly those associated with gross leg length discrepancy and distortion of the foot, are best managed by amputation and prosthetic replacement.

PRE-OPERATIVE ASSESSMENT

The prosthetic prescription is determined by a number of factors in addition to the level of amputation. For some amputees cosmesis is of paramount importance, while for others, particularly those of an independent nature who have to care for themselves, it is better to sacrifice cosmesis in favour of function or comfort. Similar factors should be allowed to influence the level of amputation. For example, disarticulation, where technically possible, may be expected to provide a more robust and comfortable stump although it is less cosmetic. Thus it is important to take a detailed social history and form an impression about the degree and direction of the patient's motivation. Where possible it should be established prior to surgery whether or not a patient is likely to be able to use a prosthesis. If it is clear that he is not, because of severe disorders of the locomotor or central nervous systems, then it is appropriate to select a proximal level of amputation where there is a good chance of primary healing and less risk of difficulties arising through joint contracture. In this it is important not to be misled by a patient who is in severe pain or who is in a toxic state due to infection.

In the dysvascular amputee the level of amputation is determined largely by criteria such as tissue appearance, hair growth, Buerger's test and a clinical assay of skin temperature. The presence or absence of peripheral pulses is generally less helpful. A number of supplementary investigations have been found valuable and one in particular is beginning to vie in importance with the clinical impression. This is the measurement of blood pressure adjacent to the proposed level of amputation using transcutaneous Doppler recordings. Techniques of determining skin blood-flow are still under assessment and they include thermography, radioactive xenon clearance and local histamine injections. Angiography is often misleading as an indicator of tissue perfusion.

With all major amputations a radiograph of the chest and a haemoglobin estimation should be available. In dysvascular cases electrocardiography together with blood urea and fasting blood sugar estimations are also desirable. Sepsis in the part to be amputated must be assumed to have led to contamination of the lymphatics at the site of amputation and cultures should be made so that the appropriate antibiotic therapy can be commenced at the time of surgery.

PREPARATION

Amputation has an irrevocable quality not shared by most other surgical procedures. It is important that the patient understands why the operation is necessary. In the case of amputations performed as an elective procedure for such conditions as chronic sepsis or congenital deformity, it is customary for the surgeon to seek a second opinion from one of his colleagues in order to confirm his decision and share the responsibility. With children great care should be taken in explaining to the parents the reason for the amputation as recriminations and feelings of guilt so often follow in the wake of a childhood amputation. The consent form must be signed. In the case of vascular disease or acute inflammation it is often desirable to obtain consent to proceed to a higher level of amputation should it prove necessary on the operating table. The limb to be amputated should be clearly marked.

Once the decision has been made to perform an amputation the patient should be encouraged to be as mobile as possible. Smoking is forbidden. Diabetes is controlled as far as possible and anaemia should be corrected. Blood should be cross-matched to cover the possibility of haemorrhage at the time of surgery and in the immediate postoperative period. On the day of surgery the skin is shaved and infected areas on the extremity are sealed off inside a polythene bag. Antibiotic therapy is commenced at the time of premedication. It is desirable to give penicillin or erythromycin to protect against clostridial infection and to supplement this with whatever antibiotics are required to deal with organisms that have been identified. Arrangements should be made for the disposal of the amputated specimen whether it is to go for histological examination or simply incineration.

General anaesthesia is preferred for all amputations other than the distal half of the digits. If this is precluded by toxaemia or other factors, epidural anaesthesia is the next best choice. Intravenous regional anaesthesia can be used for distal amputations and infiltration anaesthesia may be suitable away from an infected area, particularly with disarticulations.

Amputation surgery, except where there is marked ischaemia, is greatly facilitated by the use of a pneumatic tourniquet, especially if a myoplasty is involved. If exsanguination with an Esmarch's bandage is thought undesirable the limb can be drained satisfactorily by elevation.

MANAGEMENT OF INDIVIDUAL TISSUES

Skin

The skin flaps are conveniently marked using a throat swab dipped in Methylene blue or another dye. The bases of the flaps are generally level with the proposed bone section. Ideally, from the point of view of skin closure, the edges of the two flaps should be of roughly equal length. Where one flap is made much longer than the other it is often difficult to estimate the exact length required and so it is marked much longer than necessary and cut accurately at the time of skin closure. The skin is closed with interrupted, simple sutures. Where there is a particular risk of postoperative infection the skin edges should be opposed with two or three sutures over ribbon gauze soaked in aqueous proflavine emulsion. If at 5 days the wound is clean then the skin edges can be sutured as a delayed primary closure. If there is contamination then later secondary closure is more appropriate. Skin traction is a technique that is sometimes useful in a neglected traumatic amputation as it can draw down innervated skin, thereby preserving stump length and diminishing the need for skin grafting.

Muscle

This is handled in different ways depending on individual amputations. In general it should be cut with a raked incision, the knife being angled towards the bone at the level of section. The fibres tend to fall back towards the level of the cut end of the bone but their elasticity allows the outer fibres and the fascial coverings to be pulled down over the end of the bone and sutured to the opposing muscle groups or periosteum. The muscle should be stitched with catgut or Dexon unless an osteomyoplasty is performed, in which case monofilament nylon is preferred as it is less likely to be damaged by contact with the cut surface of the bone.

Bone

In deciding the level of bone section in the lower thigh and arm, consideration is given to the fact that there should be sufficient room between the cut end of the bone and the axis of the artificial joint immediately below the stump to accommodate a number of structures: the soft tissue covering the end of the bone, the end-socket space or padding, the socket wall and the joint mechanism itself. The axis of the artificial joint is normally set at the level of the axis of the contralateral anatomical joint. If insufficient bone is removed then either the axis of the artificial joint must be set more distally, sacrificing cosmesis, or side joints must be used which are also less cosmetic, weaker and tend to rub holes in clothes.

The level of bone section should be approached extraperiosteally. The periosteum is then divided circumferentially and the bone is cut immediately distally. In most situations the Gigli saw is much the most satisfactory tool for this purpose. The fibula, which is often a difficult bone to divide cleanly, is best cut with an oscillating saw. The cut-end of the bone should always be rounded with a sharp rasp used in such a way it does not damage the surrounding soft tissues. The latter should be prevented from coming into contact with bone dust by covering them with saline-soaked swabs and once the work has been completed on the bone the area should be irrigated with saline.

Vessels

Vessels the size of the common femoral vein and artery and larger should be doubly ligated with strong silk. The superficial femoral, the axillary and brachial vessels can be doubly ligated individually with strong catgut or Dexon and smaller vessels can be ligated as a bundle with a transfixation ligature after dissecting them away from the associated nerve.

Nerves

These are gently pulled down, divided and allowed to retract from the level of the wound. The median, sciatic and posterior tibial nerves often carry a vessel sufficiently large to cause troublesome bleeding. It should be caught and ligated before the nerve is allowed to spring out of reach.

Drainage

All but the most minor amputations should be drained with vacuum drains. These are brought out through the skin, some distance from the wound, and the dressings are arranged in such a way they are not disturbed when the drain is pulled out in a proximal direction at the end of the second postoperative day.

POSTOPERATIVE CARE

In the first 10 days gentle terminal pressure should be applied to the end of the stump to discourage the formation of a haematoma and the accumulation of an inflammatory exudate. The stump is wrapped in wool and a crêpe bandage, the dressing being pulled proximally by one of several means. In the case of the foot or a below-elbow amputation this can be achieved by a few turns of bandage round the ankle or the flexed elbow. Similarly with a short above-knee or above-elbow amputation a few turns round the trunk will suffice. Longitudinal strips of Elastoplast are also satisfactory. The best method of achieving terminal pressure for amputations below the knee and elbow and distal to those levels is a rigid dressing. It is applied immediately after surgery. The plaster is prevented from soaking into the crêpe bandage by applying a thin layer of plaster wool. The plaster is then suspended on the limb by moulding it above bony prominences such as the femoral condyles or by attaching it to the trunk with a simple harness or belt. The initial dressing is best left untouched for the first 10 – 14 days unless there is reason to suspect a wound complication. Once the wound is well on the way to being healed attention should be directed towards the shaping of the stump to fit the artificial limb. The area to be enclosed by the socket should be bandaged in such a way that there is a gradient of circumferential pressure, the maximum being at the distal end of the stump. The bandage must be kept clean by washing in soap and water and it must not tend to lose its elasticity. Ordinary crêpe bandage does not usually stand up to this treatment and an Elset bandage is preferred. In suitable cases serial plasters can be used for the same purpose. The use of a cast has the additional advantage that a foot or terminal device can be incorporated allowing an early restoration of function. Prophylactic antibiotic therapy is usually discontinued after 5 days. In the case of lower extremity amputees, mobilization should commence as soon as the drain is removed. The remaining joints in the amputated extremity should be put through a full range of movement where this is not precluded by the rigid dressing. Prone lying for 20 min twice a day helps to prevent the development of hip flexion contractures. Muscle-setting exercises help to strengthen the stump.

During the postoperative period the patient should be closely observed for the signs of infection or haematoma developing in the wound. Increasing pain, rising pulse and blood pressure, and the appearance of blood or pus oozing through the dressing all require an immediate inspection of the wound.

COMPLICATIONS

Haematoma

The presence of a haematoma in an amputation wound predisposes to infection and greatly delays prosthetic fitting. Sometimes the collection of blood can be aspirated but more often it must be drained surgically. Massive haemorrhage due to the slipping of a ligature or severe infection is nowadays uncommon. Nevertheless, those caring for the patient in the immediate postoperative period should be alert to the possibility and know how to deal with it. Should it occur the vessel must be religated and the haematoma evacuated. While preparations are being made the bleeding can usually be controlled by firm local pressure and elevation. A sphygmomanometer cuff can be used as a temporary tourniquet.

Infection

An amputation is one of the commonest wounds in surgery to become infected. This is because the tissues are often poorly vascularized, transection of the bacteria-laden lymphatics is inevitable if there is sepsis in the distal part of the extremity and finally the wound often contains dead tissue such as haematoma, denuded cortical bone, ligature material etc. When infection occurs it can sometimes be eradicated with antibiotics, together with incision and drainage of any collection of pus. But all too often a chronic sinus develops that persists until the focus is removed. This is usually found to be a small sequestrum at the cut end of the bone or ligature material. In diabetics sloughed connective tissue is often responsible. These patients should always receive antibiotic cover to avoid the hazards of gas gangrene particularly following lower limb amputations.

Necrosis

Skin flap necrosis of a minor degree occasioned by the presence of sutures may sometimes be dealt with by conservative measures. Extensive necrosis requires either a wedge resection down to and including bone or a re-amputation.

Joint contractures

Joint contractures affect particularly the knee and the hip. They are common especially in patients made immobile by old age or pain. Active and passive exercises and corrective posturing improve mild contractures. Prosthetic fitting and ambulation are also very helpful. The more severe contractures may require serial plasters or surgery. Not infrequently they may preclude the use of a prosthesis altogether.

Neuromata

The formation of stump neuromata at the cut ends of nerves is, of course, inevitable. If they become trapped in scar tissue then they may give rise to disabling pain. Treatment consists of resecting the neuroma or a length of the affected nerve away from the scarred area.

Phantom limb sensation

It is usual for an adult amputee to feel that the missing part of a limb is still present after an amputation. He should be re-assured about this strange feeling and made aware of the danger of attempting to use a limb that is not there, especially when waking at night.

Phantom pain

Occasionally amputees complain of severe pain in the phantom limb for which no local cause can be found. It does not respond even to drastic measures such as nerve division, root section or even cordotomy. The phenomenon is more common with proximal than distal amputations, when there has been much severe pain before amputation and when the amputee has been made excessively aware of the problem by being exposed to another patient with phantom pain. Hospital staff should avoid introducing the concept of phantom pain unless the patient has already complained of it. He should be given an optimistic prognosis and re-assured as far as possible. Unfortunately this highly disturbing problem can be quite relentless and on occasions has driven amputees to suicide.

AMPUTATION IN CHILDREN

Children tolerate amputations well. Phantom pain is unusual and, especially in younger children, there is very little disturbance of body image. Children are also very adept at learning to use prostheses. The main problems that arise from amputations in children are associated with subsequent growth. A mid-thigh or a forearm amputation in a child does not grow in proportion to the rest of the body. In some cases a stump that is functional initially becomes too short to be of any value at the time growth has ceased. The opposite applies to below-knee and above-elbow stumps which can start off too short and later become long enough to work a prosthesis. However, the cut end of the humerus and the tibia and particularly the fibula are prone to grow by a process of accretion to the end of the bone. This new bone is capable of ulcerating through the skin. A below-knee amputation in an infant may for this reason require three or more revisions before the cessation of growth.

AMPUTATION IN THE ELDERLY

Ninety-two per cent of those who have an amputation at the age of 60 years or older have either peripheral vascular disease or diabetes mellitus. In this group it is often difficult to decide whether to save the knee joint or not. To succeed is to halve the functional loss imposed by an above-knee amputation (in as far as it is possible to make such an assessment). To attempt a below-knee amputation and fail usually means weeks of hospitalization and further surgery and consequent lowering of the patient's morale. The decision must take account not only of clinical factors and the results of investigations but also such things as the degree to which the patient is motivated and the home circumstances. For some patients a speedy return to a caring family is more important than the preservation of maximum function and in such cases a below-knee amputation should be undertaken only if there is a high chance of success. For others the successful fitting of a below-knee amputation may make all the difference between an independent existence at home and the need for institutional care and so there is little to lose by choosing the lower level. This type of information may be difficult to elicit from a sick patient in severe pain and there should be no hesitation in consulting the patient's general practitioner and relatives to gain an insight into his needs and capabilities.

IMMEDIATE POSTOPERATIVE FITTING

The fitting of a limb around the dressing immediately after an amputation has been claimed to reduce the psychological impact of the operation and to speed rehabilitation. The procedure has been adopted in a number of centres and evaluated in others. It places considerable demands on the time of doctors and prosthetists and is practicable in only a few hospitals housing limb-fitting centres. The procedure has particular value for the patient who finds it difficult to accept the loss of an extremity and whose rehabilitation may be seriously disrupted by the sudden realization of it. The techniques, in the case of lower extremity amputations, have been fully described by Burgess, Romano and Zettl (1969).

REHABILITATION

An amputation is but the first step of a rehabilitation process that involves surgical, nursing, prosthetic, workshop and remedial therapy expertise. Ideally those involved should work in close contact with one another in the same environment. Unfortunately it is not practicable to site comprehensive prosthetic workshops in every district hospital so a schism is created which is often exacerbated by bureaucratic factors and the need for the artificial limb prescription and rehabilitation elements to be in the hands of other doctors. Even so, the surgeon is in the unique position of being able to monitor and influence the entire process and thus has a responsibility to ensure that the final outcome is, as far as possible, that planned at the time the patient consented to amputation. It follows, therefore, that a surgeon who undertakes to perform an amputation must also accept a measure of responsibility for co-ordinating the subsequent treatment.

References

Burgess, E. M. (1969). *The Below-Knee Amputation*, Inter-Clinic Information Bulletin, VIII, No. 4
Burgess, E. M., Romano, R. L. and Zettl, J. H. (1969). *The Management of Lower Extremity Amputations*, TR 10–6, August, Washington: U.S. Government Printing Office
Report of the Chief Medical Officer, Department of Health and Social Security (1977).

Amputations through the Upper Extremity

J. C. Angel, F.R.C.S.
Consultant Orthopaedic Surgeon, Royal National Orthopaedic Hospital,
Stanmore, Middlesex

PRE-OPERATIVE

Indications

The principal indication for these procedures is injury. In such patients every effort should be made to conserve tissue but where this is not possible a formal amputation must be carried out. Other indications include malignant tumours, gas gangrene, ischaemic gangrene, occasional chronic infection, deformities and congenital abnormalities.

Contra-indications

Except as a life-saving procedure formal amputation through the upper extremity should be proceeded with only after careful deliberation. Where there is no urgency it is usually wise to obtain a second and third opinion before performing such operations.

Pre-operative preparation

A general anaesthetic is preferred. As an alternative a brachial plexus block may be used. The patient lies flat on the back. A tourniquet is applied to the upper arm and the limb is placed on an arm board at just less than a right angle to the trunk. An inverted bowl is placed under the limb, just proximal to the site of amputation.

THE OPERATIONS

BELOW-ELBOW AMPUTATION

1a & b

The incision

Equal dorsal and volar skin flaps are marked out with their bases at the junction of the middle and lower thirds of the ulna (approximately 17 cm distal to the tip of the olecranon process). Care should be taken in positioning the arm to place it in supination on the arm rest without any torsional strain below the elbow joint. Otherwise the flaps, after being cut, are drawn into an oblique position by the natural elasticity of the skin. The skin flaps of the first incision should include the deep fascia.

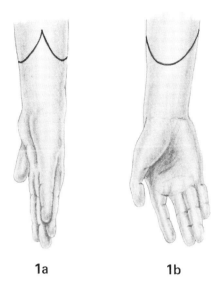

1a   **1b**

2

Exposure and division of soft tissue

The skin and fascial flaps are freed and turned back in a plane deep to the deep fascia. The tendons, muscles and other soft tissues are cut with a slightly raked incision to meet the bone at the level of bone section. In practice it is found that the most suitable site is where the majority of the muscle bellies become tendinous. The skin and fascia are retracted by an assistant.

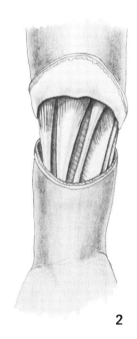

2

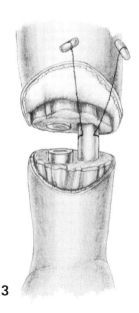

3

3

Division of radius and ulna

After division the soft tissues retract. The periosteum is incised circumferentially at the level of the section and the bones are divided with a Gigli saw. The main blood vessels are then identified and ligated and the main nerves gently pulled down and cut across as high as possible. The tourniquet is released and haemostasis is secured.

4

Closure and drainage

A suction drain is passed out through the muscle and skin on the lateral side of the forearm. The deep fascia is sutured over the ends of the bones with catgut sutures and the skin is closed with fine interrupted sutures.

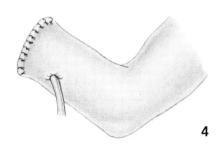

4

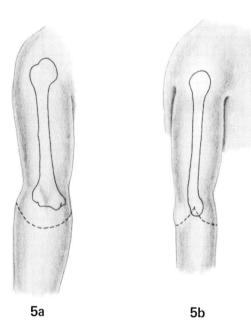

5a   **5b**

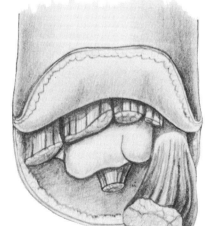

6

DISARTICULATION AT THE ELBOW

5a & b

Skin flaps

With the forearm in full supination equal anterior and posterior flaps are fashioned, their bases being level with the humeral epicondyles. The anterior flap extends to just below the bicipital insertion and the posterior flap to just below the tip of the olecranon.

6

Division of soft tissues

The skin flaps are reflected proximally to the level of the epicondyles. The bicipital aponeurosis is divided and the flexor mass arising from the medial epicondyle is detached and reflected distally. This gives access to the main neurovascular bundle lying medial to the biceps tendon. The brachial vessels are individually ligated. The main nerves are drawn down and divided with a scalpel so that they retract at least 3 cm proximal to the level of the joint line. Next the biceps tendon is detached from the radial tuberosity and the brachialis from the coronoid process of the ulna. The extensor musculature arising from the humeral epicondyle is divided at a level 6 cm distal to the joint line and reflected proximally. The triceps tendon is detached from the tip of the olecranon and the disarticulation is completed by dividing the anterior capsule and the collateral ligaments. The tourniquet is released and haemostasis is secured.

7

Provision of soft tissue covering for distal end of bone

The next task is to fashion a soft tissue covering for the distal end of the humerus, the articular surface of which is left intact. The triceps is brought forward and sutured to the distal ends of the biceps and brachialis. The remains of the extensor muscle mass is thinned by removing some of the deeper fibres and sutured to the remnant of the flexor mass at the medial epicondyle.

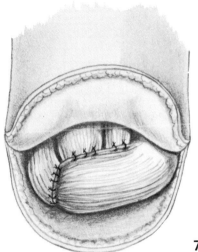

7

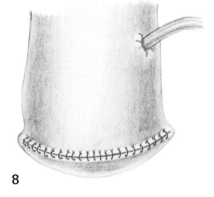

8

8

Closure

A suction drain is passed out through the skin on the lateral side of the arm, its tip being buried in contact with the articular surface. The skin flaps are closed with interrupted sutures.

ABOVE-ELBOW AMPUTATION

9

The incision

Equal anteroposterior flaps are marked out, their bases being 8 inches (20 cm) from the tip of the acromion process of the scapula. The incision outlined is the ideal one as the scar will eventually be terminal where it is free from pressure from the socket. It may be necessary to vary the shape of the incision according to the surgical requirements and the disorder for which the operation is performed.

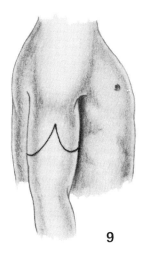

9

10

Division of soft tissues and humerus

The initial skin incision is continued through the deep fascia and then through the muscle with a slightly raked cut meeting the bone at the level of bone section. The periosteum is divided circumferentially and the bone cut with a Gigli saw.

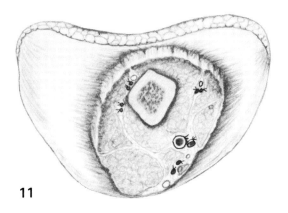

11

Haemostasis

The main vessels are now ligated and the nerves are gently pulled down and shortened by about 1 inch (2·5 cm) so that they fall back into the depths of the wound. The tourniquet is now deflated and any further bleeding controlled.

12

Closure and drainage

The deep fascia and superficial parts of the musculature are closed over the bone end using interrupted catgut sutures. The drain is brought out through the muscle and skin on the lateral side of the arm. The skin is closed with interrupted sutures.

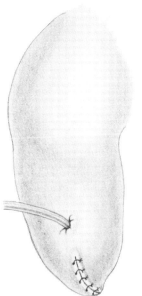

12

POSTOPERATIVE CARE

The wound is dressed and bandaged in such a way that gentle pressure is applied to the end of the stump. The drain is removed in 48 hr when physiotherapy to mobilize the remaining joints of the limb is commenced.

Prosthetics

A functioning forearm prosthesis can be fitted even if the below-elbow stump only extends 1 inch (2·5 cm) distal to the insertion of the biceps tendon. With a stump of average length the socket of the prosthesis is held in place by a harness and passes up the arm behind the back and around the root of the opposite arm. A rotary device is fitted to the bottom of the socket which allows the same function as forearm rotation. Into it can be connected a cosmetic hand, a functioning hand, a split-hook or other terminal devices. The hand or split-hook is operated by a cord

that is tensed by a forward shrugging movement of the shoulders. Also available for below-elbow amputees is a simple lightweight cosmetic hand that pulls onto the stump in much the same manner as a glove. With the above-elbow prosthesis the socket and rotary device are separated by an elbow turntable that simulates rotation in the axis of the humerus and an elbow joint that can be locked in several positions of flexion and extension.

The advantage of the through-elbow disarticulation compared with the above-elbow level is that the stump is capable of transmitting shoulder rotation to the prosthesis and also it provides a longer lever arm. The disadvantages are that jointed side steels have to be placed at either side of the rather bulky lower end of the socket and the elbow locking mechanism is less robust and less efficient. The lower level of amputation is definitely advantageous to a man who works with his hands, particularly if the dominant hand has been lost. It is less useful in women whose sleeves tend to snag on the side joints of the prosthesis causing excessive wear to garments and an uncosmetic appearance.

[*The illustrations for this Chapter on Amputations through the Upper Extremity were drawn by Mrs. A. Barrett.*]

Forequarter Amputation

Paul C. Weaver, M.D., F.R.C.S., F.R.C.S.(Ed.)
Consultant Surgeon, Portsmouth and South East Hampshire Group of Hospitals;
Clinical Teacher, University of Southampton

INTRODUCTION

The first successful forequarter or interscapulothoracic amputation was carried out in 1836. In 1887 Berger reviewed and standardized the anterior approach technique used today with some variation. In this operation the main vessels and nerves are ligated early, as opposed to the posterior or Littlewood operation in which the quarter is dissected free before the vessels and nerves are secured.

When this amputation is carried out the whole of the upper limb is removed with the scapula and outer two-thirds of the clavicle (unless this bone is involved when the clavicle is disarticulated at the sternal joint).

PRE-OPERATIVE

Indications

Forequarter amputation is performed almost exclusively for malignant disease. It can be of use in the management of tumours of the humerus, infiltrating tumours of the shoulder girdle and tumours of the axilla which invade nerves and vessels. Occasionally tumours such as soft tissue sarcomas and malignant melanoma may produce a cumbersome, painful, foul smelling and bleeding limb calling for palliative section even when non-troublesome metastases are known to be present. Trauma is a rare indication.

Contra-indications

(1) The presence of secondary deposits or the inability to remove all tumour.
(2) The patient's refusal to accept mutilation.
(3) Physical or mental unfitness for major surgery.

Pre-operative preparation

Biopsy

Unequivocal microscopic evidence is essential. Care must be taken with the biopsy not to encroach upon the skin flaps of the amputation.

Investigations

X-rays and E.M.I. scans are used to help define the limits of the disease and exclude possible metastatic spread.

Anaemia should be corrected and 6 units of blood are made available although it is seldom necessary to use more than 2 or 3 units.

Pre-operative breathing exercises are helpful in reducing postoperative respiratory problems.

Bacteriology

Pre-operative swabs are taken from any fungating lesion but, unless there is established infection, there is no need for routine antibiotic cover.

Understanding and agreement must be obtained from the patient and the treatment team.

Radiotherapy and/or chemotherapy may be given initially with their possible curative effect in mind, or to decrease tumour size and reduce the possibility of recurrence after surgery.

Anaesthesia

Endotracheal intubation is necessary. Hypotensive general anaesthesia helps reduce blood loss and contributes to the speed, accuracy and safety of surgery.

THE OPERATION

In general the classic Berger operation is used and requires a racquet-shaped incision with linear extension parallel to and above the clavicle. This is preferable to and safer than the Littlewood operation because the large vessels are controlled early, reducing blood loss and, in addition, traction on the brachial plexus is minimized.

The posterior approach can be used when there is some doubt of operability and when exploration is deemed necessary before the major vessels and nerves are divided.

ANTERIOR APPROACH (Berger)

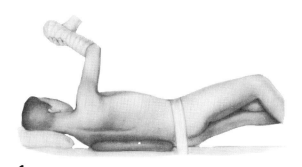

1

Position of patient

The patient is placed on the table on his side with the affected arm uppermost. A low sandbag or support is placed so that the trunk is inclined backwards to facilitate the initial approach to the clavicle and vessels. The affected arm is draped so that it is free and can be held by an assistant when required.

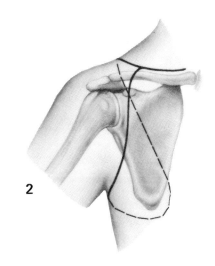

2

The incision

The skin flaps are marked out by drawing a line extending above and parallel to the inner two-thirds of the clavicle, and dividing into an anterior and posterior portion. The anterior incision passes obliquely downwards over the clavicle and coracoid process, then across the middle of the anterior axillary fold and obliquely across the axilla to the inferior angle of the scapula. The posterior portion passes over the outer part of the supraclavicular fossa and downwards across the scapula to its inferior angle. Modifications are made according to the site of the tumour and the state of the surrounding skin of the shoulder.

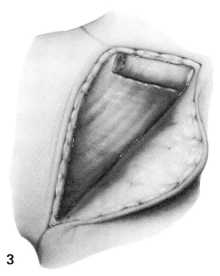

3

Division of clavicle

The supraclavicular incision is made to expose the medial two-thirds of the clavicle. The insertion of the pectoralis major and the outer edge of the sterno-mastoid are divided, using cutting diathermy; and a subperiosteal resection of the middle third of the clavicle is carried out using a Gigli saw. The axillary and subclavian vessels, and the brachial plexus, remain covered by the deep periosteum of the clavicle, axillary and cervical fascia, and the subclavius muscle.

4

Ligation of subclavian vessels and anterior dissection

The pectoralis major is now divided downwards from the clavicular bed to provide a wider exposure of the vessels. The deep periosteum and fascia are divided with care, exposing the axillary vein which is traced proximally to the first rib. Ligation of the suprascapular and cephalic veins will facilitate double ligation of the axillary vein at the level of the first rib. The axillary artery is now exposed, and after ligation of the superior thoracic and acromiothoracic vessels, the subclavian artery is doubly ligated at the level of the first rib. The trunks of the brachial plexus can now be cut across cleanly with the knife. The anterior skin incision is now completed, retracting the flap downwards and medially. The pectoral muscles are removed with the limb, dividing both pectoralis major and minor close to the chest wall. Axillary fat, lymphatics, clavipectoral fascia are dissected downwards and outwards *en bloc*.

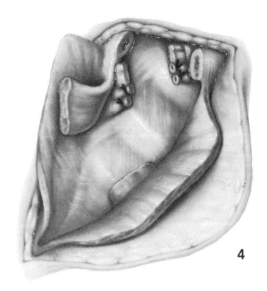

4

5 & 6

Posterior dissection

The posterior incision is made with the affected arm held forwards by an assistant. The suprascapular vessels are ligated. The flap is dissected backwards just posterior to the vertebral border of the scapula. Portions of the trapezius, latissimus dorsi and levator scapulae are resected according to the site and size of the tumour, using cutting diathermy. The rhomboid muscles, major and minor, are divided. By retracting the scapula away from the chest wall, the lower digitations of serratus anterior are divided close to the scapula. Traction on the arm is released and the patient allowed to roll gently backwards again. The arm is now lifted laterally and the upper digitations of serratus anterior and omohyoid are divided with their attached fascia.

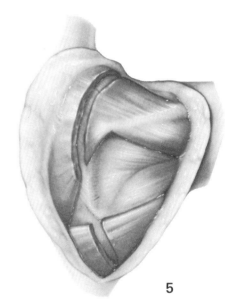

5

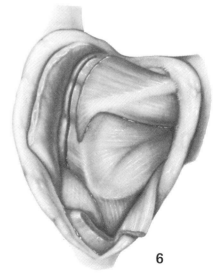

6

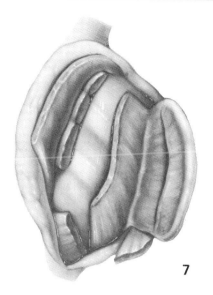

7

7 & 8

The forequarter is now removed and accurate haemostasis achieved. The wound is closed after introducing large suction drains. The skin only is closed using interrupted sutures. The drains are connected to a closed underwater seal drainage bottle and thence to a Roberts' pump. The wound is dressed with gauze, wool and strapping.

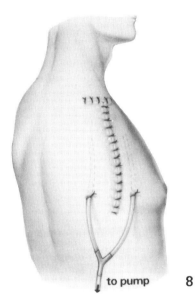

to pump   8

POSTERIOR APPROACH (Littlewood)

This operation involves dividing the same structures as described in the previous operation but in a different sequence. The operation begins with the patient rotated forwards, completing the posterior dissection as described. The upper part of the anterior incision is then made and a subperiosteal resection of the middle third of the clavicle carried out. This allows the quarter to fall away from the trunk, exposing the neurovascular bundle from behind, the limb and shoulder being supported by an assistant to prevent over-traction on the nerves. The trunks of the brachial plexus are divided, followed by ligation of the subclavian artery and vein. The anterior skin flap is then cut and the pectoral muscles are divided. The wound is closed and drained as previously described.

POSTOPERATIVE CARE

The intravenous drip is retained until it is certain that no further blood transfusion is required and all bleeding has stopped. Fluids may be given by mouth when the patient is conscious. Morphine analgesia by intramuscular injection is usually required for the first 48 hr.

Care of the wound

The suction drains are left in place on suction until drainage is less than 50 ml/24 hr and are usually removed about the fifth postoperative day, without removal of the pressure dressing which is left in place for 10 days. Sutures are removed on or about the fourteenth day, depending upon the state of the wound.

Prosthesis

Gross shoulder deformity, in order to support normal clothing, is corrected with a light shoulder piece, the preparation of which can be facilitated by taking a plaster cast before the amputation if the tumour mass permits. An artificial limb is not usually provided, and in cases where patients ask for one they frequently stop using it as the cosmetic appearance of the present prostheses is outweighed by their nuisance value.

[*The illustrations for this Chapter on Forequarter Amputation were drawn by Mr. M. J. Courtney.*]

Hindquarter Amputation

Paul C. Weaver, M.D., F.R.C.S., F.R.C.S.(Ed.)
Consultant Surgeon, Portsmouth and South East Hampshire Group of Hospitals;
Clinical Teacher, University of Southampton

INTRODUCTION

Hindquarter amputation was first carried out by Billroth in 1891 for soft tissue sarcoma; his patient died. The first recorded survival was in 1895 — a patient of Girard. The operation was developed in Britain by Sir Gordon Gordon-Taylor and the technique is based upon descriptions by Gordon-Taylor and Monro (1952) and Westbury (1967). When the amputation is carried out part of the pelvic girdle and the whole lower limb are removed from the body.

PRE-OPERATIVE

Indications

Hindquarter and hip amputations are performed almost exclusively for malignant disease of the bone or soft tissues of the pelvis or thigh (and rarely for malignant melanoma). In the main it is used as an attempt to cure the patient though it can be of value in palliation when pain and massive fungation makes management impossible. This radical surgery is used most frequently following or in association with radiotherapy and/or chemotherapy.

Very occasionally this major procedure is indicated for congenital malformations or chronic infections involving the hip. A few cases of traumatic hindquarter amputation are on record (McLean, 1962). Extended hemipelvectomy in continuity with adherent pelvic visceral cancer is described by Brunschwig (1962).

Contra-indications

(1) The presence of secondary deposits or inability to remove all tumour. (2) The patient's refusal to accept mutilation. (3) Physical or mental unfitness for major surgery.

Pre-operative preparation

Biopsy

Unequivocal microscopic evidence is essential. Care must be taken with a biopsy incision not to encroach upon the skin flaps or the amputation.

Investigations

X-rays and scans are used to help define the limits of the disease and exclude possible metastatic spread. Anaemia should be corrected and 6 units of blood made available though it is seldom necessary to use more than 2 or 3 units.

Bacteriology

Pre-operative swabs are taken from any fungating lesion and from the perineum. The main bacterial worry of high lower limb amputations is contamination with clostridial bacteria from the bowel. Where there is no known allergy intramuscular penicillin is given, starting with the anaesthetic premedication, to protect against this infection. Other antibiotics can be added or held in reserve as the situation merits.

An enema or rectal washout is given prior to surgery to prevent early bowel evacuation and dressing contamination. If iodine is to be used as a skin preparation (it is one of the most effective agents against clostridial contamination), a patch test is worthwhile.

Understanding and agreement must be obtained with the treatment team and the patient. If time permits, arm exercises are started and the patient is introduced to walking aids. The case is discussed with a 'Limb Fitting Surgeon' who can introduce the patient to other similar amputees and demonstrate their prosthetic limbs.

Anaesthesia

Hypotensive anaesthesia sometimes with additional spinal or epidural block helps reduce blood loss and contributes to the speed, accuracy and safety of surgery.

After anaesthetic induction and establishment of an intravenous line, a Foley catheter is passed to empty the bladder and is left in place. The anus is excluded by a small woolpad and sealed round the natal cleft by an adhesive surgical drape.

THE OPERATION

1

Position of patient

The patient is positioned on his back with a long, narrow sandbag under the shoulder and buttock of the affected side. This gives good access to the major, anterior, extraperitoneal part of the dissection and an assistant holding the leg can roll the patient towards the lateral position for the short time needed to cut the posterior flap and muscles.

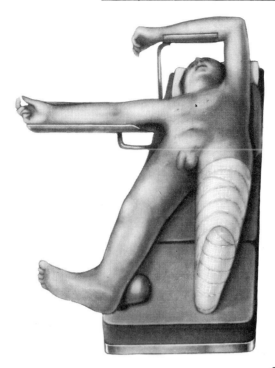

1

2

The incision

The outline of the skin flaps is drawn. The anterior line passes immediately above and parallel to the inguinal ligament. The backwards extent depends upon the proposed site of section of the posterior pelvis. The posterior incision, made later in the operation, curves over the buttock in front of the greater trochanter, across the ischial tuberosity into the crease between the genitals and the thigh. Modifications are made where tumour is close and to avoid skin damaged by radiotherapy or by previous biopsy.

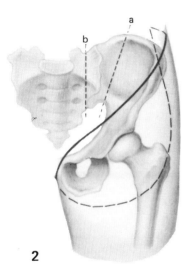

2

3

Exposure of iliac vessels and pubic disarticulation

The anterior incision is made and deepened through the abdominal wall muscles. The peritoneum of the iliac fossa is stripped medially and operability confirmed. The deep epigastric vessels are divided and the spermatic cord is mobilized and pushed medially. The rectus abdominis is cut across just above the pubis. The symphysis is divided at this stage, using a solid scalpel helped by a few blows with the osteotome. Monro's tubercle, the vertical ridge on the posterior aspect of the symphysis, is an invaluable guide to the plane of the articular cartilage.

After dividing the suprapubic ligament, with regard to the underlying membranous urethra, the symphysis opens. A gauze pack controls any venous oozing from this region while attention is turned to the crucial phase of the operation, division of the vascular pedicle of the limb. The peritoneum and ureter are swept medially to expose the iliac bifurcation.

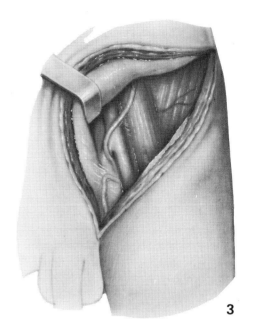

3

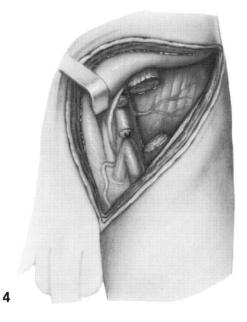

4

4

Ligation of common iliac artery and vein

The common iliac artery is divided between silk ligatures followed by division of the psoas muscle with cutting diathermy. The nerves, femoral, obturator and lateral cutaneous nerve of the thigh (not shown) are cut cleanly with a knife. The ends of the psoas retract revealing the iliolumbar tributaries of the common iliac vein. These branches, between one and four in number, tether the main vein and must be divided carefully between silk ligatures, to permit the safe mobilization and ligation of the common iliac. If this step is omitted, the iliolumbar veins will tear out with the possibility of disastrous haemorrhage.

5a & b

Division of the posterior ilium

The posterior flap is developed, preserving a variable portion of gluteus maximus according to the site of the lesion. The divided vascular pedicle is gently pushed downwards to expose the greater sciatic notch. Both sides of the notch are now exposed and a large artery forceps is passed underneath this to draw through the end of a Gigli saw. The site of the pelvic section depends on the location and nature of the pathology. Division of the posterior part of the ilium involves minimal blood loss; the projecting remnant can be trimmed when the specimen is removed. Where necessary, section can be made through the ala of the sacrum in preference to sacro-iliac disarticulation. The hindquarter is now lifted away from the trunk and the remaining soft structures divided: levator ani, perineal membrane, branches of the internal iliac vessels, sciatic nerve, piriformis, sacrotuberous and sacrospinous ligaments. Bleeding from the veins of the prostatic plexus and cavernous tissue may be troublesome and are best controlled by catgut stitches.

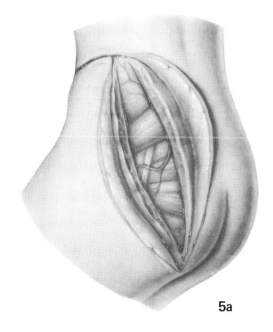

5a

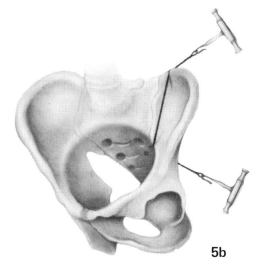

5b

6

Wound closure

The wound is closed with skin sutures only and suction drainage (via underwater seal drainage bottle and a Roberts' pump) applied for 5–6 days. The bladder catheter is removed on the fifth postoperative morning. The wound is supported with gauze wool and strapping.

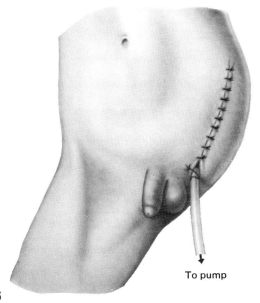

To pump

6

POSTOPERATIVE CARE

General nursing

After the first 24 hr the patient's position is changed 4-hourly. Analgesia is given as frequently as necessary to keep the patient comfortable. Fluids and food can be given by mouth after 24 hr. An orthopaedic lifting chair is provided and active movement encouraged on the third day. Increased mobility is not encouraged until the drains are removed and these should be taken out with as little disturbance as possible to the support dressing, which is untouched for 14 days providing there is no unexplained pyrexia or excessive pain. Sutures are frequently left for 21 days as healing is slower than with most other wounds, particularly after radiotherapy.

After 14 days walking with crutches is started where possible and a wheelchair is provided. After the removal of the sutures the possibility of a prosthesis is reviewed and ordered if necessary.

References

Brunschwig, A. (1962). 'Hemipelvectomy in combination with partial pelvic exenteration for uncontrolled recurrent and metastatic cancer of the cervix, 5 year survival.' *Surgery* **52**, 299

Gordon-Taylor, Sir G. and Monro, R. (1962). 'Technique and management of the hindquarter amputation.' *Br. J. Surg.* **39**, 536

McLean, E. M. (1962). 'Avulsion of the hindquarter.' *J. Bone Jt Surg.* **44B**, 384

Westbury, G. (1967). 'Hindquarter and hip amputation.' *Ann. R. Coll. Surg.* **40**, 226

[*The illustrations for this Chapter on Hindquarter Amputation were drawn by Mr. M. J. Courtney.*]

Disarticulation at the Hip

J. C. Angel, F.R.C.S.
Consultant Orthopaedic Surgeon, Royal National Orthopaedic Hospital,
Stanmore, Middlesex

PRE-OPERATIVE

Indications

The main indication for disarticulation at the hip is malignant disease that cannot safely be dealt with by amputation above the knee. Occasionally it may be called for in severe trauma, vascular disease and infection.

Pre-operative preparation

General anaesthesia is essential. The patient lies supine with the sacrum elevated on a large sandbag.

THE OPERATION

1

The incision

The incision commences just lateral to the anterior superior iliac spine, descends a short distance and then turns medially, running parallel to the inguinal ligament, to reach the medial side of the thigh 5 cm below the root of the limb. Continuing posteriorly, it descends to a level 5 cm below the ischial tuberosity and sweeps in a broad curve 8 cm below the base of the greater trochanter. Thence it ascends to the starting point next to the anterior superior iliac spine.

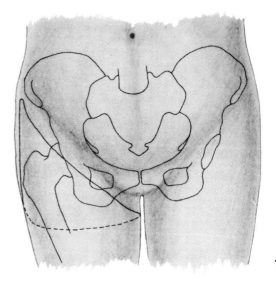

1

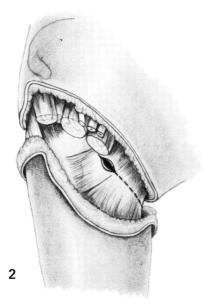

2

Dissection

2

The femoral vessels are exposed and ligated. The femoral nerve is divided. The limb is externally rotated and abducted and the flexors and adductors are divided in the line of the incision.

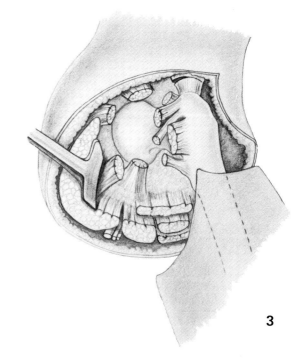

3

3

Next the limb is internally rotated and the gluteus medius and minimus are detached from the greater trochanter. The fascia lata and the distal fibres of gluteus maximus are divided in the line of the skin incision. The tendon of gluteus maximus is released from its attachment to the linea aspera. The sciatic nerve is divided. The short rotators are detached from the region of the greater trochanter and the hip is disarticulated.

4

Subtrochanteric amputation

Alternatively if a subtrochanteric amputation is desired, the skin and muscle flaps can be cut slightly longer and the bone is sectioned below the level of the lesser trochanter. Gluteus medius and minimus and the short rotators can be left intact.

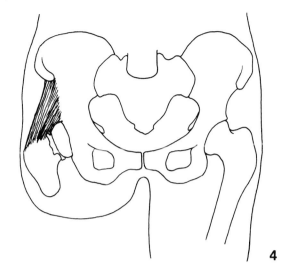

4

5

Closure

The muscle and fascia of the posterior flap is brought anteriorly and sutured to the pectineus and adductor muscles. Two large suction drains are placed under the skin flaps and brought out laterally.

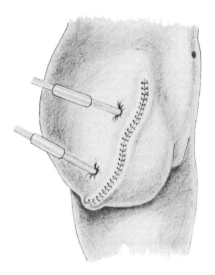

5

POSTOPERATIVE CARE

The wound is dressed and supported with bulky cotton wool and firm crêpe bandaging. The drains are removed after 2 days and the stitches can usually come out at about the fourteenth day.

Prosthetics

The wound is not usually sufficiently mature for a cast to be taken before the end of the first month. The leather or plastic socket is designed to fit snugly round the pelvis, most of the body weight being transmitted through the ischial tuberosity. For this reason it is of vital importance to avoid scars in this area. Of the two types of prosthesis available the conventional limb has certain advantages of lightness and stability but, because the artificial hip projects below the socket, sitting is uncomfortable. The Canadian limb, with its anteriorly placed hip, allows comfortable sitting and a 15° arc of hip movement during walking which provides a more natural gait. It must be remembered that the energy required to use these so called 'tilting table' prostheses greatly exceeds the requirements of crutch-walking so that few elderly people are able to use them.

[*The illustrations for this Chapter on Disarticulation at the Hip were drawn by Mrs. A. Barrett.*]

Amputation above the Knee

J. C. Angel, F.R.C.S.
Consultant Orthopaedic Surgeon, Royal National Orthopaedic Hospital,
Stanmore, Middlesex

PRE-OPERATIVE

Indications

Amputation above the knee is usually the next level to be considered whenever a below-knee amputation is precluded by the nature or extent of the pathological process involved. Occasionally intervening levels such as through-knee or supracondylar amputations, may provide a suitable alternative but the decision to use them must be taken with due regard to prosthetic considerations.

Contra-indications

The operation is contra-indicated in children if it is possible, by any measure, to save the growing lower end of the femur.

Pre-operative preparation

Both hips should be examined for fixed deformity, the presence of which may require a shorter stump to be fashioned in order that the deformity may be accommodated in the socket of the artificial limb. A hip with a very restricted movement in a patient too frail to become a prosthetic user, necessitates an amputation sufficiently high to allow comfortable sitting.

It is re-assuring to have a tourniquet round the root of the limb in case of emergency, although this may not be practicable with a short conical thigh where it might encroach upon the operative area. The buttock is elevated on a sandbag.

Operating from the opposite side of the table will give improved access and facilitate elevation of the stump throughout the operation.

THE OPERATION

MYOPLASTIC ABOVE-KNEE AMPUTATION

1

The incision

Equal anterior and posterior flaps are marked, their bases being level with the proposed bone section. Their combined lengths should slightly exceed the diameter of the thigh and they should be well rounded in shape rather than pointed. The position of the flaps may have to be adjusted to take account of the scars of previous surgery.

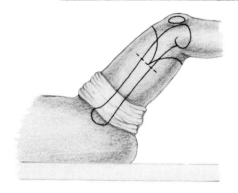

2

Dissection

The incision is taken down to deep fascia allowing the skin to retract slightly. From the level to which the skin flaps have retracted the muscle is divided with a raking cut that meets the bone precisely at the level of section. The femoral vessels are encountered beneath the sartorius muscle and these should be divided between clamps and doubly ligated with 1/0 Dexon. The deeper posterior muscles and the profunda vessels are conveniently dealt with after cutting the bone.

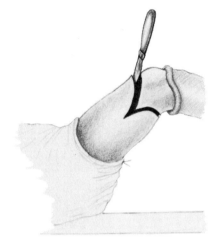

3 & 4

Bone section

The precise level (*see* page 303) is measured from the distal aspect of the lateral femoral condyle which is easily palpated in the flexed knee. The periosteum is divided circumferentially at the same point in order to prevent it from being stripped, and the bone is divided with a Gigli saw. A bone hook is inserted in the distal femur and used to apply traction while the profunda vessels are sought and ligated in the tissues immediately posterior to the bone. The sciatic nerve is gently pulled down and its epineurium is held with forceps while the arteria nervi ischiadii is caught and ligated with fine catgut. The remaining musculature is divided, allowing the amputated limb to be removed. Haemostasis is secured. The cut end of the femur is rounded with a rasp and a slight bevel is produced over the anterolateral aspect.

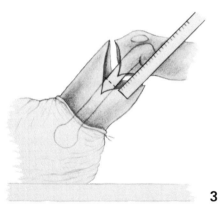

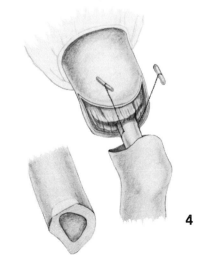

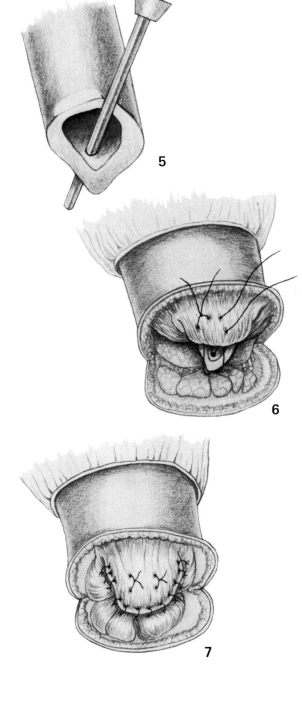

5, 6 & 7

Myodesis

A small hole is drilled through the posterior cortex of the femur. Two mattress sutures of 1/0 Dexon are passed through it and used to anchor the quadriceps over the end of the bone. The remaining muscles are sutured to the quadriceps. The aim is to have each muscle group under slight tension with the hip in the neutral position and to achieve this a secondary trimming of the muscles may be necessary.

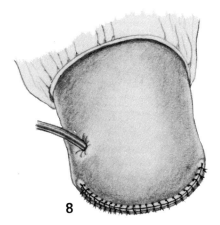

8

Closure

A suction drain is inserted under the skin flaps and brought out on the lateral side of the thigh. The skin is closed with interrupted sutures.

POSTOPERATIVE CARE

Gauze is placed along the incision and a firm pressure dressing is applied using sterile orthopaedic wool and 6 inch (15 cm) crêpe bandage. This can be held in place either by means of adhesive strapping or by wrapping two turns of bandage around the waist. The drain is removed after 2 days and the patient is then encouraged to be as mobile as possible. Prone lying for 15 min twice a day prevents the development of a flexion-contracture of the hip. Even after the wound has healed the stump must be bandaged to prepare it for limb fitting. It is important that the bandage should apply a gradient of pressure that decreases proximally, and extends right to the root of the limb.

Prosthetics

Provided wound healing is by primary intention the dimensions of the stump usually stabilize sufficiently by the third or fourth week to allow the fitting of a temporary limb or pylon. Measurements for the definitive limb are usually taken between the sixth and twelfth week.

Suction Socket and Stabilized Knee

Simple Socket and Semi-Automatic Knee Lock

13·5cm

6·2cm

9

Most above-knee amputees of both sexes, up to the age of fifty, have the strength and agility to take advantage of a limb fitted with a stabilized knee mechanism, which prevents the joint from buckling when the weight is applied in a bent position, and a suction socket. To don the latter the amputee must stand on his sound leg and draw down his stump. Such refinements necessitate the removal of 13·5 cm of bone from the distal end of the femur. Insufficient clearance will make it necessary either to lower the centre of the artificial knee, which is undesirable from the cosmetic point of view, or to modify the prosthetic prescription.

Older people require less sophisticated mechanisms, generally preferring the security of a fixed knee. Less clearance is needed and so a longer stump can be fashioned. This point is illustrated in the accompanying diagram in which it must be stressed that the minimum amount of clearance has been shown. A little extra room for the knee mechanism eases the task of the prosthetist.

Notes

(*1*) The depth of the soft tissue distal to the end of the bone is determined by the thickness of the subcutaneous layer and the myoplastic technique.

(*2*) The prolonged use of a suction socket tends to draw down and increase the length of the soft tissues.

(*3*) The axis of the artificial knee is set at the level of the contralateral joint line.

[The illustrations for this Chapter on Amputation above the Knee were drawn by Mrs. A. Barrett.]

Disarticulation at the Knee

J. C. Angel, F.R.C.S.
Consultant Orthopaedic Surgeon, Royal National Orthopaedic Hospital,
Stanmore, Middlesex

PRE-OPERATIVE

Disarticulation at the knee has advantages and disadvantages compared with amputation above the knee. It provides a robust stump that may be capable of full end-bearing. In some cases it is possible to suspend the prosthesis on the protuberant femoral condyles doing away with the need for a waistband. However, healing is not as reliable, the jointed side-steels of the prosthesis are uncosmetic and it is difficult to fit control mechanisms for either the swing or stance phase of gait.

Indications

It is indicated in geriatric patients who are expected to require a locked knee prosthesis and for whom function is very much more important than cosmesis. Its terminal load-carrying properties are useful where there is scarring at the root of the limb, particularly in the region of the ischial tuberosity where weight is normally borne in the above-knee amputee. It is also useful in very ill patients as it can be performed very rapidly, if necessary, under infiltration anaesthesia.

Contra-indications

The operation should not be performed in a patient who could subsequently benefit by being fitted with a free knee and appropriate controlling mechanisms. It is rarely indicated in peripheral vascular disease as the small extra risks of a below-knee amputation are amply justified by the potential rewards. Where a below-knee amputation has failed in atherosclerosis a through-knee disarticulation is unlikely to do any better.

Pre-operative preparation

General anaesthesia is preferred although epidural anaesthesia is an alternative. If a tourniquet is used it should be inflated with the knee flexed to 90°. The operation is most easily performed in the prone position unless there is a hip flexion-contracture.

304

THE OPERATION

THROUGH-KNEE AMPUTATION USING LATERAL FLAPS

1

The incision

From a point mid-way between the lower pole of the patella and the tibial tubercle, the lateral incision is curved downwards to mark a flap that extends 5 cm below the joint line. The line then curves proximally to a point in the mid-line of the popliteal fossa 2·5 cm above the joint line with the knee extended. The medial flap needs to be 2 cm longer to cover the larger medial femoral condyle.

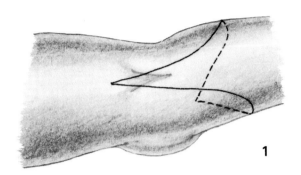

2

Deep tissues

The incisions are carried down through skin, sub-cutaneous tissue and fascia and the flaps are raised, keeping close to bone. The patellar tendon is dissected off the tibial tubercle. The medial and lateral hamstrings are divided close to their insertions. The main vessels are sought and ligated. The medial and lateral popliteal nerves are divided and the gastrocnemius is sectioned close to its origin. The joint capsule is dissected from the tibia and the knee joint is entered on the under-surface of the menisci. The cruciates are divided and the limb is finally severed by dividing the popliteus tendon close to the femur. Haemostasis is secured after releasing the tourniquet.

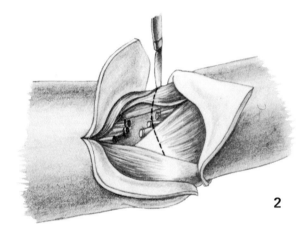

3 & 4

Closure

Next the patellar tendon is sutured to the cruciate ligaments with thick 2/0 nylon mattress sutures and the retinaculae either side of the tendon are stitched to the hamstrings. The menisci should be removed if there is a particular risk of sepsis but otherwise they may assist in covering the femoral condyle. As with any disarticulation the patient's comfort depends on what measure of success the surgeon has in cushioning the articular surface with soft tissue.

A suction drain is passed out laterally through the skin proximal to the level of the wound and the skin is closed with interrupted sutures.

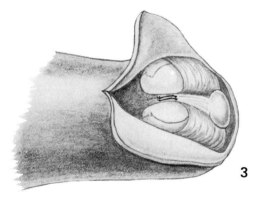

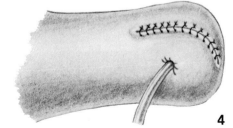

POSTOPERATIVE CARE

The wound is then covered with gauze and the stump is bandaged with orthopaedic wool. The patient is returned to the supine position and a snug-fitting plaster is applied to the stump and firmly moulded just above the femoral condyles in order to prevent it from slipping distally. The suction drain projects from the top of the cast in such a way that it can be easily withdrawn after 48 hr without disturbing any part of the dressing.

Prosthetics

The prosthesis has a moulded leather thigh corset. It can be provided with a tuber-bearing seat if required.

[*The illustrations for this Chapter on Disarticulation at the Knee were drawn by Mrs. A. Barrett.*]

The Gritti-Stokes Amputation

J. C. Angel, F.R.C.S.
Consultant Orthopaedic Surgeon, Royal National Orthopaedic Hospital,
Stanmore, Middlesex

PRE-OPERATIVE

Indications

In the Gritti-Stokes amputation the femur is sectioned immediately proximal to the femoral condyles, the cut end of the bone being capped with the anterior half of the patella. It heals well from the point of view of the skin wound although some series have reported a high incidence of non-union of the patella. The operation produces a long strong stump that is suitable for elderly patients who are too frail to graduate from a light pylon to an artificial limb. It is also of value in the bilateral amputee and the patient who is confined to bed or a wheelchair.

Contra-indications

Apart from being contra-indicated in potential prosthesis users the operation should also be avoided in the presence of a hip flexion contracture because of the long stump, in severe osteoporosis because of the need for internal bony fixation and in infection because of the presence of foreign material buried in the stump.

Pre-operative preparation

General anaesthesia is preferred although an epidural anaesthetic may be a suitable alternative. A tourniquet should be applied to the root of the limb and inflated after the final skin preparation.

THE OPERATION

1

The incision

The centre point of each femoral condyle is marked, as is the centre of the tibial tubercle. The anterior incision is elliptical and passes through these three points. The posterior incision is a straight line joining the centre point of each condyle.

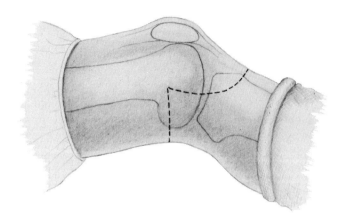

1

2

Skin flaps

An anterior flap only is raised and the anterior incision is made down to bone with one bold sweep. Consisting of skin, fascia, patellar ligament and capsule of knee joint, it is reflected upwards taking the patella with it thus exposing the knee joint and the anterior surface of the femoral shaft.

The posterior incision should be made down to and including the deep fascia overlying the hamstrings. No flap is raised.

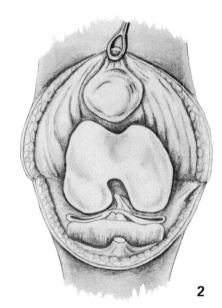

2

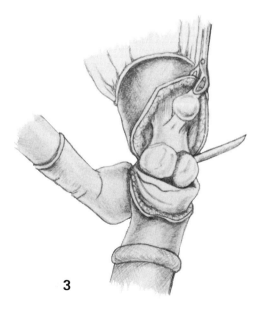

3

3

Division of soft tissues and femur

The soft tissues behind the femur are divided with one sweep of the amputation knife at the level of the posterior skin incision. The main vessels should be secured individually with 1/0 Dexon after preliminary dissection. If a tourniquet has been employed it should be released at this stage and haemostasis secured. The femur is divided with an oscillating saw immediately above the condyles. The site should be selected so that the cut end of the femur is slightly larger than the proposed cut surface of the patella.

4

Preparation of the patella

The articular surface of the patella is removed with an oscillating saw. For this purpose the soft tissues surrounding the patella should be grasped firmly in a large swab in order to hold the patella steady. A smooth flat surface should be left at this stage, which is the most difficult part of the operation.

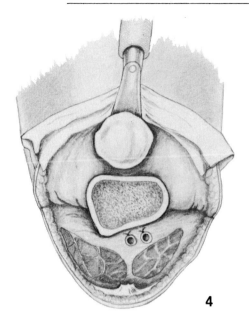

4

5

Attachment of patella to femur

A hole is drilled transversely across the patella, two-thirds of the way down its length. Two more are drilled obliquely from the cut surface of the femur out to the posterior aspect. A length of 20-gauge stainless steel wire is passed through the holes and used to fix the patella firmly on the femur. A proper fix cannot be obtained without the use of wire tighteners. The twisted ends are cut off and buried in the femur with a punch.

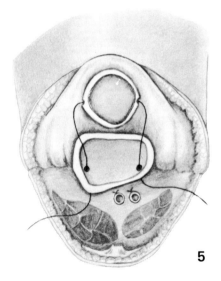

5

6

Closure of wound

A suction drain is passed through the substance of vastus lateralis and out through the skin on the lateral side of the thigh. The quadriceps expansion and the capsule of the knee joint are then sutured to the deep fascia of the posterior compartment of the thigh with interrupted sutures of 1/0 Dexon. No subcutaneous fat sutures should be used. The skin is closed with fine interrupted sutures.

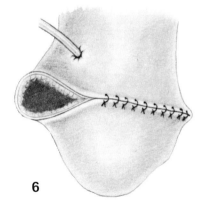

6

POSTOPERATIVE CARE

A dry dressing is applied to the wound and the stump is wrapped in wool and bandaged. To ensure that the dressing is not displaced it is attached to the skin of the thigh with long pieces of strapping, one extending from the anterior aspect of the thigh and abdomen over the end of the stump and upwards to the skin of the posterior thigh and buttock and the other from the medial aspect of the thigh in the groin, round the end of the stump and upwards over the lateral aspect. The dressing should not be disturbed until the removal of sutures unless a haematoma or infection is suspected.

Prosthetics

The length of the Gritti-Stokes stump is such that if it is fitted with a definitive artificial limb the knee centre has to be lowered by 2·5 inches (7 cm). This represents a considerable cosmetic disadvantage although there may be instances where it is offset by the improved function of the stump compared with the above-knee level. Many elderly patients are too frail to graduate from a light pylon to a definitive artificial limb and for them the extra stump length presents no problem.

For those who are unable to walk at all the stump offers improved sitting balance and better mobility in bed.

[*The illustrations for this Chapter on The Gritti-Stokes Amputation were drawn by Mrs. A. Barrett.*]

Amputation below the Knee

J. C. Angel, F.R.C.S.
Consultant Orthopaedic Surgeon, Royal National Orthopaedic Hospital,
Stanmore, Middlesex

PRE - OPERATIVE

Indications

Amputation below the knee is indicated in peripheral vascular disease, trauma, chronic infection and certain deformities. In these conditions the long posterior flap operation is generally suitable. Below-knee amputation is also indicated for severe acute infection and tumours but here equal flaps are normally preferred.

Contra-indications

The operation is generally contra-indicated if other disorders of the locomotor or nervous system preclude the future use of a prosthesis, if the resulting tibial stump is less than 5 cm long, if there is an uncorrectable flexion deformity of more than 30° or if the range of knee movement is severely restricted.

Pre-operative preparation

If the foot is grossly contaminated it should be sealed inside a polythene bag.

General anaesthesia is preferred but where this is not suitable epidural anaesthesia can be used.

The performance of the operation is greatly simplified by the use of a tourniquet, although it is usually avoided in peripheral vascular disease.

Once the skin has been prepared and the area draped, the limb should be supported on an inverted bowl placed under the proximal third of the leg.

THE OPERATIONS

THE LONG POSTERIOR FLAP BELOW-KNEE AMPUTATION

1

The incision

The anterior flap is marked by the anterior two-thirds of the circumference of the limb at a level 14 cm from the knee joint line. This is also the level of bone section. The edges of the posterior flap curve forwards slightly and then descend distally to be connected by a posterior incision. The posterior flap is essentially rectangular and fashioned initially too long so that it can be accurately trimmed later. A common error is to inadvertently taper the sides.

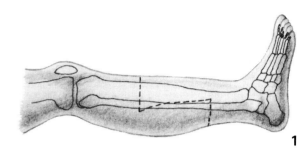

1

2

Dividing the bones

The lateral incisions are deepened to include the deep fascia. The anterior incision is taken cleanly down to bone and interosseous membrane, ligating the anterior vessels on the way. The periosteum on the front of the tibia is raised proximally for a short distance and a Gigli saw is used to divide the tibia. During the last half of the cut the handles are gradually angled towards the knee so as to produce a bevel. The fibula is also conveniently divided at the same level bearing in mind that a further 15 mm require to be trimmed at a later stage.

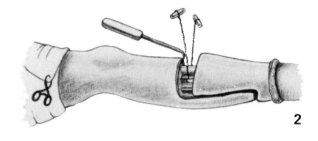

2

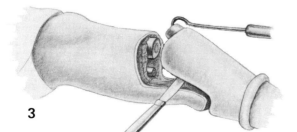

3

3

Removal of the limb

A bone hook, inserted into the cut end of the tibia, is used to apply traction to the distal part of the limb. The deep muscles of the calf are sectioned at the same level as the tibia and the posterior tibial and peroneal vessels are ligated and the posterior tibial nerve is divided. A long raking cut is then made through the soleus and gastrocnemius muscles with Syme's amputation knife. It emerges from the muscle at the level of the musculotendinous junction, finally severing the limb.

4

Shaping the bone

The distal end of the tibia is sculptured with an osteotome and then a rasp. The fibula is cut cleanly with either a Gigli saw or an oscillating saw and bevelled laterally. Usually a bone nibbler is convenient for this purpose.

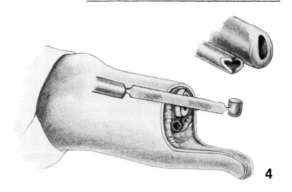

4

5

Trimming the muscle

The gastrocnemius is held up under slight tension and cut level with the deep fascia and periosteum of the anterior flap. Further trimming of the sides of the long muscle flap and the peronei may be required to give the stump a rounded, non-bulbous shape.

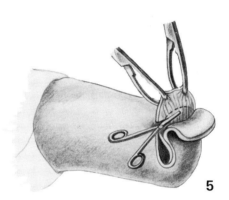

5

6

Trimming the skin and closure

The tourniquet is released and the bleeding controlled. A suction drain is passed up in the peroneal compartment and brought out through the skin some 8 cm above the wound. The deep fascial-periosteal layer is closed with Dexon sutures. The skin of the posterior flap is laid over the front of the shin and trimmed level with the opposing skin edge. Skin closure is performed with a fine material using interrupted sutures.

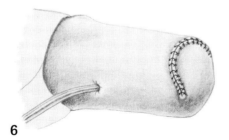

6

BELOW-KNEE AMPUTATION WITH EQUAL ANTERIOR AND POSTERIOR FLAPS

7

The incision

Equal anterior and posterior flaps are marked with their bases 14 cm below the joint line and their lengths half the diameter of the limb. The skin flaps are taken down to include the deep fascia and are raised to the level of the apex of the incisions. The deep fascia is incised as a continuous layer to include the periosteum of the tibia as it merges with it. The periosteum is stripped with a rugine and the combined layer of periosteum and deep fascia is raised off the bone to the point where it is proposed that the bone will be divided.

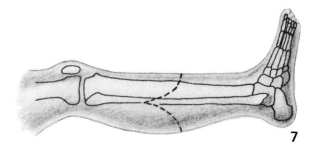

7

8

Deep tissues

The muscles are divided to allow them to retract to the level of bone section. The bones, vessels and nerves are handled in much the same way as for the long posterior flap operation.

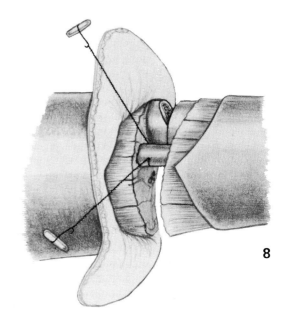

8

9

9

Closure

The deep fascia is sutured with interrupted catgut or Dexon and the skin is closed with interrupted sutures.

POSTOPERATIVE CARE
10

The rigid plaster dressing

Dry gauze is placed over the wound and the limb is bandaged up to mid-thigh with sterile plaster wool. A 10 cm wide crêpe bandage is wrapped over the end of the stump. Plaster can be prevented from soaking into the bandage by covering it with a thin layer of wool; this greatly facilitates removal at a later date. A snug-fitting plaster cast is then applied to mid-thigh level. As it is setting it is firmly moulded just proximal to the femoral condyles in order to provide suspension. The drain emerges at the top of the cast underneath the wool.

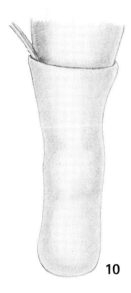

10

The patient should remain in bed for the first 48 hr with the stump elevated on pillows. At the end of this time the drain is pulled out and progressive mobilization is commenced. The cast need not be disturbed for 14 days unless the development of pain, discharge or pyrexia indicate a need to look at the wound. If, at the end of this time the wound appears to be healing satisfactorily plans can be made to construct some form of temporary walking device. The precise nature of this will depend on the expertise and facilities available. It should be as near to the patellar tendon-bearing principle as possible as this will give the maximum stimulus to the quadriceps and shape the stump. If there is delay in wound healing or the patient has not reached the stage of independence with crutches, hopping on the sound limb, it is likely that an ischial-bearing pylon with a thigh corset will be required.

The stitches can be removed at 2 weeks except in the case of peripheral vascular disease when they may need to remain for up to 4 weeks.

Once out of the rigid dressing, the stump should be bandaged until its shape has become stable. Great care must be taken to ensure that a full range of hip and knee flexion is maintained.

Prosthetics

The below-knee stump provides proprioception and good control over the position of the foot, something that is denied the above-knee amputee. From the functional point of view, the difference between the below-knee amputation and the above-knee is as great as that between having an intact limb and a below-knee amputation.

The below-knee stump is usually fitted with a patellar tendon-bearing prosthesis. The walls of the snug-fitting socket are made so as to direct pressure to those areas that are best able to withstand it such as the lower pole of the patella, the medial tibial condyle and the popliteal fossa. The prosthesis is suspended by a leather cuff that grips the femoral condyles.

Another type of prosthesis is available for those engaged in heavy manual labour on rough ground, those who need to kneel to do their work and for patients with unstable knees. This consists of a thigh corset which receives most of the body weight from the inverted cone of the thigh, jointed side steels and a below-knee socket that plays a relatively small part in load transmission although it is important in detecting and controlling the position of the foot.

[The illustrations for this Chapter on Amputation below the Knee were drawn by Mrs. A. Barrett.]

Syme's Amputation

J. C. Angel, F.R.C.S.
Consultant Orthopaedic Surgeon, Royal National Orthopaedic Hospital, Stanmore, Middlesex

PRE - OPERATIVE

Syme's amputation produces a stump with end-bearing properties and good proprioception. It allows ambulation with a lower energy consumption. Some patients are able to walk without a prosthesis. These points add up to a clear functional advantage over the below-knee amputation.

Indications

It is indicated in trauma, diabetes, other vascular disorders involving the distal vascular tree and congenital deformities associated with gross shortening.

Contra-indications

These include ulceration of the heel and atherosclerosis (except in cases of residual forefoot gangrene after the relief of a proximal arterial block). For cosmetic reasons it is not generally suitable for women.

Pre-operative preparation

The operation is performed with the patient supine. A sandbag is placed under the mid-calf.

THE OPERATION

1a & b

The incision

Two points are marked; one at the tip of the lateral malleolus and the other 2 cm below the tip of the medial malleolus. They mark the junction of a plantar incision, which runs in a plane perpendicular to the sole of the foot, and an anterior incision that takes the shortest distance across the front of the ankle.

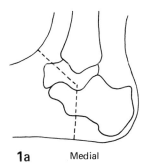 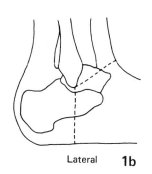

1a   Medial   Lateral   **1b**

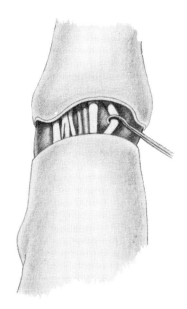

2

2

The extensor tendons

The plantar incision is deepened directly down to bone. Anteriorly, the extensor retinaculum is divided transversely. The extensor tendons are each pulled down and divided as high as possible. The distal stumps of the tendons are also cut off to prevent them from getting in the way. The ankle joint is then entered through the anterior capsule and the medial and lateral ligaments divided from within.

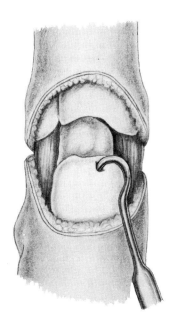

3

3

Dissecting off the heel pad

Attention is then turned to the posterior flap. Subperiosteal dissection of the os calcis is begun and continued posteriorly as far as it comfortably can be. Returning to the dorsal incision, the posterior capsule of the ankle is divided and the dorsal surface of the os calcis is exposed, taking care to keep close to bone. This part of the dissection can be facilitated by drawing the tarsus forward with a bone hook driven first into the dome of the talus and then into the back of the os calcis. As the posterior pole is approached the heel pad is gradually dissected off the bone by working from the sides and from above and below in a systematic manner. After removing the foot the malleoli are cleared of soft tissue.

4

Bone section

Next the medial and lateral plantar and the anterior tibial vascular bundles are ligated, the tourniquet is released and the bleeding is controlled. The nerves are pulled down a short distance and cut. A tenon saw is used to cut off the malleoli and the distal end of the tibia. Great care is taken to ensure that the plane of section is at right-angles to the long axis of the tibia. The level is such as to just remove all the articular cartilage. The cut edges are lightly smoothed with a file.

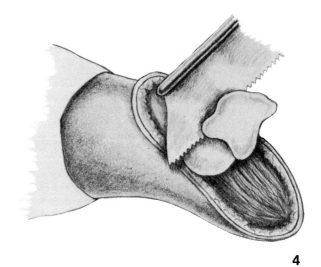

4

5

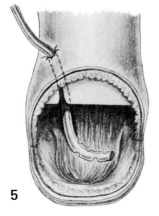

5

Preparing the flaps

The tendons are pulled down and divided as high as possible. The flap is fitted and if necessary raked slightly to allow the skin edges to meet easily. Loose pedicles of fibrous tissue are trimmed. The remaining muscle fibres in the heel pad are left as intact as possible. A suction drain is driven up behind the inferior tibiofibular joint and brought out on the posterolateral aspect of the leg 3 inches (7·5 cm) above the level of the wound.

6

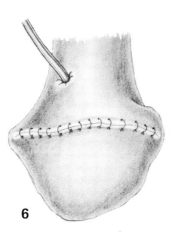

6

Closure

The plantar fascia is sutured to the soft tissue on the front of the tibia with absorbable sutures making sure that the heel pad is located centrally on the cut surface of the bone. Skin closure must be meticulous despite the difference in thickness in the two flaps. The wound is dressed and bandaged in such a way as to avoid undue pressure on the protuberant corners of the wound.

POSTOPERATIVE CARE

The drain is removed after 48 hr. At 7 days the stump is wrapped in a plaster cast moulded to maintain the correct position of the heel pad. In the third week a rocker can be added to the bottom of the cast to allow weight-bearing. The heel pad is vulnerable to displacement during the first 6 weeks. Vigilance and correct cast-management are necessary to prevent this.

The Syme's prosthesis, in accommodating the bulb of the stump, usually has an unsightly appearance. The exceptions to this occur in those cases of congenital deformity where the overall shortening allows the bulb to be accommodated in the calf of the prosthesis. An artificial limb with side-steels and a leather lace-up corset is durable and also capable of off-loading some of the weight from the end of the stump. However, a better cosmetic appearance and ease of donning and doffing is provided by another type of prosthesis with an enclosed plastic socket and an inner liner.

TWO-STAGE SYME'S AMPUTATION

7

The two-stage Syme's amputation has proved successful in the management of diabetes (Wagner *et al.*, 1973). The first stage, which can be undertaken even in the presence of gross sepsis, is a simple disarticulation through the ankle. The second stage performed about 6 weeks later removes the malleoli and also part of the malleolar flares. It is performed through elliptical incisions on either side of the ankle.

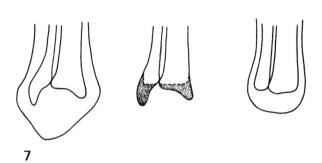

7

Reference

Wagner, F. W., Brodie, I., Mooney, V. and Nickel, V. L. (1973). 'Syme's amputation done in 2 stages.' *J. Bone Jt Surg.* **55A**, 1970

[*The illustrations for this Chapter on Syme's Amputation were drawn by Mrs. A. Barrett.*]

Transmetatarsal Amputation

J. C. Angel, F.R.C.S.
Consultant Orthopaedic Surgeon, Royal National Orthopaedic Hospital,
Stanmore, Middlesex

PRE- OPERATIVE

Indications

Transmetatarsal amputation is indicated for severe trauma involving the toes and forefoot. It is important that there should be sufficient plantar skin to turn up over the cut ends of the metatarsal shafts. Occasionally it is indicated in diabetes mellitus.

Contra-indications

The operation should not be performed for gangrene if the major cause is a proximal arterial block.

Pre-operative preparation

Local infection should be controlled as far as possible. In the case of frostbite, ample time should be allowed for a line of demarcation to appear. A pneumatic tourniquet is applied to the root of the leg and a sandbag placed under the right buttock helps to control the position of the foot. The operator sits at the end of the table.

THE OPERATION
1 & 2

The incision

The dorsal incision commences mid-way between the dorsal and plantar surfaces of the foot and passes convexly across the dorsum, just distal to the anticipated level of bone section. The plantar incision fashions a longer flap that extends parallel to the flexion crease of the toes and, ideally, 1 cm proximal to it. The plantar flap has to be slightly longer medially in order to cover the greater thickness of the foot on this side.

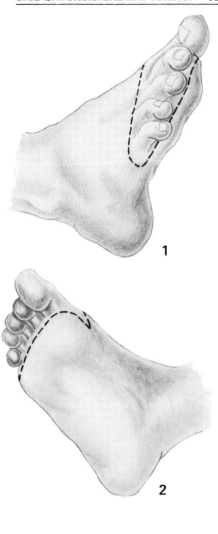

1

2

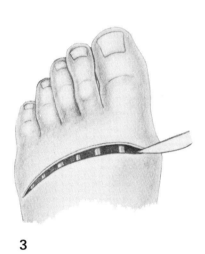

3

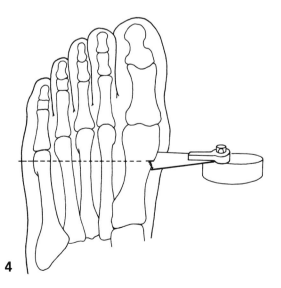

4

3 & 4

Dissection and bone section

The plantar incision is carried down to bone and a short flap is raised back to the level of bone section. The dorsal incision is made down to bone, but no attempt to raise a flap is made. Using a power saw, the metatarsal bones are divided at a level suitable for closure of the flaps. The section is made parallel to the tarsometatarsal joints but the fifth metatarsal bone is shortened and the outer side bevelled.

5

Cutting of extensor and flexor tendons

The extensor and flexor tendons are grasped with forceps, pulled down and cut short with scissors.

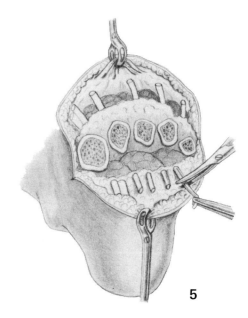

5

6

Closure

The deep fascia is sutured with interrupted catgut sutures and the skin closed with nylon. No drains should be used.

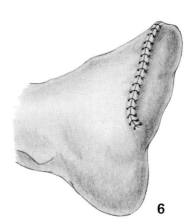

6

POSTOPERATIVE CARE

The postoperative care is the same as for a ray resection (*see* page 327).

[*The illustrations for this Chapter on Transmetatarsal Amputation were drawn by Mrs. A. Barrett.*]

Ray Resections in the Foot

J. C. Angel, F.R.C.S.
Consultant Orthopaedic Surgeon, Royal National Orthopaedic Hospital,
Stanmore, Middlesex

PRE-OPERATIVE

Indications

Ray resections in the foot are indicated when small-vessel disease has caused gangrene that has spread almost to the web of the affected digit. The operations are also useful in the management of diabetes complicated by the sequence of perforating ulcer leading to septic arthritis, digital artery involvement and gangrene of the distal part of the toe. They are contra-indicated in the absence of a vigorous inflammatory reaction at the line of demarcation, healing being dependent on a fairly good blood supply.

Pre-operative preparation

Diabetes should be stabilized as far as is possible in the presence of infection. Surgery should be performed under antibiotic cover, the choice of drug being dependent on prior sensitivity studies.

Because the extent of necrosis in the deep tissues can only be determined during the course of the operation it is wise to obtain consent for more extensive procedures should these prove necessary.

An adequate debridement is helped by the use of a tourniquet. In the case of lateral resections, a sandbag placed under the ipsilateral buttock helps to control the position of the foot.

THE OPERATIONS

RESECTION OF SECOND, THIRD OR FOURTH RAY

1

The incision

A circular incision is made around the dorsal aspect of the affected toe and the two cuts of the incision gradually converge on the plantar surface of the foot to meet at about the centre. The incision is then extended backwards almost to the heel.

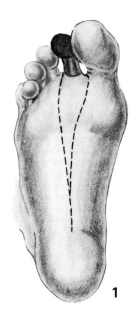

2

Division of metatarsal ligaments

The incisions are deepened down to the metatarsal arch on either side of the affected toe and metatarsal bone. The toe is then grasped firmly with one hand and the ligaments connecting the metatarsal head to the adjacent metatarsals are divided. The soft tissues on either side of the metatarsal bone are divided, isolating the long and short flexor tendons of the affected toe.

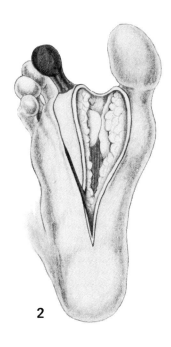

3

Metatarsal bone disarticulated

The base of the metatarsal bone is then disarticulated with a sharp scalpel so that with a few cuts the entire toe and metatarsal with its accompanying flexor tendons, the lumbrical muscle and interosseous muscle origins are removed. At this point a meticulous search is made for necrotic and infected material. The tourniquet is then released, allowing poorly vascularized areas to be identified and further trimmed back.

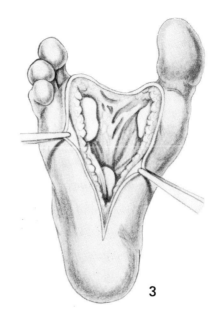

3

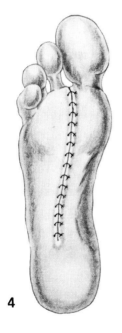

4

4

Wound closure

All bleeding points are carefully secured. Haemorrhage may be brisk from vessels in the plantar arch or one of the metatarsal arches and they should be ligated with fine absorbable material. The soft tissues may then be drawn together with a few interrupted catgut mattress sutures. The skin is closed with interrupted nylon or silk sutures leaving a narrow foot. Exact skin apposition is essential and no drain should be used.

RESECTION OF FOURTH AND FIFTH RAYS TOGETHER

5

The incision

The incisions start in the cleft between the third and fourth toes and pass obliquely across the dorsum and plantar aspects of the foot to meet on the lateral border at the prominence indicated by the base of the fifth metatarsal bone. The incision across the sole of the foot is more laterally placed than that on the dorsum.

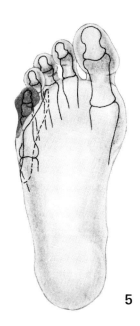

5

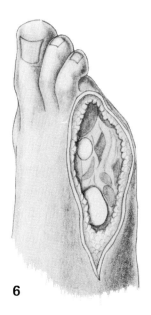

6

6

Disarticulation

The incisions are deepened down to bone and the head of the fourth metatarsal is disconnected from its attachments to the third metatarsal head. The soft tissues between the third and fourth metatarsal bones are then divided, care being taken not to damage the plantar arch, but only to divide its metatarsal branches. The base of the fifth and fourth metatarsal bones are then disarticulated from the cuboid bone and the side of the third cuneiform and metatarsal. All bleeding points are carefully secured and ligated.

7

Skin sutures

The skin is then closed with interrupted nylon sutures to leave a dorsal scar. No drain is necessary.

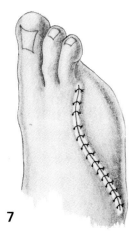

7

POSTOPERATIVE CARE

Gauze is applied to the wound and the foot is wrapped in sterile orthopaedic wool and a 4 inch (10 cm) crêpe bandage. The surgeon should be alert to the possible development of skin flap necrosis and infection, both of which are common complications of these procedures. If all is well after several days, a below-knee walking cast should be applied and the patient allowed to take progressively more weight on the amputated limb. After the removal of the sutures during the third week the plaster can be exchanged for footwear that incorporates a deep moulded Plastazote insole designed to distribute pressure as evenly as possible over the remaining part of the foot. The patient who has a peripheral neuropathy should be made aware of the lifelong risk of pressure ulceration occurring beneath the remaining metatarsal heads.

[*The illustrations for this Chapter on Ray Resections in the Foot were drawn by Mrs. A. Barrett.*]

Amputation of the Lesser Toes

J. C. Angel, F.R.C.S.
Consultant Orthopaedic Surgeon, Royal National Orthopaedic Hospital,
Stanmore, Middlesex

PRE-OPERATIVE

Indications

One or more of the lesser toes may need to be amputated for diabetic gangrene, deformity, severe bony infection, and trauma including frostbite.

Collectively the lesser toes are important in running and in balancing in the squatting position. Individually they are of minimal biomechanical importance but single toes cannot be amputated with impunity because of the tendency for secondary deformities to develop. Amputation of the second toe very commonly leads to the development of hallux valgus despite efforts to fill the gap with a toe spacer. Removal of the fifth toe leaves the fifth metatarsal head exposed to mechanical trauma and predisposes to the formation of a tender bursa. Partial amputation of the lesser toes is often followed by a deformity in the remaining stump: hammer toe developing in a middle phalanx amputation and an extension deformity of the metatarsophalangeal joint developing in amputations through the proximal phalanx. These deformities can, of course, be dealt with as they arise and, particularly in the case of the second toe, it may be preferable to do this rather than remove the whole toe.

An amputation through the base of the proximal phalanx has the advantage of leaving a small wound cavity that heals rapidly and also it causes the least interference with the metatarsal ligaments. The base of the phalanx, should it become deformed, is too short to cause any problems.

THE OPERATION

1

The incision

For this operation a racquet incision is made. In the second, third and fourth toes the handle of the racquet is placed in the middle line of the dorsum of the toe at least 1 inch (2·5 cm) proximal to the web, enabling the blade of the racquet to encircle the toe just distal to the web. In the case of the little toe the handle of the racquet is placed nearer the mid-line of the foot so that the scar is out of the way of pressure from the shoe.

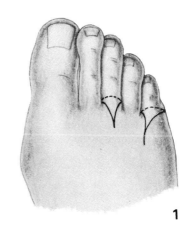

1

2 & 3

Dissection

The flaps are taken straight down to bone and then dissected off the proximal phalanx. Where possible the base of the phalanx is preserved and the bone is divided just distal to the capsular insertion. Otherwise a disarticulation is performed with care being taken to divide the capsule of the metatarsophalangeal joint as distally as possible in order to retain the transverse metatarsal ligaments.

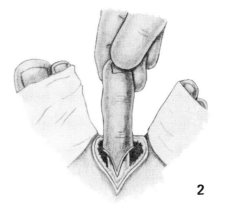

2

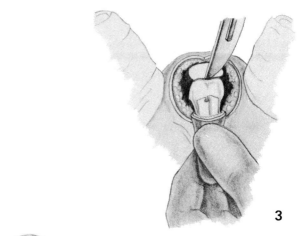

3

4

Closure

Haemostasis is secured. The wound edges should be sutured only if the case is clean.

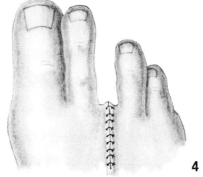

4

POSTOPERATIVE CARE

Tulle gras and gauze are applied to the wound and the foot is wrapped in sterile orthopaedic wool and bandaged. A few turns round the ankle help to hold the dressing in place and apply gentle pressure to the amputation site.

If stitches have been inserted they can usually be removed by the tenth day. Where the wound has been left open it will be found to have healed with a linear scar in the same interval.

The tendency for secondary deformities to occur in the remaining toes may be diminished by the use of a toe spacer for which the patient may be referred to a chiropodist.

[The illustrations for this Chapter on Amputation of the Lesser Toes were drawn by Mrs. A. Barrett.]

Techniques of Bone Biopsy

J. Chalmers, M.D., F.R.C.S.(Eng.), F.R.C.S.(Ed.)
Consultant Orthopaedic Surgeon, Royal Infirmary
and Princess Margaret Rose Orthopaedic Hospital, Edinburgh

BONE BIOPSY FOR SYSTEMIC SKELETAL DISORDERS

Introduction

Bone biopsy is frequently required for the investigation of systemic skeletal disorders such as osteoporosis, osteomalacia, hyperparathyroidism and renal osteodystrophy each of which may be diagnosed by their characteristic histological appearance. For some purposes such as the diagnosis of osteomalacia, undecalcified bone is essential, while for other purposes decalcified tissue is preferred. Biopsies intended for undecalcified histology should be fixed in neutral fixative such as buffered formalin. If in doubt it is wise to contact the pathologist before biopsy to ascertain his requirements.

In systemic disease all parts of the skeleton are involved and the site for biopsy can be selected on grounds of convenience and least discomfort to the patient. In general, cancellous bone is preferred by the pathologist as it is easier to prepare than cortical bone. The iliac crest affords a convenient site. The operation can be done painlessly under local anaesthesia as an out-patient procedure.

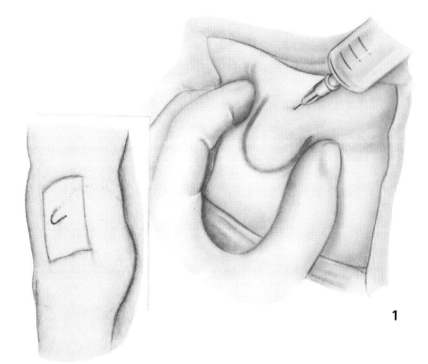

TECHNIQUE OF ILIAC CREST BIOPSY

1 & 2

The crest is gently gripped through the soft tissues just behind the anterior superior spine. The skin and periosteum are infiltrated with 1 per cent lignocaine with adrenaline and further local anaesthetic is injected down the inner and outer surfaces of the crest for about 3 cm.

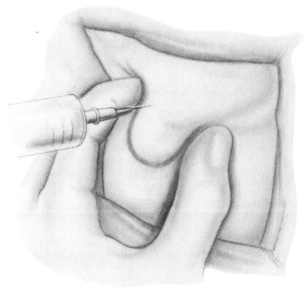

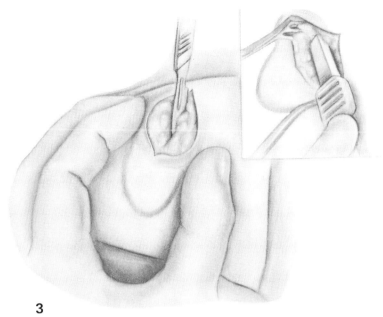

3

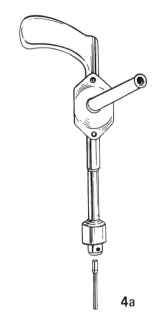

4a

The 6 mm scaphoid trephine (Stryker catalogue No. 1108—6)

3, 4 & 5

An incision 2—3 cm in length is made along the margin of the crest and is deepened to periosteum. A self-retaining retractor is inserted and the periosteum is elevated from the margin of the crest for 2 cm. The biopsy is taken with a trephine of which there are a variety available. The 6 mm scaphoid trephine used with a hand drill is simple and atraumatic. The trephine is entered through the margin of the crest and is directed caudally and medially for about 2 cm between the cortical surfaces. The instrument is then gently rocked to fracture the trabeculae at the limit of penetration and to allow the plug to be withdrawn. The plug is then gently pressed from the trephine using the obturator provided or the reverse end of a drill bit. Two plugs of bone should be obtained in this way. Careful suture of the periosteum limits bleeding from the bone. The skin may be closed with subcutaneous absorbable sutures.

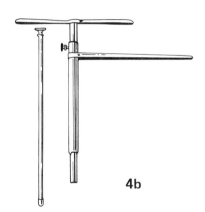

4b

The Royal National Orthopaedic Hospital iliac crest trephine (Downs catalogue No. AG 325—01—R)

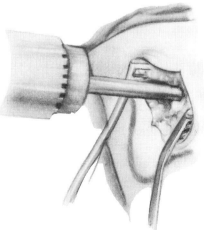

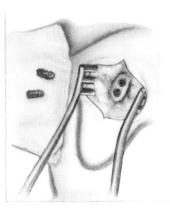

5

BIOPSY OF LOCALIZED SKELETAL DISORDERS

Bone biopsy is commonly required for the diagnosis of localized skeletal pathologies and is mandatory before radical treatment of malignant bone tumours can be undertaken. Bone biopsy may be purely diagnostic and is then aimed at obtaining a representative sample of tissue for examination or it may combine diagnosis with an attempt at cure — an *excision biopsy*. It is prudent to make a routine of sending biopsy material both for pathological and bacteriological examination in every instance because infection and malignancy can mimic each other closely both in clinical presentation and radiological appearance. Only by taking this simple precaution in every case will misdiagnosis be prevented.

Frozen section or routine histology?

Frozen sections which permit immediate diagnosis are of great value in many areas of surgery such as breast and lung cancer and it is tempting to apply this technique also to bone pathology so that definitive treatment can be planned under one anaesthetic. There are, however, particular difficulties in connection with bone. Most bone tumours are uncommon and correspondingly less familiar to the pathologist. It can prove extremely difficult for example to distinguish between osteosarcoma and early fracture callus, or between benign and malignant cartilaginous tumours. Most bone lesions also will contain some bone tissue which presents technical problems in frozen sectioning. For these reasons frozen sections should not be requested on bone biopsies, except perhaps in specialist centres with exceptional experience. It is much better to await the deliberate study of a routinely prepared section even if it means a few days' delay, rather than risk the disaster of an unnecessary radical operation for a benign disorder. The responsibility for diagnosis in difficult cases should be shared between the surgeon, radiologist, and pathologist in consultation.

Open biopsy or needle biopsy?

Needle biopsy is theoretically attractive in that it is a limited procedure that can often be done under local anaesthesia. Many bone tumours, however, have a variable cellular differentiation at different sites and the limited material obtained by needle may be so unrepresentative as to be misleading. In general, pathologists prefer more generous samples obtained by open biopsy and needle biopsy should be reserved for areas such as the vertebral bodies where open access involves a major exposure; but no part of the skeleton is surgically inaccessible if needle biopsy fails.

TECHNIQUE OF OPEN BIOPSY

Where possible a tourniquet should be used. The skin incision should be placed such that the biopsy wound may be completely excised if further surgery is required. If the lesion is large several specimens should be obtained from different sites and depths. Reactive areas of new bone formation at the margins of a bone lesion (e.g. the Codman's triangle) are best avoided as they present difficulty in histological interpretation. In lesions of long bones which have not breached the cortex it is best to avoid osteotomes or chisels to gain access because these may initiate stress cracks which can subsequently lead to fracture. It is much safer to use a drill or trephine such as those described for the iliac crest biopsy. If it is difficult to locate the site for biopsy in the case of small intra-osseous lesions operative x-rays should be used. Some bone lesions including aneurysmal bone cysts and many malignant tumours may give rise to troublesome bleeding which may not be controllable by diathermy or ligature. When faced with a tumour which is large, cystic and in an area where a tourniquet cannot be applied it is prudent to have the patient prepared for blood transfusion.

Excision biopsy

Diagnostic biopsy may be combined with total excision of the lesion. This procedure should be used only in circumstances in which there is good clinical and radiological evidence that the lesion is circumscribed and benign such as osteochondroma, chondroma or osteoid osteoma. In potentially malignant disorders, it is wiser to await the result of a diagnostic biopsy before attempting excision, as the choice of treatment and extent of surgical excision will depend on the nature of the tumour. The temptation to enucleate or scrape out with a curette, lesions of yet undiagnosed nature should be avoided as such procedures may needlessly disseminate tumour cells and make subsequent definitive treatment more difficult. Excision biopsy is inevitably a 'one off' procedure and there can be no standard operative description. Each operation should be carefully planned with a view to preserving important anatomical structures bearing in mind that anatomy may be disturbed by the presence of the lesion. With tumours closely related to major vessels a pre-operative arteriogram may help in planning the operative approach. Care should be taken with benign cartilaginous tumours to avoid leaving behind fragments of cartilage as they have a capacity for resuming growth. If excision biopsy leaves a defect in bone of such a size as to require bone grafting, it is important that the bone graft should be obtained from the donor site as a separate surgical procedure using fresh instruments, drapes and gloves to avoid the possibility of transfer of tumour cells to the donor site.

NEEDLE BIOPSY

The advantages and disadvantages of needle biopsy have been discussed on page 334. Although the technique of vertebral body biopsy only will be described here, similar methods may be applied to any part of the skeleton using the same instruments. The procedure may be done under local or general anaesthesia.

Choice of biopsy needles

Several needles and trephines are available for vertebral body biopsy. Needles have the advantage of being relatively atraumatic, but they have a narrow bore and limited ability to penetrate bone and so may only succeed in obtaining a specimen if the tissue is soft or purulent. Trephines have wider bores and obtain a better bone sample but carry greater potential risk of damaging important structures.

Closed or needle approaches to all segments of the spine have been described (Valls et al., 1948; Craig, 1956, Ottolenghi, 1967; Debnam and Staple, 1975; Evarts, 1975). In the cervical and thoracic spine down to the tenth thoracic vertebra the close relationship of important anatomical structures is such that these procedures should not be done by the occasional operator. Below the tenth thoracic vertebra the approach is safe provided the correct procedure is followed. X-ray guidance is essential. Two-plane image intensification is ideal and greatly shortens the operation time.

6

Technique of needle biopsy of the vertebra, from T10-L5 using the Craig trephine

The patient lies prone on the x-ray table. The safe access to these vertebrae passes obliquely through the erector spinae muscle. A track is infiltrated with 1 per cent lignocaine from a point 6–7 cm lateral to the appropriate spinous process passing medially at an angle of 35° from the vertical.

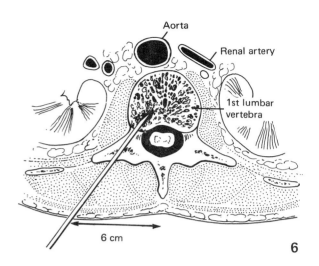

6

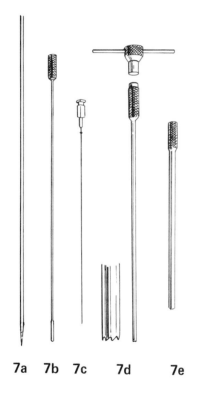

7a 7b 7c 7d 7e

7a-e

Valls, Ottolenghi and Schajowicz (1948) describe a guide to facilitate this stage but with the help of image intensification the guide is not essential. If a transverse process is encountered the needle (*c*) is moved to pass above or below and is then advanced to strike the vertebral body. When the position has been confirmed by x-ray the blunt trochar (*a*) is then inserted alongside the needle through a stab skin incision. The position is again checked by x-ray. The ideal point of contact with the vertebrae is the dorsolateral aspect. The cannula (*e*) is then passed over the trochar which is removed. More local anaesthetic is injected and the cutting trephine (*d*) is then inserted through the cannula and rotated into the bone. The degree of penetration can be gauged by using the blunt stylet (*b*) which is included in the set or by x-ray. The plug of bone is then withdrawn with the help of syringe suction. Slight repositioning of the cannula allows two or three samples to be obtained. If necessary Gelfoam may be passed through the cannula to control local bleeding.

8

Technique for the thoracic vertebrae T1-T10

The approach is similar and the same instruments may be used. However, at this level the needle is inserted 4 cm lateral to the spinous process or just medial to the angle of the rib. Again the needle is advanced at an angle of 35° to the vertical infiltrating with local anaesthetic as it is inserted. If a rib is encountered the needle is redirected to pass below. If radicular pain is experienced it is important to remove the syringe and observe for cerebrospinal fluid leakage. The needle should not be advanced more than 7 cm as deeper penetration endangers the major vessels. It is helpful therefore to use a needle on which the centimetres are marked. Use of the needle rather than trephine at the thoracic level is safer because if the pleura or a major vessel is accidently penetrated the damage is likely to be less.

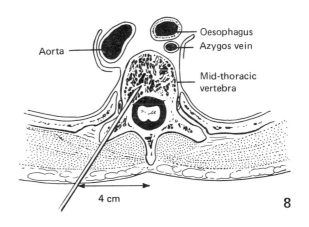

Aorta
Oesophagus
Azygos vein
Mid-thoracic vertebra
4 cm
8

9

Cervical spine, cervical vertebrae from C1-C3

Cervical vertebrae 1–3 are best approached through the posterior pharyngeal wall in the mid-line. These vertebral bodies are too closely surrounded by major vessels and nerves to permit a lateral blind approach. The lower cervical vertebrae can be reached through a lateral approach which passes behind the sternomastoid muscle in a line running vertically downwards from the mastoid process. The needle is then passed medially behind the carotid sheath and should reach the vertebral bodies at a depth of 3·5 cm. As the illustration demonstrates, the vertebral artery and branches of the brachial plexus are at hazard in this approach and it is wise, therefore, to use a relatively small calibre needle. If a larger biopsy is required it is probably easier and safer to carry out open biopsy of the lower cervical vertebrae through the standard lateral or anterolateral approaches.

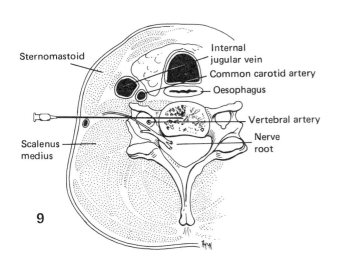

Sternomastoid
Internal jugular vein
Common carotid artery
Oesophagus
Vertebral artery
Nerve root
Scalenus medius
9

References

Craig, F. S. (1956). 'Vertebral body biopsy'. *J. Bone Jt Surg.* **38A,** 93
Debnam, J. W. and Staple, T. W. (1975). 'Needle biopsy of bone.' *Radiol. Clins N. Am.* **13,** 157
Evarts, C. M. (1975). 'Diagnostic techniques: Closed biopsy of bone.' *Clin. Orthop.* **107,** 100
Ottolenghi, C. E. (1967). 'Aspiration biopsy of the spine.' *J. Bone Jt Surg* **49A,** 1479
Valls, J. Ottolenghi, C. E. and Schajowicz, F. (1948). 'Aspiration biopsy in diagnosis of lesions of vertebral bodies.' *J. Am. med. Ass.* **136,** 376

[*The illustrations for this Chapter on Techniques of Bone Biopsy were drawn by Miss A. McNeil.*]

Division of Sternomastoid Muscle for Congenital Torticollis

Sir Henry Osmond-Clarke, K.C.V.O., C.B.E., F.R.C.S.(I.), F.R.C.S.(Eng.)
Former Orthopaedic Surgeon to her Majesty Queen Elizabeth II;
Consulting Orthopaedic Surgeon, The London Hospital and
Robert Jones and Agnes Hunt Orthopaedic Hospital, Oswestry;
Honorary Civilian Consultant in Orthopaedics, The Royal Air Force;
Consultant in Orthopaedic Surgery, King Edward VII's Hospital for Officers;
Chairman of Consultants at Osborne House

PRE - OPERATIVE

Indications

Division of the sternomastoid muscle is indicated in the presence of deformity from a contracted sterno-cleidomastoid muscle which is producing a cosmetic blemish sufficient to distress parents or patient.

Contra-indications

It is wise always to examine the cervical spine by radiography: if there are bony abnormalities (as in the Klippel-Feil syndrome) division of the sterno-mastoid muscle is unlikely to help; furthermore, stretching and manipulating the neck under anaesthesia might cause serious neurological complications.

The best time for operation is somewhere between 3 and 10 years of age; in adults little correction can be hoped for because there are secondary contractures of the other soft tissue structures.

Anaesthesia

General anaesthesia with endotracheal tube is recommended.

Position of patient

A low pillow is placed between the shoulder-blades, and the chin is kept rotated to the opposite side. After the skin has been prepared two towels are placed under the head, the top towel being folded over to cover the head completely from the point of the chin upwards. Other towels are arranged appropriately.

THE OPERATIONS

The muscle may be divided at its lower or upper attachment. Division at the lower end is the easier, but it leaves a scar which may cause some distress to a girl.

DIVISION OF LOWER ATTACHMENT

1

The incision

A transverse incision is made about 1 inch (2·5 cm) above the clavicle. It is helpful to pull the skin down until the area to be divided lies over the clavicle; skin and platysma can then be cut through neatly in one stroke.

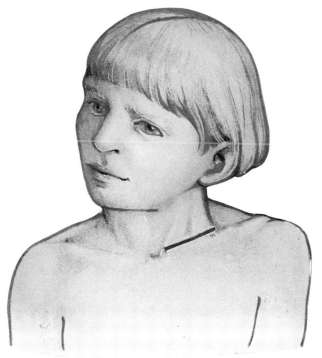

1

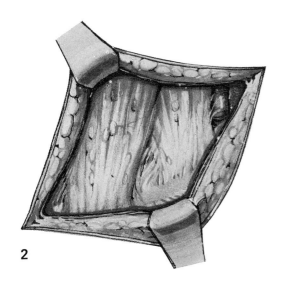

2

2

Exposure

The skin and platysma are divided, exposing the taut sternal and clavicular heads of the sternomastoid muscle covered by fascia. The external jugular vein presents near to the posterior margin of the muscle.

3

Passage of dissector

The fascia covering the sternomastoid muscle is cleaned off and the anterior and posterior surfaces of this muscle are clearly exposed by blunt dissection. The dissector is passed behind the muscle, working alternatively from the medial and from the lateral sides, always keeping close to the deep surface of the muscle.

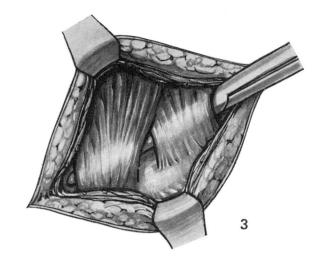

4

Division of muscle

The muscle is divided about 1 inch (2·5 cm) above the clavicle; it is unwise to detach it from the bone because ossification, producing an unsightly protuberance, may occur if a haematoma forms. If the muscle is divided by a series of cuts intramuscular vessels can be caught as they are cut, and ligated or cauterized before the muscle retracts on complete division.

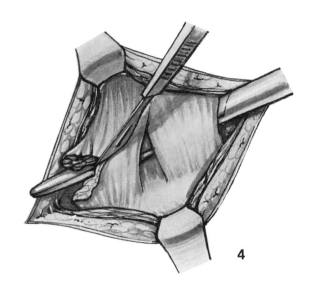

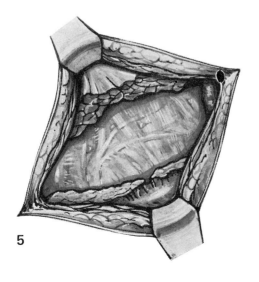

5

Inspection of operation area

After complete division of the sternomastoid muscle its posterior sheath, the deep cervical fascia and the large vessels deep to it are inspected.

6

Division of posterior sheath and deep cervical fascia

The posterior sheath and the deep cervical fascia are usually contracted and should be divided. Because of the immediate proximity of the internal jugular vein, the thyrocervical axis with its transverse cervical and transverse scapular branches, and the subclavian artery and vein, this step of the operation should be performed with great care. The proximity of these important structures indicates the dangers which could be encountered by subcutaneous tenotomy of the muscle, a procedure which is still practised by some.

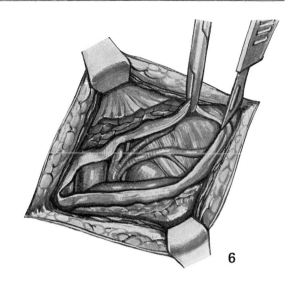

6

7

Correction of deformity

Before the platysma and skin are closed the deformity is overcome by gentle manipulation, bending the head towards the opposite shoulder and rotating the chin towards the side of operation. After this the wound is closed and the head is held in the corrected position by a head band attached to a pillow fixed by sandbags.

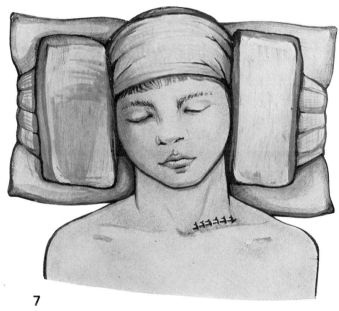

7

DIVISION OF UPPER ATTACHMENT

8

The incision

Division of the sternomastoid at its upper attachment has the advantage that the scar can be hidden above the hair-line, but the operation is more difficult than division of the lower attachment. If correction of torticollis has been delayed until late adolescence or early adult life it is wise to divide the muscle at both ends (and wise to correct gradually by continuous halter or skull traction rather than by a vigorous manipulation under anaesthesia which may damage important structures such as the brachial plexus). After shaving the area an incision is made beginning behind the pinna at the level of the lower margin of the external auditory meatus, the incision curves upwards and backwards across the base of the mastoid process and extends backwards along the anterior one-third of the superior nuchal line.

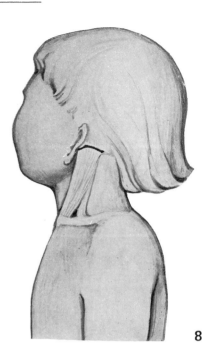

8

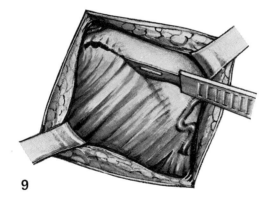

9

9

Division of muscle

The skin and subcutaneous tissues are divided and the muscle is detached close to its bony attachment. Care should be taken to avoid the main stems of two branches of the external carotid artery—the posterior auricular in front and the occipital behind. The former is liable to injury in dividing those fibres of the sternomastoid which are inserted into the anterior margin of the mastoid process (*see Illustration 11*).

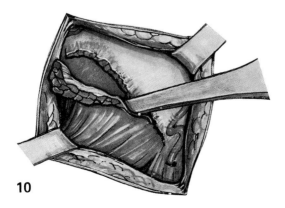

10

10

Detachment from bone

The remainder of the muscle is detached from the skull by a rugine. The deformity is overcome by manipulation (or by traction) and the wound is closed. After-treatment is the same as for division at the lower end.

11

Anatomical relationships

This illustration shows the important vessels and nerves in the area. Note the close relationship of the accessory nerve—hence the wisdom of dividing the muscle at its bony attachment. The posterior auricular and occipital arteries and the jugular vein are clearly shown, with the facial nerve lying deep to the anterior border of the muscle.

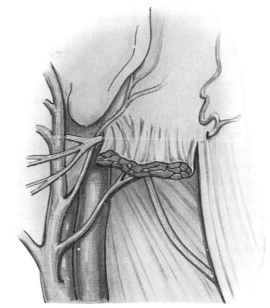

11

12

Application of rigid collar

When the stitches are removed in 5—7 days a plaster-of-Paris collar is applied, with care to ensure that the deformity is slightly over-corrected.

POSTOPERATIVE CARE

The plaster or other rigid collar is retained for 6 weeks. Thereafter a prolonged period (up to 1 year) of re-education in maintaining correct head and neck posture is required. The older the child the more necessary and the more rigorous this course must be.

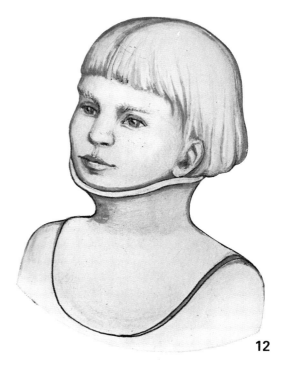

12

[*The illustrations for this Chapter on Division of Sternomastoid Muscle for Congenital Torticollis were drawn by Miss C. M. Lamb.*]

Operation for Cervical Rib and Scalene Syndrome

David L. Hamblen, Ph.D., F.R.C.S.
Professor of Orthopaedic Surgery, Western Infirmary, Glasgow

INTRODUCTION

The scalene or 'thoracic outlet' syndrome is sometimes associated with the presence of a cervical rib. This is seen on x-ray as a rudimentary costal element articulating with the transverse process of the seventh vertebra and possibly extending distally as far as the first rib. The syndrome, which is ill-defined and difficult to diagnose, may also occur in the absence of a cervical rib from pressure of a fibrous band or accessory scalene muscle.

The majority of patients present with an irritative lesion of the lower trunk of the brachial plexus causing radiating pain following a vascular pattern. The pain and paraesthesia are referred to the medial aspect of the forearm and ulnar two digits and are increased by lifting or carrying heavy weights. In more severe obstruction there may be associated weakness and wasting of the small muscles of the hand.

A less common presentation, but one which may accompany nerve root compression, results from acute or intermittent obstruction to the subclavian artery as it crosses the first rib. This may lead to weakening or obliteration of the radial pulse when the neck is extended and rotated to the opposite side.

PRE - OPERATIVE

Indications

Surgical exploration should only be undertaken when the symptoms of thoracic outlet compression, either neurological or vascular, fail to respond to adequate conservative treatment by shoulder-girdle strengthening exercises. Other causes of nerve compression in the neck and upper limb should be excluded by plain x-rays, myelography and nerve conduction studies. Arteriography may confirm compression of the subclavian artery when vascular symptoms are present.

When the vascular symptoms predominate in the absence of a cervical rib, exploration and excision of the first rib through the axilla as described by Roos (1966) may be preferred to the supraclavicular approach.

Anaesthesia

General anaesthesia with endotracheal intubation is routine to allow adequate preparation and draping of the skin over the base of the neck and shoulder.

Position of patient

The patient is placed in the supine position with a sandbag between the shoulders and the head turned to the opposite side.

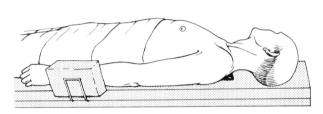

1

THE OPERATION

2

The incision

An obliquely transverse skin incision is made 2 cm above the clavicle, extending 5 cm back from its medial end. This is continued down through the underlying platysma muscle and the lateral clavicular origin of the sternomastoid.

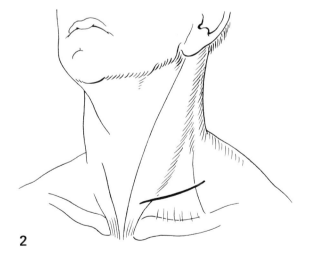

2

3

Exposure of the neurovascular structures

The transverse cervical and suprascapular vessels lie deep to the sternomastoid and may require ligation. The omohyoid muscle is next divided to expose the scalenus anterior muscle, which must be clearly identified and differentiated from the upper roots of the brachial plexus. The phrenic nerve will be identified on its anterior surface and should be carefully preserved. A blunt dissector is passed gently under the scalenus anterior from its lateral side and the muscle fibres divided under direct vision. This exposes the lower trunk of the plexus and the sub-clavian artery lying on the scalenus medius muscle.

4

Relief of obstruction

The pressure on the plexus and artery may be relieved by division of the scalenus anterior alone, but a careful search should always be made for other pathology. The nerve trunk and artery are carefully mobilized from the suprapleural membrane to visualize the front of the scalenus medius. Any rudimentary cervical rib or fibrous band running from the transverse process of C7 to the upper border of the first rib can then be excised under direct vision. At the completion of the procedure there should be no pressure on the nerve trunk or artery in the angle between the scalenus medius muscle and first rib when the arm is pulled down at the side.

Wound closure

The wound is closed with suction drainage, which is used for 24 hr to minimize wound haematoma formation. No deep sutures are required, but to achieve maximal cosmesis the platysma should be closed as a separate layer and a subcuticular suture used in the skin.

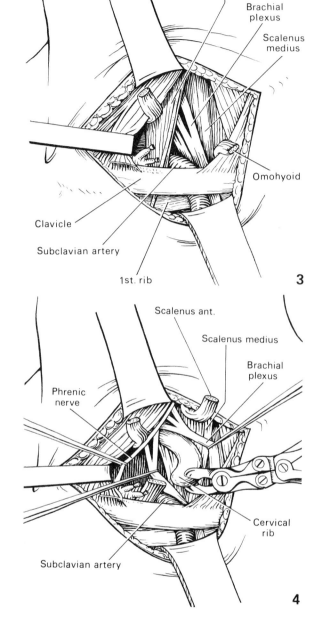

POSTOPERATIVE CARE

The patient may be allowed to mobilize with a light dressing once the drain has been removed. An arm sling used for the first few days helps to relieve local pain in the wound.

Reference

Roos, D. B. (1966). 'Transaxillary approach for first rib resection to relieve thoracic outlet syndrome.' *Ann. Surg.* **163,** 354

[The illustrations for this Chapter on Operation for Cervical Rib and Scalene Syndrome were drawn by Mrs. P. Miles.]

Anterior Fusion of the Cervical Spine

David L. Hamblen, Ph.D., F.R.C.S.
Professor of Orthopaedic Surgery, Western Infirmary, Glasgow

INTRODUCTION

The anterior approach to the cervical spine allows the use of direct interbody fusion techniques as well as permitting clearance of degenerate disc material from the intervertebral space and spinal canal. The anatomy of the region permits easy anterolateral exposure to the bodies of the third to seventh vertebrae. Three techniques of interbody fusion have been described using this common approach. They utilize cortico-cancellous bone from the iliac crest in the form of a block (Robinson and Smith, 1955), a dowel (Cloward, 1959) or a 'keystone' strut graft (Bailey and Badgley, 1960).

Above and below these levels the approach to the bodies is technically more difficult and requires a direct anterior transpharyngeal or trans-sternal approach as described by Fang *et al.* (1964). These serious operations should not be used routinely and will not be described further.

PRE - OPERATIVE

Indications

(*1*) To achieve intervertebral stability following removal of degenerate disc material or posterolateral osteophytes through an anterior approach.

(*2*) Post-traumatic instability following hyper-flexion fractures or fracture-dislocations.

(*3*) Cervical spondylosis confined to one or two levels associated with progressive neurological impairment from cord or root compression.

(*4*) Following resection of major portions of one or more vertebral bodies involved by infections or tumours of benign or low-grade malignancy.

(*5*) To correct and stabilize late hyperflexion deformities following extensive posterior surgical laminectomies.

General considerations

The selection of the level, or levels, for fusion is usually based on the clinical features together with routine x-rays, including lateral views in maximum flexion and extension. Occasionally special investigations, such as myelography or discography, may be indicated when the level of disc degeneration is uncertain. They are not recommended as routine since they are difficult to perform and even more difficult to interpret.

When excessive spinal instability is present as a result of trauma or disease, fusion may be preceded by the application of skeletal traction through skull calipers. This may sometimes be required to achieve reduction of dislocated articular facets in acute injuries.

Anaesthesia

General anaesthesia is preferred as a routine and the insertion of an armoured endotracheal tube facilitates mobilization and handling of the tracheo-oesophageal structures while preventing obstruction to the airway. It also allows more adequate skin preparation and draping of the patient.

THE OPERATIONS

Special instruments

Special instrumentation is only required for the Cloward dowel graft fusion. The other techniques of interbody fusion use general orthopaedic instrumentation. Useful additions are blunt-ended self-retaining retractors, a range of curettes, fine pituitary rongeurs, a laminar spreader, angled osteotomes and a bone punch.

1

Position of patient

The patient is placed in the supine position with a small sandbag between the shoulders. The head is supported in a cerebellar head rest in slight extension with the chin turned away from the side of operation. Either side may be used, but the left is usually preferred because of the smaller risk of damage to the recurrent laryngeal nerve. However, the presence of the thoracic duct on the left should be kept in mind during the procedure. After preparation of the skin a standard thyroid drape is used, which allows the anaesthetist access to the face if necessary. The iliac crest on the same side should be prepared and draped for removal of the bone graft.

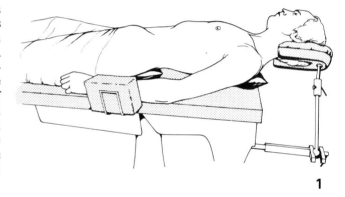

1

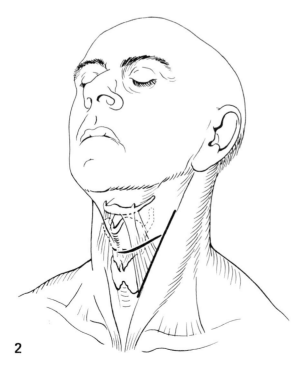

2

2

The incision

The level and technique of fusion determines the type of skin incision used. An incision in a skin crease, running from the mid-line to the anterior border of the sternomastoid at the level of the lower border of the thyroid cartilage gives the best cosmetic result. For a more extensive exposure to allow clearance of bone disease, or to permit multiple level fusion, a vertical incision along the line of the anterior border of the sternomastoid is recommended. This begins 2 cm below the mastoid process and ends just above the sternum.

3

Exposure of the spine

The thin muscular layer of the platysma is divided in the line of the skin incision but preserved as a separate layer for repair. The flaps are retracted proximally and distally to allow vertical incision of the fascia along the anterior border of the sternomastoid muscle. Blunt dissection is used to develop the space between the strap muscles medially and the sternomastoid laterally after retraction or division of the omohyoid muscle distally. Deep to the sternomastoid the carotid artery can be easily palpated and gently retracted laterally with the other contents of a carotid sheath. The trachea and oesophagus are separated from the prevertebral fascia and mobilized medially to allow the finger to palpate the anterior surfaces of the bodies of the mid-cervical vertebrae. Normally only the middle thyroid vein requires ligation and division. In high exposure it may be necessary to ligate the superior thyroid artery and vein, with care to avoid damage to the superior laryngeal nerve running down the lateral wall of the pharynx.

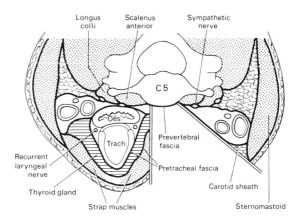

3

4

Identification of vertebral level

The mid-line of the bodies is easily recognized as a fascial strip between the two vertebral longus colli muscles. At this stage it is essential to confirm the proposed level of fusion using radiological control. A 26-gauge hypodermic needle is inserted into the selected intervertebral space and its position checked with a lateral x-ray or the image intensifier. The angle of the space is also revealed by the position of the needle, which tends to run upwards from the neutral position. After identification of the correct level, or levels, the longus colli muscles can be stripped laterally to allow wider exposure of the intervertebral space prior to disc removal.

5

Disc excision

Using a long-handled scalpel the anterior ligament and annulus are excised over the front of the intervertebral space to allow clearance of disc material with curettes and rongeurs. Care must be taken not to dissect into the space to a depth greater than 1·25 cm to avoid entering the spinal canal with the risk of damage to its contents. The vertebral end-plates should be left intact to prevent collapse of the vertebral bodies around the graft. The further stages in the operative procedure depend on the type of fusion undertaken.

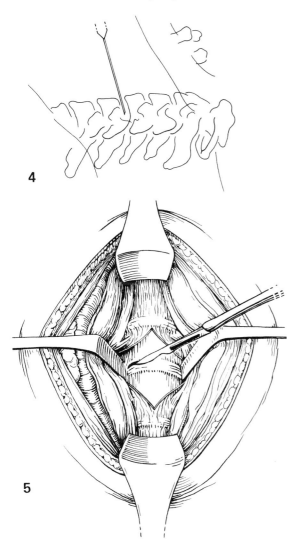

4

5

THE CLOWARD DOWEL PROCEDURE

Preparation of vertebral cavity

6a, b & c

After clearance of disc material the special drill guard (*a*) is inserted in the mid-line over the inter-vertebral space by tapping the teeth on its footplate into the bone of the two adjacent vertebrae. The broad 14 mm drill (*b*), which has a collar at its base, can then be passed down the adjustable guard so that the tip passes through the hole in the footplate and a shallow 1 cm hole cut. To run in the line of the inter-vertebral space the hole should have the disc running across its centre. The screw thread on the drill guard is advanced 1–2 mm at a time to allow gradual deepening of the hole. Each time the drill is removed bony debris are cleared and the depth tested with the graduated guide (*c*) to avoid accidental penetration of the spinal canal. When the cortical wall is breached any remaining fragments of bone and disc can be removed from the canal with fine pituitary rongeurs.

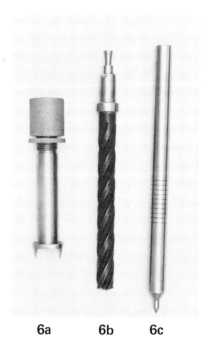

6a   6b   6c

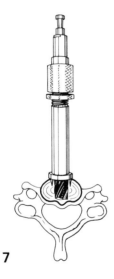

7

7

Occasionally, prominent posterolateral osteophytes cause nerve root compression and may require removal. The Cloward instruments include a specially angulated guard to allow these to be undermined with a drill burr. Its routine use is not recommended since osteophytes may resolve spontaneously following interbody fusion due to distraction of the interverte-bral space and elimination of movement.

8

Removal of dowel graft

The outer table of the anterior portion of the iliac crest is exposed through a short transverse incision and the periosteum stripped from its surface. The special dowel cutter is introduced on a Hudson brace and drilled completely through the ilium to give a cylindrical plug with a cortical surface at both ends. This is trimmed to size by reducing its length to 2 mm less than the depth of the drill hole, which can be measured from the graduations on the drill guide (*see Illustration 6c*).

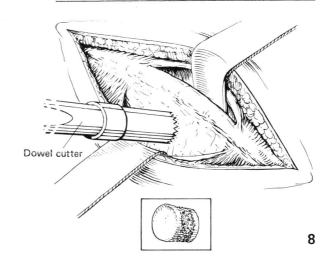

Dowel cutter

8

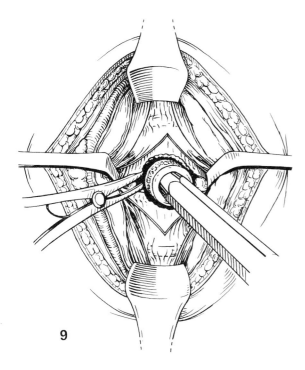

9

9

Insertion of dowel graft

The intervertebral space is distracted by traction on the head and insertion of the laminar spreaders. This allows the cylindrical graft to be tapped into the prepared cavity with a punch. It should be countersunk to a depth of 1 mm below the surface of the bodies to minimize risk of extrusion. When two adjacent spaces are to be fused the cavities are drilled off centre deliberately so that they do not communicate and thereby predispose to dowel extrusion.

THE ROBINSON BLOCK GRAFT TECHNIQUE

10

Preparation of intervertebral space

After complete removal of the intervertebral disc the laminar spreaders are inserted and the cartilaginous end-plates are curetted out, leaving the subchondral bone-plates largely intact. These may be perforated at a few sites to encourage bone ingrowth into the graft.

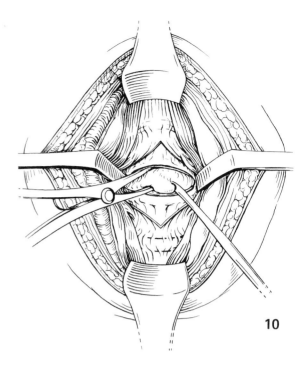

10

11

Removal of block graft

A full-thickness bone graft is removed from the anterior end of the iliac crest using two parallel cuts into its superior border. These should measure 1 cm in width and 2 cm in depth. The cortex is left intact on the superficial and deep surfaces of the graft as well as on its free edge. The graft is then trimmed to be 5 mm less than the measured depth of the intervertebral space.

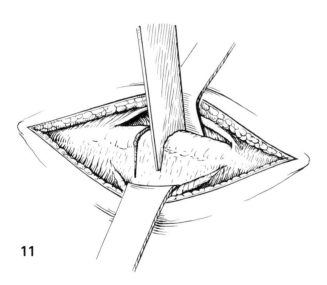

11

12

Insertion of block graft

The intervertebral space is distracted to its maximum extent by the insertion of laminar spreaders or by the anaesthetist pulling on the head. The graft is positioned in the mid-line of the space with its cortical surfaces lying vertically on each side to provide maximum resistance to collapse. It is tapped into position with a punch until it is countersunk 1—2 mm and the traction is then released to lock it under compression.

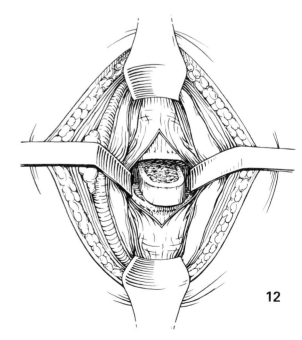

12

THE BAILEY STRUT GRAFT TECHNIQUE

13

Preparation of graft bed

After routine clearance of the intervertebral disc the bed for the graft is prepared by cutting an anterior trough in the bodies to be fused. When neoplastic or infective tissue is to be removed this is included in the excised area. The proximal and distal ends of the trough are bevelled into the posterior bone of the vertebral body to produce a 'keystone' effect.

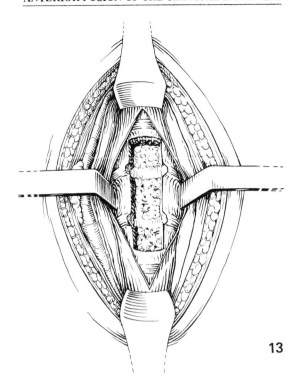

13

14

Removal of strut graft

A suitable slightly oversized rectangular cortico-cancellous graft is then removed from the outer table of the iliac crest together with some cancellous bone chips.

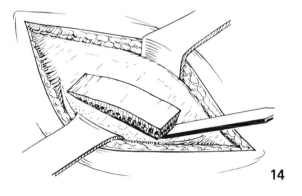

14

15

Insertion of strut graft

After the cancellous chips are packed into the base of the trough and the intervertebral space, the vertebrae are distracted by traction and the rectangular graft tapped into position with a punch. The cortical surface should lie anteriorly and is locked in position by the anterior edges of the vertebrae proximally and distally once traction has been released.

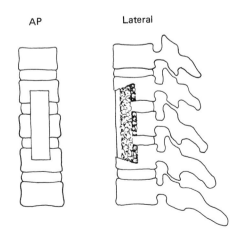

AP   Lateral

15

Wound closure

The same wound closure is used following each type of intervertebral fusion. A single suction drain should be used for 24 hr to minimize wound haematoma formation. No deep sutures are needed unless the longus colli muscle and prevertebral fascia require closure. For optimum cosmesis, the platysma muscle should be repaired as a separate layer and the skin closed with a subcuticular suture.

POSTOPERATIVE CARE

This is dependent on the pathology present and the stability achieved following the insertion of the graft. Following fractures and dislocations, or where portions of several vertebral bodies have been removed, it may be necessary to use a rigid cervicodorsal brace for a few weeks until early radiological fusion is apparent. In the majority of patients a soft rubber collar may be required until the wound is healed and splintage can then be discarded and normal mobility allowed.

References

Bailey, R. W. and Badgley, C. E. (1960). 'Stabilization of the cervical spine by anterior fusion.' *J. Bone Jt Surg.* **42A,** 565
Cloward, R. B. (1959). 'Vertebral body fusion for ruptured cervical discs. Description of instruments and operative technic. *Am. J. Surg.* **98,** 722
Fang, H. S. Y., Ong, G. B. and Hodgson, A. R. (1964). 'Anterior spinal fusion – the operative approaches.' *Clin. Orthop. Related Res.* **35,** 16
Robinson, R. A. and Smith, G. W. (1955). 'Antero-lateral cervical disc removal and interbody fusion for cervical disc syndrome. *Bull. Johns Hopkins Hosp.* **96,** 223

[*The illustrations for this Chapter on Anterior Fusion of the Cervical Spine were drawn by Mrs. P. Miles.*]

Posterior Fusions of the Cervical Spine

David L. Hamblen, Ph.D., F.R.C.S.
Professor of Orthopaedic Surgery, Western Infirmary, Glasgow

INTRODUCTION

The posterior aspect of the cervical spine is readily accessible from the occiput to the cervicodorsal junction. This approach allows fusion from the atlas to the seventh cervical vertebrae and permits the fusion mass to be carried up onto the occiput or down to the first thoracic vertebra. Using a mid-line incision, the ligaments and muscles are stripped subperiosteally from the spinous processes and laminae. No dangerous structures are encountered except at the upper end of the spine where the vertebral arteries and dural sinuses are at risk.

Four basic types of fusion can be performed using this posterior approach. They are occipitocervical fusion, atlanto-axial fusion, interspinous fusion, and posterolateral facet fusion. The indications and techniques for each procedure differ but the pre-operative care, anaesthesia and positioning is common to all.

Pre-operative

Posterior fusions are frequently preceded by the application of skeletal traction to reduce dislocations or subluxations and to maintain stability. Either conventional skull calipers or a halo splint can be utilized and provide easy control of the position of head and neck when the patient is turned from the supine to the prone position.

Anaesthesia

General anaesthesia is routinely used and demands considerable skill to achieve endotracheal intubation while avoiding excessive flexion or extension of the cervical spine. An armoured, non-kinkable endotracheal tube must be used in all cases.

1

Position of patient

After induction of anaesthesia the patient is placed in the prone position with the head supported by a neurosurgical cerebellar head rest. This permits easy adjustment of the position of the spine in any plane while permitting access to the face for anaesthetic purposes. The spine is normally placed in slight extension from the neutral position. Though some flexion permits easier access, this is likely to result in redisplacement of vertebrae. The final position should be checked with a lateral x-ray before surgery is commenced.

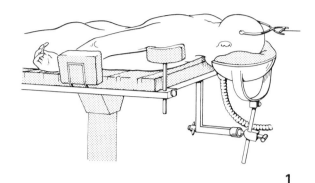

1

OCCIPITOCERVICAL FUSION

Indications

Fusion from the upper cervical vertebrae to the occiput may occasionally be required for the following indications.

(*1*) Comminuted bursting fracture of the ring of the atlas (Jefferson fracture).

(*2*) Atlanto-axial instability complicating rheumatoid arthritis or local sepsis where access to the posterior arch of the atlas is inadequate to permit atlanto-axial fusion.

(*3*) Following posterior surgical decompression for congenital anomalies in the craniovertebral region or for unreduced atlanto-axial dislocation.

Special instruments

Stainless steel wire of 18–20 s.w.g. is used to provide stability in all posterior fusions. Wire handling instruments are required including passers, tighteners and cutters. A small air drill facilitates the placement of holes for vertebral wiring and can also be used with a dental burr for rapid decortication. If the graft is to be wired to the occiput, instruments for neurosurgical burr holes will be required and the assistance of a neurosurgeon, if available, is ideal.

THE OPERATION

2

The incision

A longitudinal mid-line incision is used extending from the external occipital protuberance to the spinous process of the most distal vertebra in the fusion. Occasionally when access to the suboccipital region is difficult, this can be extended as a T-shaped Cushing incision at its upper end for 5 cm on each side.

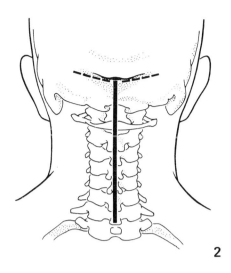

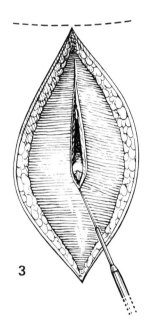

3

Division of ligamentum nuchae

Using cutting diathermy the dense ligamentum nuchae and intermuscular septum is incised to expose the occipital protuberance and the tips of the spinous processes. Care should be taken to remain in the mid-line as this will minimize bleeding.

4

Muscle-stripping from bone surfaces

Using a broad Cobb elevator the muscles are stripped subperiosteally from the spinous processes and laminae. Care must be taken not to carry the dissection out laterally for more than 1·5 cm from the mid-line of the arch of the atlas to avoid damage to the vertebral arteries. To minimize bleeding, muscle-stripping and packing with gauze swabs should be performed alternately on each side.

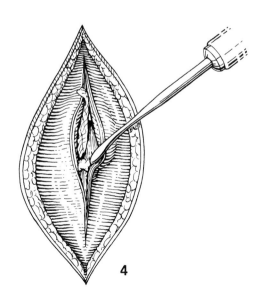

5

Exposure of bony surfaces

Self-retaining retractors are now inserted to expose the posterior aspect of the occiput up to the external protuberance, the posterior arch of the atlas, and the spinous processes and laminae of the distal vertebrae. Any remaining muscle and interspinous ligament can be removed with nibbling forceps prior to placement of the wires.

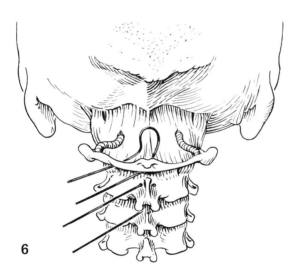

5

6

6

Placement of vertebral wires

By careful dissection of the posterior atlanto-occipital membrane from the anterior aspect of the posterior arch of the atlas it should be possible to pass a wire loop around the bone. This can then be divided to provide a wire on each side of the mid-line. Distally it is more difficult to pass wires around the laminae and these may be passed through drill holes in the base of the spinous process on each side.

7

Placement of occipital wires

Proximal wiring of the graft to the occiput is not routinely used. Normally the grafts can be shaped to lie against the rawed surface of the occiput and would become incorporated after 2–3 months. When immediate stability is required wires can be passed through occipital burr holes to anchor the graft proximally. Two burr holes are made on each side, at least 1 cm from the mid-line to avoid the dural sinuses. The alternative use of a single hole on each side to allow the wire to be passed into the epidural space and out over the posterior lip of the foramen magnum demands more difficult dissection and is not recommended.

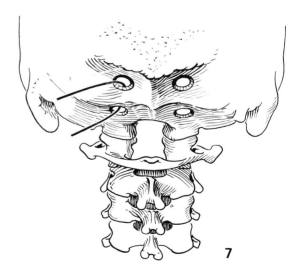

7

8

Removal of bone graft

The bone graft can be removed from the posterior iliac crest without altering the position of the patient. Through a curved incision along the iliac crest the muscles are stripped from the lateral aspect of the ilium. Using several broad osteotomes, the outer table is removed as a large corticocancellous graft. The rectangular graft measuring about 8 cm × 5 cm can be split into two longitudinally, after preliminary holes for the wires have been made with an awl. Additional cancellous chips are removed prior to wound closure over a suction drain.

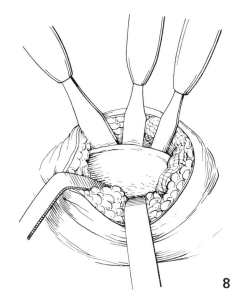

8

9

Preparation of graft bed

With the wires in position the bone in the fusion bed is cleaned of all soft tissue and cancellous bone exposed. On the occiput the bone can be rawed with a dental burr or an air drill, but for the laminae and spinous processes rongeurs are much safer.

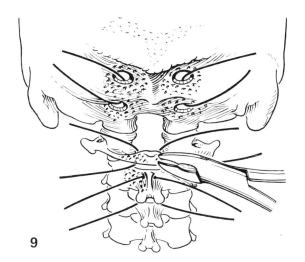

9

10

Fixation of graft

The two corticocancellous grafts are then placed in position after the wires have been passed through the prepared holes. The natural curve of the ilium allows these to conform to the laminae and spinous processes on each side of the mid-line. The wires are then tightened and twisted with suitable wire tighteners. The additional cancellous bone chips are then inserted around the main graft to re-inforce the fusion mass. They should not be used where wide laminectomy has been performed to avoid any risk of cord compression.

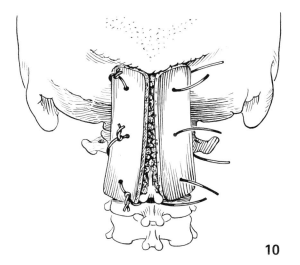

10

Wound closure

The wound is closed in layers using absorbable sutures to close the muscles taking care to cover the graft completely. A single suction drain used for 24 hr will reduce wound haematoma formation, which might lead to cord compression or wound breakdown.

Postoperative care

Skull traction is continued normally for 2 weeks until the wound is healed. During this period the patient is nursed on a turning frame or in a split cardiac bed with a traction pulley placed at its head. If x-ray shows satisfactory stability at this stage the patient can be sat up for application of a moulded minerva plaster jacket. When a halo splint has been used in combination with a plaster or polythene body jacket earlier ambulation may be permitted. After 3 months the jacket can be changed to a deep moulded plastazote cervicodorsal support with polythene re-inforcements, which is worn until radiological union is complete.

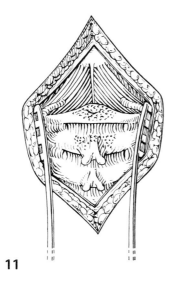

11

ATLANTO-AXIAL FUSION

Indications

A localized posterior fusion of atlas to axis is indicated for:

(*1*) Unstable fractures through the base of the odontoid process, except in the very young or very old where conservative treatment will suffice.

(*2*) Congenital anomalies of the odontoid such as hypoplasia, absence or separation, which may result in atlanto-axial dislocation.

(*3*) Atlanto-axial dislocation from rupture or softening of the transverse ligament associated with chronic rheumatoid disease, or more rarely following local sepsis. Surgical stabilization is usually reserved for dislocations complicated by signs of spinal cord compression or vertebral artery ischaemia.

Special instruments

As for occipitocervical fusion.

THE OPERATION

The incision

A mid-line incision is used, extending from the occipital protuberance to the mid-cervical region. The ligamentum nuchae is incised and the muscles stripped subperiosteally from the first three cervical vertebrae as in the occipitocervical fusion.

11

Exposure of atlas and axis

The posterior arch of the atlas may be very thin and needs to be exposed with care. Dissection is carried laterally from the tubercle with a small periosteal elevator for no more than 1 cm to avoid damage to the vertebral arteries. These can normally be palpated as they emerge above the arch about 1·5 cm from the mid-line. The spinous process and laminae of the axis are then cleared of soft tissue and nibbled down to expose raw cancellous bone.

12

Placement of wire loop around atlas

The posterior atlanto-occipital membrane is carefully dissected from the superior and inferior margins of the posterior arch of the atlas in the mid-line. A loop of 18–20 s.w.g. stainless steel wire can then be inserted from below to pass anterior to the arch and posterior to the membrane. The wire can be drawn out above the arch with fine curved forceps and looped back down over the spinous process of the axis to lie around its base.

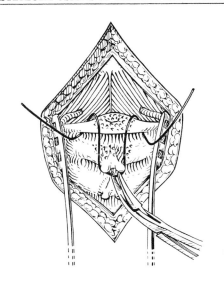

12

13

Fixation of graft

A corticocancellous graft measuring approximately 3 cm × 4 cm is removed from the posterior iliac crest using the technique described for occipitocervical fusion. It is trimmed and a notch cut on its inferior edge to allow it to sit securely on the spinous process of the axis. Two shallow notches cut in the lateral edges will allow the free ends of the wire to be tied over the graft without slipping. Extra cancellous bone chips are packed under the main graft before final tightening of the wire.

Wound closure

Closure in layers as for occipitocervical fusion.

Postoperative care

When skull traction is used pre-operatively it is continued after surgery until the wound is healed. If fixation appears satisfactory on x-ray the patient can be mobilized wearing a moulded re-inforced plastazote support or a rigid cervicodorsal brace.

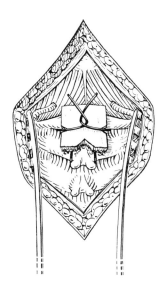

13

INTERSPINOUS FUSION

Indications

Stabilization of the posterior vertebral complex is most efficiently achieved by interspinous fusion and is indicated for instability following:

(*1*) Fracture and fracture-dislocations of the cervical vertebrae associated with gross disruption of the posterior ligamentous complex, or where open reduction is required for locked facets.

(*2*) Limited decompressive laminectomy at one level.

(*3*) Failed anterior interbody fusion.

(*4*) Multiple level subluxation due to rheumatoid arthritis or other inflammatory disease when associated with neurological impairment.

THE OPERATION

The incision

A mid-line incision is used along the tips of the spinous processes from one level above to one level below the fusion. A lateral x-ray with a wire marker should be used if the vertebral level is in doubt.

14

Exposure of spinous processes

After incision of the ligamentum nuchae in the line of the incision, the muscles are stripped subperiosteally from the spinous process and laminae on each side. Dissection is carried out laterally to the articular facet joints and self-retaining retractors inserted. The posterior elements are cleared of all soft tissue including the interspinous ligaments over the segment to be fused.

15

Drilling of spinous processes

Drill holes are made through the cortical bone at the base of the mid-portion of the spinous processes on each side. The holes are joined transversely by the use of a wire passer or sharp towel clip. The use of a hollow wire passer facilitates the introduction of the steel wires across the mid-line. One loop of wire is used for each two consecutive vertebrae to be included in the fusion mass. When more than three levels are to be fused an additional wire is used to encircle the whole length passing through the spinous processes of the proximal and distal vertebrae. The wires are then tightened and twisted to secure fixation.

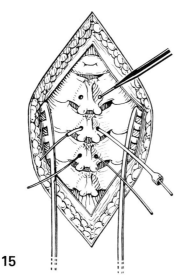

14

15

16

Decortication of fusion bed

It is preferable to defer decortication until the wires have been inserted and tightened. This provides more stability and resistance, as well as ensuring that the sites of cortical bony support for the wire are not prejudiced. The cortical bone of the lamina is removed conveniently with fine nibbling forceps or rongeurs down to bleeding cancellous bone. For the spinous processes this can be performed more speedily with a dental burr on an air drill with less risk of accidental cord damage.

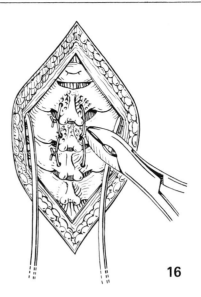

16

17

Insertion of bone graft

As the wires provide stability in the interspinous fusion the use of corticocancellous strips and chips is preferred to large grafts. These can be conveniently removed from the posterior iliac crest and provide the best osteogenic stimulus to fusion. They are packed on and around the prepared laminae and spinous processes.

Wound closure

The wound is closed in layers over the graft with suction drainage to limit haematoma formation.

Postoperative care

Skull traction, when used, is continued until the wound has healed and x-rays have shown intact wires giving satisfactory stability. The patient can then be mobilized in an extended plaster, or re-inforced Plastazote, collar until radiological union is complete. When a halo splint is used with a body corset earlier ambulation may be permitted.

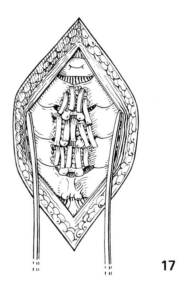

17

POSTEROLATERAL FACET FUSION

Indications

Posterolateral facet fusion is mechanically less efficient and technically more difficult than interspinous fusion but is indicated for:

(*1*) Primary stabilization immediately following extensive decompressive laminectomy for cord compression at multiple levels.

(*2*) Late instability following previous multiple level laminectomy when this causes severe pain or neurological impairment.

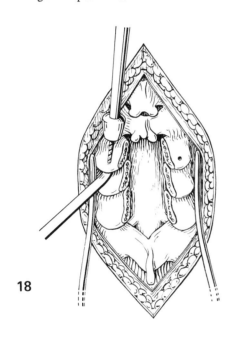

18

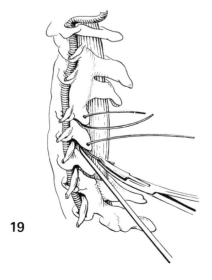

19

THE OPERATION

The incision

A long mid-line incision is used to allow generous exposure of the area, particularly for revision surgery. When previous laminectomy has been performed great care is required in deepening the incision because of the danger of damage to a dural prolapse or the underlying cord. If possible the dissection should begin proximally and distally from any intact spinous processes until the margins of the laminectomy defect can be defined. The central soft tissues are left undisturbed and subperiosteal clearance of the lateral remnants of the laminae and facet joints can be performed without risk.

18

Preparation of facet joints

The articular facet joints are exposed from one level above to one level below the laminectomy defect. The capsule is excised to permit distraction of each joint by insertion of a narrow osteotome or dissector. The articular cartilage can then be curetted from the surface of the facets. A 7/64 inch drill hole is made through the centre of each inferior facet at right angles to the plane of the joint.

19

Insertion of wires

An 18–20 s.w.g. wire loop is then passed through the hole in each inferior facet to provide anchorage for the graft. To facilitate this the joint is again distracted by 2–3 mm to allow the insertion of the jaws of fine artery forceps to seize the end of the wire as it is passed through the hole.

20

Insertion of bone grafts

A large corticocancellous graft is obtained from the posterior iliac crest using the technique described for occipitocervical fusion. This is split longitudinally and trimmed to appropriate length for the number of joints to be fused. Before insertion the remnants of the laminae and the facets are decorticated as much as possible without prejudicing the wire flexion. The two grafts are placed in position laterally and the wire loop in each facet tightened and twisted over them and then cut short.

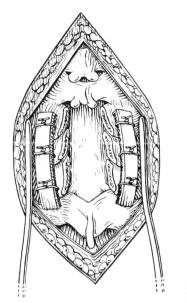

20

Wound closure

Wound closure is routine in layers with suction drainage.

Postoperative care

Because of the poor mechanical stability more rigid postoperative splintage is required than with interspinous fusion. When skull traction is used pre-operatively it can be continued for up to 4 weeks and the patient then mobilized with a rigid cervicodorsal plaster cast or brace. This immobilization is continued until radiological union occurs, which may take 3—4 months.

References

Hamblen, D. L. (1967). 'Occipito-cervical fusion.' *J. Bone Jt Surg.* **49B,** 33
Robinson, R. A. (1964). 'Anterior and posterior cervical spine fusions.' *Clin. Orthop.* **35,** 34
McGraw, R. W. and Rusch, R. M. (1973). 'Atlanto-axial arthrodesis.' *J. Bone Jt Surg.* **55B,** 482

[*The illustrations for this Chapter on Posterior Fusions of the Cervical Spine were drawn by Mrs. P. Miles.*]

Operations for Infections of the Spine

Robert Roaf, M.Ch.(Orth.), F.R.C.S.(Ed.), F.R.C.S.(Eng.)
Emeritus Professor of Orthopaedic Surgery, University of Liverpool;
Consultant Orthopaedic Surgeon, United Liverpool Hospitals
and Robert Jones and Agnes Hunt Orthopaedic Hospital, Oswestry

INTRODUCTION

Forty years ago two main types of spinal infection were generally recognized — tuberculosis of the spine and acute staphylococcal infections which usually manifested themselves as extradural abscesses and frequently led to the rapid onset of paraplegia. Occasional rarities such as actinomycosis and hydatid disease occurred but these were often only diagnosed at autopsy.

The treatment of spinal tuberculosis was usually conservative. The results of laminectomy in the early part of this century had been almost uniformly disastrous. Costotransversectomy for an enlarging mediastinal abscess was occasionally performed but with variable results. The merits and demerits of aspirating cold abscesses, e.g. a psoas abscess were debated but there was no uniform concensus of opinion.

A few surgeons — notably in Japan and the U.S.S.R. — had reported direct anterior or anterolateral approaches to the spine for progressive Pott's disease but it was not until Dott (1947) and Alexander (1946) published their results of anterolateral decompression for tuberculous paraplegia that any widespread interest in operations for spinal infections was aroused.

Their outstanding results were achieved before the introduction of streptomycin but it is pertinent to point out that some of their success might have been due to the use of skeletal traction to the skull. Following their work there was a widespread use of anterolateral decompression for Pott's paraplegia.

Later, with the introduction of specific antituberculous therapy, operative excision of caseous and necrotic material was also widely used for tuberculosis of the spine without paraplegia. A further development was the transpleural approach to the thoracic spine advocated by Hodgson and Stock (1956).

Since then there have been widespread variations in opinion about the role of surgical intervention in spinal infections. Konstam and Konstam (1958) and others have claimed that conservative measures yield equally good results and recent developments in specific antituberculous measures do much to substantiate their claims. At the same time it has come to be recognized that there are many types of non-tuberculous spinal infections both acute and subacute which may become chronic and mimic tuberculosis.

Sophisticated techniques such as tomography, isotope scanning and a variety of serological tests have improved diagnostic accuracy.

PRE-OPERATIVE

Indications for operation

Operative intervention for spinal infections may be indicated for five main reasons.

(*1*) For diagnosis.

(*2*) When the disease does not respond to specific antibiotics or chemotherapy.

(*3*) Where an expanding abscess is threatening vital structures, e.g. trachea, oesophagus, aorta or spinal cord.

(*4*) For progressive paraplegia or when a significant paraplegia does not respond to conservative measures.

(*5*) To stabilize an unstable kyphotic spine.

Indication 1

It is usually possible to make a diagnosis without resorting to operation. Nevertheless, sometimes it is difficult to differentiate infections and tumours or it may be desirable to determine the organism and its sensitivity either by aspiration under radiological control or by open operation.

Indication 2

Most surgeons nowadays would treat early spinal infections conservatively with the appropriate antibiotic and chemotherapeutic regime. If, however, there is already widespread tissue destruction with necrotic bone and disc material there is some evidence that removal of such material accelerates healing. On the other hand if there are multiple tortuous sinuses and 'honeycombing' of the spine surgical excision of all affected tissue is not feasible.

Indication 3

Dyspnoea due to pressure of an abscess on the trachea or bronchus obviously requires urgent relief.

Indication 4

Paraplegia secondary to tuberculosis of the spine is classified into two main groups.

(*a*) Early onset paraplegia, i.e. the paraplegia manifests itself at the same time as the spinal disease. This type of early onset paraplegia usually recovers with conservative treatment.

(*b*) Late onset paraplegia, i.e. the paraplegia appears in a patient who has had spinal tuberculosis for a number of years. There are two types of late onset paraplegia with quite different causes and indications for treatment.

Type 2a. In this type the paraplegia is basically due to a recrudescence of active infection. Here the prognosis with conservative treatment is not quite so good. Many such paraplegias recover with control of the infection but deformity, caseous matter, necrotic bone and disc material are usually still present and may press on the cord and therefore their removal may be required with stabilization of the spine.

Type 2b. In this type there is no evidence of recurrence of infection, there is a marked kyphosis with an internal gibbus over which a flattened attenuated spinal cord is stretched. Often there is bony ankylosis. The cause is progressive ischaemia of the spinal cord. The value of intervention in such patients is debatable. Removing the bony prominence will of course remove pressure on the cord and sometimes this will lead to recovery of the paraplegia. On the other hand there is a risk of further damaging the already precarious blood supply to the spinal cord and making a partial paraplegia worse. Even spinal arteriograms may not reveal the degree of risk involved. On the whole if the paraplegia is not too severe, i.e. the patient can walk but with a spastic gait and has control of the sphincters it is probably best to treat such patients conservatively. However, if the patient is becoming rapidly worse the surgeon should discuss the possible risks of operation and, if the future is otherwise bleak, suggest operation.

Indication 5

Clearly if the spine is not ankylosed and there is a progressive kyphosis, relief of this, e.g. by a split plaster bed and skull traction should be tried first. Then the spine should be stabilized.

Other causes of tuberculous paraplegia such as extradural granulation tissue and extradural fibrosis are often associated with neural arch infections. If they are diagnosed with certainty and do not respond to conservative measures they are best treated by laminectomy and stripping of the fibrous tissue off the dura. Most spinal infections, however, start in the bodies of the vertebra close to the intervertebral discs into which the infection rapidly spreads. Non-tuberculous infections are brought by the extravertebral venous sinuses usually from the pelvis or abdomen. It is important that the spinal stability due to the intact laminae and posterior articulations should be maintained and therefore operations for spinal infections should usually be by an anterior or anterolateral approach.

It cannot be overemphasized that early diagnosis and appropriate conservative treatment of spinal infections are better than major operations performed at an advanced stage.

Pre-operative preparation

Clearly, whenever possible anaemia, protein and vitamin deficiency should be corrected — occasional emergency situations may preclude this.

For small children we still find a plaster bed convenient for nursing. Both the bed and the turning case should be made beforehand and whenever possible the patient should have become accustomed to both. For older children and adults recumbency on a Stoke Mandeville turning bed is a very safe and acceptable nursing regimen which may be supplemented by skull traction by tongs or 'halo' in cervical or upper thoracic lesions.

Both pyogenic and tuberculous infections occur in the neck. In the initial stages treatment by skull traction and the appropriate antibiotic usually cures but if there is already evidence of abscess formation it is easy to obtain a sample of pus in order to identify the organism and establish its sensitivities and this should be done before starting antibiotic treatment. Treatment should of course be started on the 'best guess' principle immediately after the sample has been obtained and before the laboratory results are available.

Anaesthesia

The importance of good anaesthesia cannot be overstressed. The difficulties of spinal surgery are almost entirely due to bleeding. Careful attention to posture, absence of pressure on the abdomen, low intrathoracic pressure, unobstructed airway and controlled hypotension combine to make these operations relatively simple. The reverse makes them impossible. Adequate blood replacement is of course essential but over-replacement during operation is a mistake. In many hospitals 20 per cent of the blood volume is drawn off before operation and replaced by the same volume of normal saline. The patient's blood is then given back to them at the end of operation. Naturally these techniques require careful monitoring by ECG and EEG as well as blood pressure, pulse and respiration recording.

Finally after any spinal surgery on a non-paraplegic patient in which the spinal alignment has been altered during the operation the patient must be seen to move his feet before he leaves the operating theatre.

THE OPERATIONS

CERVICAL SPINE

Facilities

Adequate radiology during the operation is essential.

Position of patient

Supine with the table tilted 'feet down' and the patient's head turned to the left for a right-sided approach, and vice versa.

The incision

For a right-handed surgeon access via the right side of the neck is usually easier. Naturally, special features, e.g. a large abscess, may indicate a left-sided approach.

1

Although it is possible to reach the cervical spine by a short horizontal incision, better and easier access is obtained by a longitudinal incision, at least 10 cm long, along the anterior border of the sternomastoid muscle. For extensive procedures such as multiple level bone grafting the incision may need to be longer. The superficial fascia and platysma are divided in the line of the skin incision.

Deep dissection

2 & 3

The sternomastoid muscle is now displayed. Easy access to almost the whole of the cervical spine can be obtained by dividing the sternomastoid muscle transversely — the two ends are now retracted upwards and downwards by stay sutures through the muscle. The carotid sheath is gently retracted medially and the prevertebral fascia is incised longitudinally in the mid-line.

4 & 5

The prevertebral muscles are stripped off the vertebral bodies using a periosteal elevator. At this stage an abscess may be encountered and pus should be collected for culture and sensitivity tests. The level should not be checked by lateral radiography with a metal marker. The affected intervertebral disc is now gently opened and curetted and the material sent for histology and culture. If the decision is made to graft the spine the best technique is an inlay graft of iliac bone.

The inner table taken from just below the iliac crest and leaving the crest intact is a satisfactory relatively non-traumatic source of suitable bone.

The wound is closed in layers with low suction drainage. Skull traction is maintained for 7 days after which a simple support collar is sufficient.

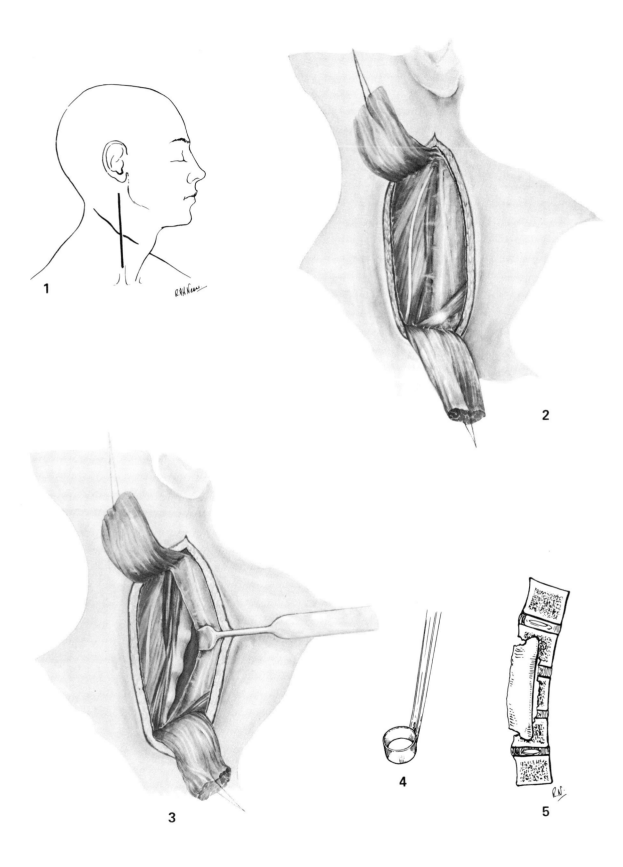

THORACIC SPINE

Anterolateral decompression

6

Position of patient

The patient lies prone with the abdomen free of pressure, the legs can with advantage be dependent; this provides an additional reservoir of blood in an emergency.

The incision

This is usually made on the side with the larger abscess shadow. A longitudinal curved incision about 18 cm long convex laterally with the centre at the level of the apex of the gibbus gives good access. The skin flap is raised and retracted medially. The trapezius and rhomboid muscles are divided longitudinally 3 cm from the spine and retracted laterally.

7

Three ribs at the apex of the kyphos are displayed and stripped and divided at the costotransverse joint level and also 5 cm laterally.

8

Two adjacent intercostal nerves are now identified and traced medially. This is the most important step in the operation. The nerves are traced medially as far as two adjacent intervertebral foramina. It is usually necessary to nibble away the related transverse processes and rib heads. During this stage of the procedure tuberculous granulation tissue, caseous material, or frank pus may be encountered and is sent to the laboratory for histological examination, bacteriological culture and sensitivity tests. This is important as other infections may mimic tuberculosis.

The pedicle between the two intervertebral foramina is now seen and carefully removed with bone nibblers.

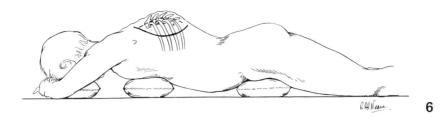

6

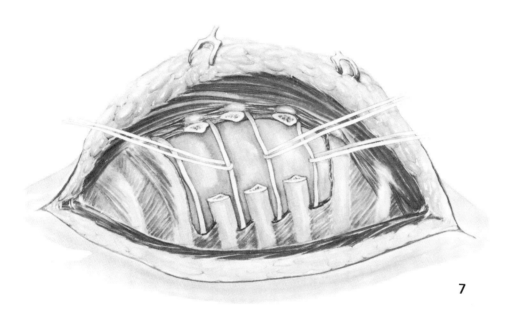

7

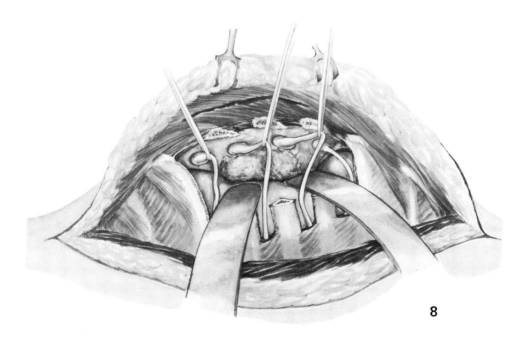

8

9

It is desirable not to tear the dural sleeves on the nerve roots.

The dura mater is now visible and it is possible to assess the mechanical factors responsible for pressure on the spinal cord. Pus, granulation tissue, caseous material, bony sequestra and necrotic disc material are easily removed without the risk of damaging the spinal cord or its blood supply. If the patient is paraplegic, bone etc. is removed until the dura is clearly seen to be free from compression.

10&11

If the disease is extensive there may be an abscess on the other side of the spine. This can usually be satisfactorily evacuated through the same approach but occasionally it is desirable to do a second operation on the other side at a later date. After removing all necrotic material there is usually a considerable gap in the anterior column of the spine but the posterior joints are often found to have ankylosed spontaneously. It is important to preserve the integrity of the posterior structures. At this stage some surgeons insert a body-to-body bone graft — the excised ribs make a convenient source. Others use the ribs for transverse process-to-transverse process grafts; others prefer to wait until all infection has been overcome before inserting free bone grafts.

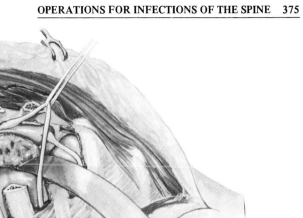

9

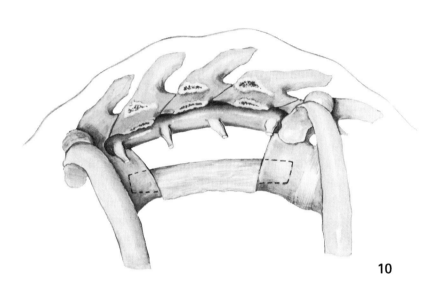

10

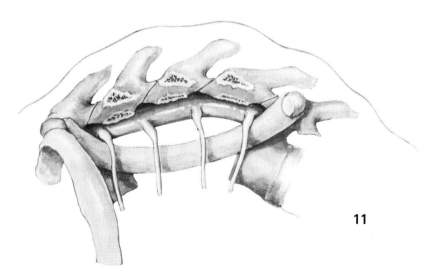

11

12

If, on opening the spinal canal, the surgeon finds that there is no evidence of active infection but that the spinal cord is flat and attenuated and stretched over a hard bony ridge, he has to make a difficult decision. In the author's experience removing the bony ridge — even if it is performed with great care using pneumatic burrs to undercut the bony prominence — is as likely to do harm as good: there must already be some impairment of the blood supply of the spinal cord and it is easy to impair the blood supply still further. On the whole if the paraplegia is still incomplete and the patient has control of his sphincters it is better to do nothing more.

The wound is irrigated thoroughly with normal saline and then closed in layers with suction drainage. If the pleura has been damaged the author inserts an underwater intrapleural drain.

Postoperative care

This depends partly on the estimate of spinal stability. If the spine was clinically stable as tested at operation, then recumbency on a turning bed such as the Egerton-Stoke Mandeville spinal bed is all that is required. If the spine appears unstable, then a halo splint applied to the skull and with 4 kg of cord and pulley traction is used.

If there was evidence of continued activity of the infection, a full antituberculous regimen is continued (*see* below). Drainage tubes can usually be removed after 48 hr and this is a convenient time to check the haemoglobin and electrolytes. During the first 48 hr it is often wise to continue with the intravenous infusion as some degree of ileus is not uncommon after spinal operations.

Any neurological complications, e.g. bladder dystonia are treated on routine lines.

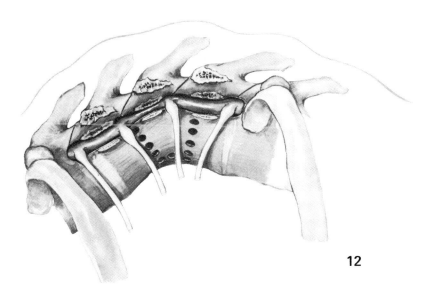

12

Later treatment

On present evidence, prolonged recumbency, e.g. on a plaster bed which was once the mainstay of treatment of spinal tuberculosis, offers no special benefit and does not improve the cure rate. The author's after-treatment is a compromise — 1 month in recumbency with skull traction if the spine is unstable, followed by wearing a posterior spinal support for 3 months. If the spine was stable the patient gets up as soon as he has recovered from the operation. A posterior spinal support is a useful reminder to go slowly. These regimens are, however, tentative and may need modification in the future. In the case of children, longer recumbency is sometimes wise as once a child is allowed to get up he tends to be overactive. Although he worked long before modern drugs were known, Hugh Owen Thomas said he welcomed the onset of paraplegia in an unruly child with Pott's disease as this gave him a chance to keep the child at rest and cure the disease.

Although it is out of fashion at the moment, rest of an infected spine may still prove to be of benefit.

Antituberculous regimens

Many alternative regimens are now available and each has its advocates. For this reason it is important to determine the drug sensitivities of the organisms to ensure that the correct drugs are being given. Provided the organisms are sensitive, streptomycin and Isoniazid for 12 months is usually an effective regimen, with ethambucil and rifampicin as second choices if there is drug resistance to streptomycin.

Transpleural approach

13

Position of patient

The patient lies on his side.

The incision

A long incision in the line of a rib corresponding to a vertebra two segments above the site of disease and extending from the costotransverse joint to the nipple line.

14 & 15

Procedure

The underlying rib is excised as far back as the transverse process. The chest wall is opened by a rib spreader and the lateral parietal pleura incised, the lung is retracted manually and the posterior parietal pleura incised. Any intercostal vessels which may interfere with access are now ligated close to the aorta. Pus, debris, caseous material, necrotic disc material and sequestra are removed. Necrotic or heavily infected bone is now removed until both cephalic and caudal vertebral bodies display healthy vascular bone. If paraplegia is present, bone is removed until the dura is clearly seen to be free of compression. A bone strut is now inserted between these two vertebrae. Rib may be used for this or bone obtained from the iliac crest. The wound is closed in layers with underwater drainage of the pleural cavity and suction drainage of the extrapleural space.

After-treatment is as for anterolateral decompression but convalescence is usually more stormy and some assistance to respiration may be required for a few days.

16

Late stabilization

In the presence of marked kyphosis but quiescent or cured infection, spinal stabilization may be required. Posterior laminal fusion is usually ineffective and some type of anterior strut is required. The author has found bilateral intertransverse rib struts to be effective and to be a relatively minor procedure which does not carry the risk of impairing the blood supply to the cord as direct anterior fusions may have.

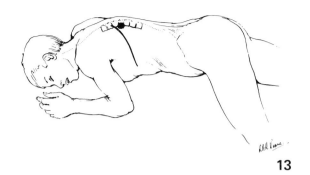

13

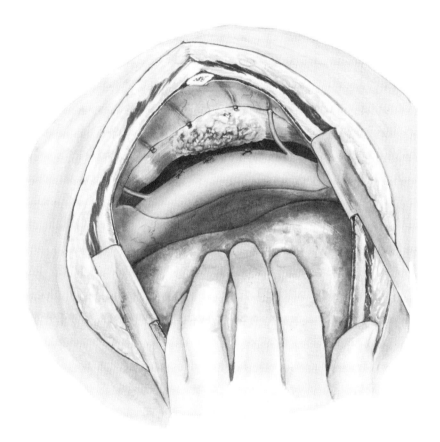

14

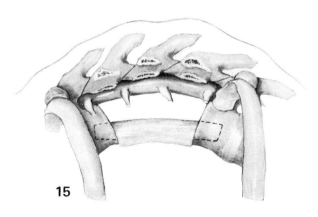

15

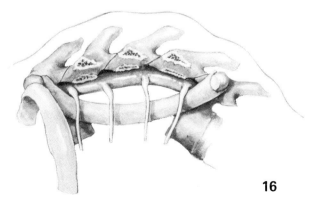

16

LUMBAR SPINE

Anterior approach

17a & b

Position of patient

Approach on the left side is preferred unless there is a right-sided abscess. The patient is placed supine, head down, and tilted to the right or lying on his side with head-down tilt.

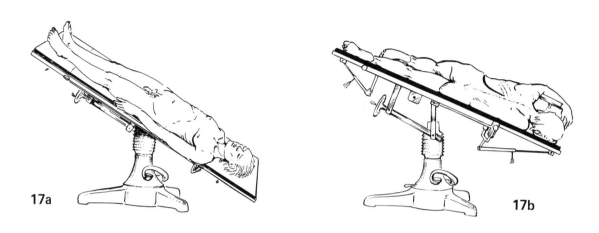

17a

17b

18a & b

The incisions

Simple procedures may be easily performed through a short oblique incision in the flank but for more extensive procedures, e.g. multiple level fusions, a J-shaped incision gives better access when the lateral posture is preferred.

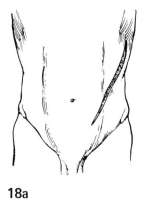

18a

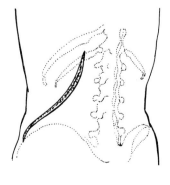

18b

Procedure

19

The abdominal muscles are divided in the line of the skin incision. The peritoneum with the ureter adherent is now seen and pushed gently towards the mid-line. Any abscess is now opened and the material sent for laboratory examination. The sulcus between the vertebral bodies and the psoas muscle is now identified. The sympathetic chain is seen and identified. For better access to the vertebral bodies, the lumbar arteries and veins are seen, isolated and doubly ligated.

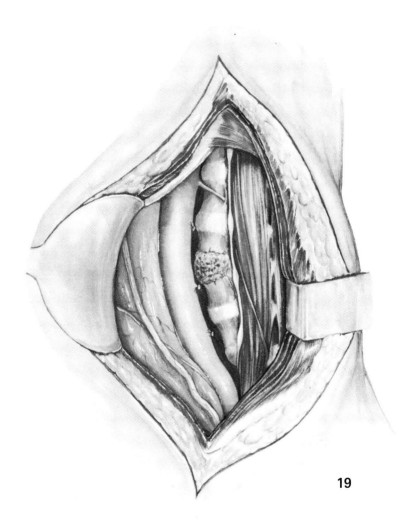

19

20a,b&c

Necrotic disc material, dead bone and granulation tissue are now removed. If it is decided to graft the spine, a bone graft which may be rib, tibia or iliac crest is inlaid into the anterolateral aspect of the vertebral bodies.
The wound is closed with drainage of the extraperitoneal space.

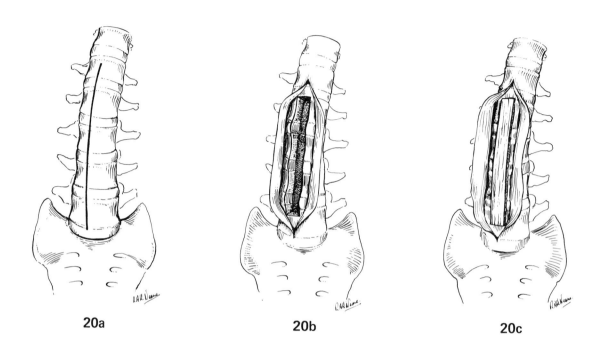

| 20a | 20b | 20c |

Postoperative care

Ileus and urinary retention may occur; some unintentional and temporary damage to the sympathetic chain is not uncommon. The patient may complain of throbbing in the affected leg.

Simple recumbency for 10–14 days is usually enough, at the end of which time a well-fitting Goldthwait support usually provides enough restriction of movement for bony fusion to occur.

Caution

While this is usually an easy operation, two conditions may make it difficult. Repeated and continued infection may lead to extensive fibrosis with adherence of the peritoneum, the muscles and great vessels. Secondly, anomalies of the great vessels occasionally make access to the lower lumbar vertebrae extremely difficult.

References

Alexander, G. L. (1946). 'Neurological complications of spinal tuberculosis.' *Proc. R. Soc. Med.* **39**, 730
Capener, N. (1954). 'Evolution of lateral rhachotomy.' *J. Bone Jt Surg.* **36B**, 173
Dott, N. M. (1947). 'Skeletal traction and antero-lateral decompression in Pott's paraplegia.' *Edin. med. J.* **54**, 620
Hodgson, A. R. and Stock, F. E. (1956). 'Anterior spinal fusion.' *Br. J. Surg.* **44**, 226
Kirkaldy Willis, W. H., Roaf, R. and Cathro, A. J. M. (1959). *Surgical Treatment of Bone and Joint Tuberculosis.* Edinburgh: Livingstone
Konstam, P. and Konstam, S. T. (1958). 'Spinal tuberculosis in Southern Nigeria.' *J. Bone Jt Surg.* **40B**, 26
Roaf, R. (1976). *Spinal Deformities.* London: Pitman
Seddon, H. J., Griffiths, D. Ll. and Roaf, R. (1956). *Pott's Paraplegia.* Oxford: Oxford University Press

[*The illustrations for this Chapter on Operations for Infections of the Spine were drawn by Mr. R. A. H. Neave.*]

Halopelvic Distraction

M. A. Edgar, M.Chir., F.R.C.S.
Consultant Orthopaedic Surgeon, The Middlesex Hospital, London,
and Royal National Orthopaedic Hospital, London

INTRODUCTION

The indications for the use of this technique for pre-operative correction of spinal deformities are discussed on page 389. It is most useful in the severe rigid scoliosis or kyphoscoliosis, particularly if this is placed in the upper or mid-thoracic spine.

The advantage of this technique is that the patient can be up and mobile whilst the correction is being carried out. In addition, if anterior decompression of the spine is required as a first-stage procedure then the halopelvic device does provide a rigid support.

Anaesthesia can be routine although intravenous ketamine in young patients is an advantage.

A full set of instruments are required as recommended by Zimmer U.S.A., Athrodax U.K., Down Bros., London or the Royal National Orthopaedic Hospital, London. These include a torque screwdriver and four halo screws and nuts, insertion jig, turning brace and metal cutters for the threaded pelvic pins.

PROCEDURE

Application of halo

The patient is placed in the supine position with a pillow under the shoulders and the occipital region of the skull supported by an assistant. Another assistant gently holds the eyelids closed so that the frontalis muscle is pulled down when the anterior halo pins are inserted into the skull. It is also important to check that the face is looking directly upwards and the skull is not rotated laterally.

1-3

The halo is placed on the skull with the screws loose. In the lateral view the halo is placed just below the maximum circumference formed by the parietal eminence, i.e. about 2 cm above the orbital margin which is about 1 cm above the top of the ears. The screw points are arranged so that they locate the frontal bosses and the lower part of the parietal eminences with the nuts loose. The halo is held in position while each screw is screwed through the outer cortex of the skull with a torque screwdriver adjusted to the 5 lb/inch^2. When the screwdriver slips on all four screws, the nuts are tightened.

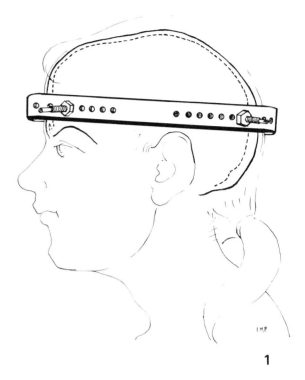

1

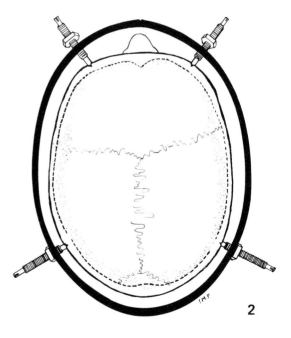

2

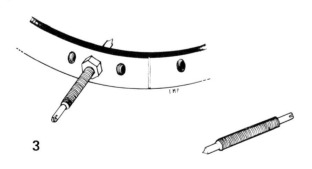

3

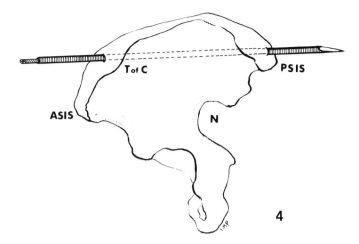

4

Insertion of threaded pelvic rods

4 & 5

With the patient in the lateral position a 2 cm incision is made over the tubercle of the upper iliac crest (T of C). The jig is then clamped between the tubercle of the crest and the posterior superior iliac spine (PSIS). This is the optimum position to allow the threaded pelvic rod to pass between the outer and inner cortices of the ilium.

It is most important that the pelvic rod is not inserted through the anterior superior iliac spine (ASIS) as it will then bow-string across the inner wall of the ilium with the danger of impaling a loop of bowel.

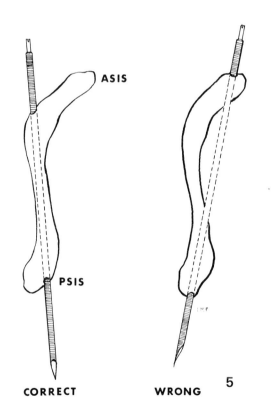

CORRECT   WRONG   5

6

A Steinmann pin is used as an introducer to make an initial hole in the tubercle of the iliac crest. The threaded rod is put in by means of the hand-turning brace. The anterior iliac crest should be carefully palpated to make sure that the rod is not deviating out through the medial side of the iliac bone. When the point of the rod appears through the posterior superior iliac spine a relieving incision is made in the skin. The jig is removed and the turning continued until 6 or 7 inches (15 or 17·5 cm) of rod has appeared. The sharp point is then cut off and the wounds dressed.

The patient is carefully turned into the other lateral position and the procedure repeated. If the pelvis is small or deformed the incision over the tubercle of the crest can be enlarged to admit a finger. The inner wall of the ilium can then be palpated more definitely.

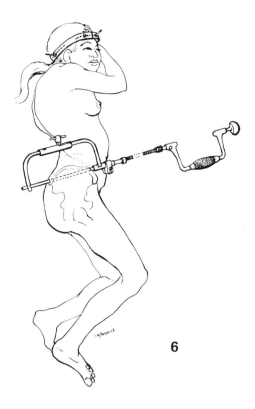

6

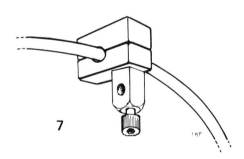

7

7

Attachment of the pelvic hoop to the threaded rods

Using the clamps, which are fitted with an Allen key notch, the hoop is fixed to the pelvic pins so that the hoop lies in a symmetrical position. Posteriorly, where the pelvic rods cross over each other in the mid-line, different size blocks and clamps may be required.

POSTOPERATIVE CARE

The four distraction bars are not set up until 48 hr after operation.

Initially, after operation, the patient should be nursed on a mattress consisting of several foam blocks so that the hoop can lie comfortably between blocks. Apart from the routine postoperative care, it is wise to palpate the abdomen for any tenderness after the first postoperative day.

8&9

On the third postoperative day the sprung distraction bars are set up. The patient is seated with the halo connected to a vertical traction cord with an upward pull of some 25 lb (12 kg). (This will vary according to the size of the patient and should not exceed one-third of the body weight.) The clamps for the distraction bars are then fixed to the halo and the sprung bars applied.

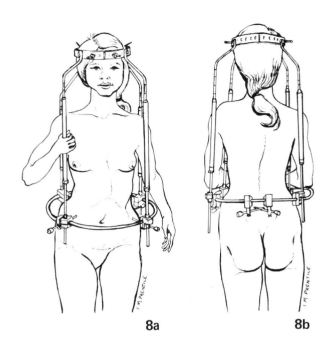

8a   8b

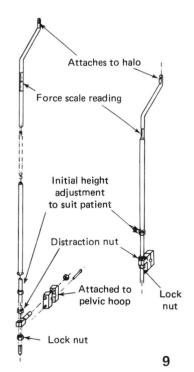

Attaches to halo

Force scale reading

Initial height adjustment to suit patient

Distraction nut

Attached to pelvic hoop

Lock nut

Lock nut

9

Distraction

Depending on the type of distraction system the bars are elongated about 2 mm each day until the summation of the distraction is half the body weight, and in any case should not exceed 40 lb (20 kg). This usually takes about 6 weeks.

It is most important that the patient is carefully observed daily. In the event of increasing neck pain, neurological signs in the cranial nerves, peripheral nerves of the upper limbs or long tract involvement, of the lower limbs, the traction force should be reduced immediately. The halo pins should be tightened with a 5 lb/inch^2 torque screwdriver twice a week. The pelvic rod wounds should be inspected once a week.

After distraction is complete, if the Stanmore system is used, each rod should be clamped to stabilize it prior to fusion

References

O'Brien, J. P. (1975). 'Halo-pelvic apparatus'. *Acta orthop. scand.* Suppl. **1**, 163
Ransford, A. O. and Manning, C.W.S.F. (1975). 'Complications of halo-pelvic distraction in scoliosis.' *J. Bone Jt Surg.* **57B**, 131

[*The illustrations for this Chapter on Halopelvic Distraction were drawn by Mrs. I. M. Prentice.*]

Surgical Procedures for Idiopathic Scoliosis

M. A. Edgar, M.Chir., F.R.C.S.
Consultant Orthopaedic Surgeon, The Middlesex Hospital, London
and Royal National Orthopaedic Hospital, London

PRE-OPERATIVE

Indications

Correction and spinal fusion in idiopathic scoliosis is indicated in three groups:

(1) Adolescent patients who have a thoracic curve with a Cobb angle over 50° particularly if there is further skeletal growth left and the deformity is not being controlled by a Milwaukee brace, or where the deformity is not cosmetically acceptable.

(2) Curves over 60° including double structural and lumbar curves. Even if maturity has been reached these deformities should be corrected and fused because there is evidence that the scoliosis can slowly deteriorrate during adult life.

(3) Patients with a scoliosis over 90° from the age of 10 upwards. This category of deformity often requires a careful and prolonged correction pre-operatively and the halopelvic device described on page 383 is valuable.

Posterior spinal fusion and internal fixation with a Harrington rod is the standard surgical procedure in idiopathic scoliosis. Such a method is contra-indicated if there is a true kyphosis present of more than 60°, but this is unusual in idiopathic cases.

In thoracolumbar and lumbar curves, particularly if there is an associated lordosis, the Dwyer anterior method (*see* pages 398–403) is useful. In the moderately severe curve of 50°–80° this has the advantage of achieving almost a complete correction, both of the lateral curvature and rotation. The fusion area is shorter than with a posterior fusion and more vertebrae remain mobile.

Kyphoscoliosis, where the kyphotic curve is over 60°, requires anterior fusion with the use of a strut of autogenous iliac bone graft. Such deformities are mostly osteogenic or due to neurofibromatosis, although occasionally a severe infantile idiopathic curve falls into this group. The procedure is not described.

1

Length of spinal fusion

From the pre-operative erect anteroposterior spinal x-ray the maximum Cobb angle of the curve is measured. In posterior fusion and Harrington instrumentation the fusion area generally extends two vertebrae above and below these levels. The end-vertebrae in the fusion should be neutral in rotation. In double structural curves the fusion extends across both curves using the above principle with one rod in a 'dollar sign' manner.

The Dwyer anterior fusion is confined to the five or six vertebrae spanned by the Cobb angle on the erect anteroposterior x-ray. Vertebrae which are almost neutral in rotation at each end of the curve can usually be excluded from the fusion area.

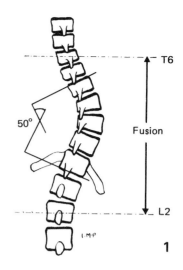

1

Pre-operative correction and preparation

Mild curves of 50° which are demonstrably mobile may be corrected with care at operation using a Harrington distraction rod. Curves which are more severe should be managed pre-operatively with a week's course of Cotrel traction followed by an x-ray during maximum dynamic traction. This method mobilizes the scoliosis and is an indication of its correctability. The Dwyer anterior method for the thoracolumbar region can be performed directly or after a week of mobilization by Cotrel dynamic traction.

Halotibial or halofemoral traction on a Stryker frame with distraction up to half the body weight over a period of 2 weeks is useful particularly in double structural curves. The Risser localizer cast or turn-buckle jacket is an alternative method in moderate single curves. In severe rigid curves over 90° or associated with kyphosis, halopelvic traction is the method of choice.

In all patients a pre-operative x-ray is taken with a small lead strip overlying an indelible skin mark placed transversely over one of the lower dorsal spines. This marker film allows the fusion levels to be determined accurately at the start of the operation.

Anaesthesia

These patients require intermittent positive-pressure ventilation and muscle relaxants during general anaesthesia. Endotracheal intubation of a patient in a localizer cast or in halopelvic traction may be difficult, requiring some adjustment to the cast or traction apparatus. A ganglion-blocking agent which induces hypotension lowers the peroperative blood loss, which may otherwise be 25—40 per cent of the circulating blood volume.

Monitoring during surgery should include ECG, arterial blood pressure (in hypotension an intra-arterial cannula and pressure transducer should be used) and rectal temperature. The operative blood loss must be carefully measured.

Careful pre-operative respiratory assessment, including FVC, FEV_1, and PF is important. Post-operatively breathing is impaired largely through pain and the patient may be near respiratory inadequacy. The FVC is usually less than 25 per cent of the pre-operative value. Therefore, a patient-triggered ventilator such as the Bird, should be used after operation, the patient having been given pre-operative instruction.

POSTERIOR FUSION AND HARRINGTON ROD INSERTION

2

Position of patient

The patient is placed prone on a double Denton rest, Toronto support or Montreal mattress. It is important to ensure that the abdomen is free from pressure. The supports are adjusted so that the area of spinal fusion does not sag into lordosis. The arms should be placed alongside the proximal support with the shoulders flexed no more than 90°.

Patients being operated on in a plaster body jacket should have the cast bivalved so that the posterior half of the shell can be removed, or else a large posterior window should be cut out to allow access to one posterior iliac crest.

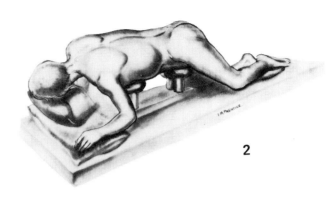

2

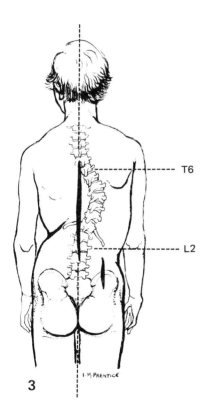

3

3

The incision

Using the indelible skin mark as a reference point, the spines along the length of fusion are palpated. A straight longitudinal incision is made over this zone in the mid-line of the back. It is useful to extend the incision proximally to the spine above the fusion level to help the exposure.

4a&b

Splitting of the cartilaginous tips of the spinous processes

After exposure of the deep fascia and supraspinatus ligament, the epiphyseal caps on the tips of the spines are split longitudinally with a scalpel or cutting diathermy. The intervening supraspinatus and interspinous ligaments are similarly divided. Each half of the epiphyseal cap is then pulled off the underlying spinous process using a Cobb spinal elevator. This process strips the periosteum of the spinous process, allowing the spinal elevator to slide into the subperiosteal plane. Stripping at this stage is continued to the base of the spinous process. It is then useful to check that the exposure is over the correct levels.

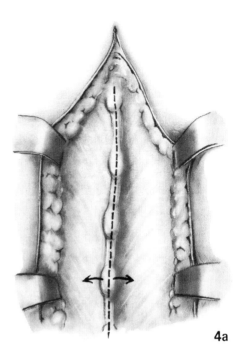

4a

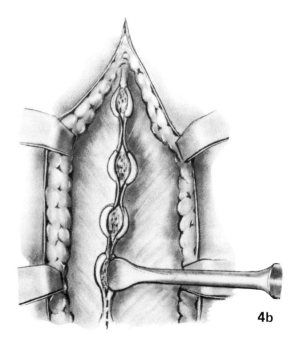

4b

5a&b

Exposure of laminae and transverse processes

Starting at one end of the incision, the spinal elevator is used to extend the periosteal stripping. In the thoracic region the exposure is continued on to the lamina and transverse process in one gentle sweep. At the tip of the transverse process there is a small cartilage cap and this is carefully pulled off. In the lumbar region, the periosteal dissection also extends out to include the transverse processes.

As each level is stripped the space which is opened up is packed with a swab to help haemostasis. Attachments of the sacrospinalis and multifidus muscles to the distal 'trailing' edge of the spines and laminae can be carefully dissected off with a scalpel.

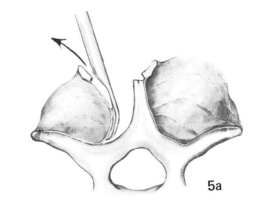

5a

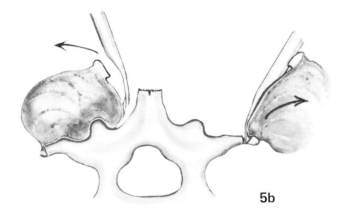

5b

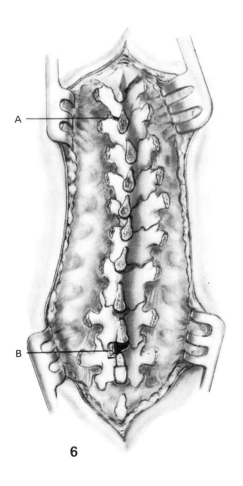

6

6

In the lumbar region the facet joint capsule is incised longitudinally and each half of the capsule together with a small underlying cartilaginous cap is removed from the posterior projection of the facet joints. Self-retaining retractors are placed at each end of the wound and any soft tissue remnants are cleared along the spine. A and B in the illustration denote the prepared sites for the upper and lower hooks (*see* pages 395 and 396).

7

Removal of autogenous graft from posterior iliac bone

A longitudinal incision, just lateral to the postero-superior iliac spine, is made as shown. The sub-cutaneous fat is divided in line with the incision and the plane just superficial to the iliac crest and gluteal fascia is developed. The gluteal fascia is divided just distal to the crest, which is not disturbed, and the periosteum is stripped over the outer aspect of the posterior ilium. Cortical bone is removed and placed up on one side. Cancellous bone is then excised in strips. Some of these are reduced to 0·5—1 cm diameter for the Moe fusion.

The posterior iliac incision is closed with a suction drain.

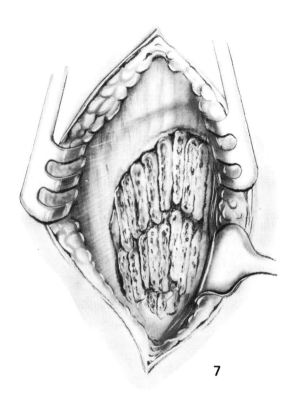

7

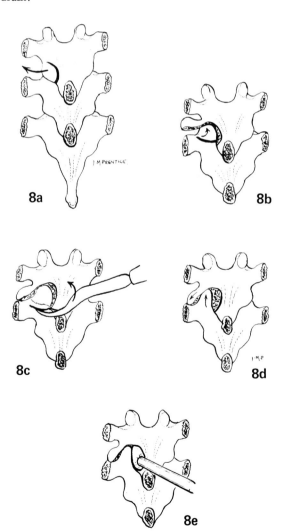

8a   **8b**

8c   **8d**

8e

8a-e

Moe fusion of the thoracic facet joints

The inferior facet is identified as a rounded prominence in the angle between the bases of the transverse and spinous processes. A small Capener or Moe gouge is used to form a flap, which is hinged laterally as shown (*a*). The flap is swung laterally to reveal the articular cartilage of the underlying superior facetal process. Starting at the base of the transverse process of this distal vertebra (*b*) the gouge is used to raise another flap consisting of the articular cartilage and subchondral bone of the superior facet (*c*). This flap is hinged similarly on the base of the transverse process and is swung laterally. A small pyramidal socket has been developed between the facetal processes and the two vertebrae with the lateral wall formed by the flaps (*d*). An appropriately sized piece of autogenous bone graft is then punched in (*e*).

A Moe fusion is not performed at the proximal joint on the concave side as the top Harrington hook is inserted.

9a,b&c

Moe fusion of the lumbar facet joints

The lumbar facet joints almost lie in a sagittal plane, compared with the transverse thoracic facets. The articular surfaces of these facet joints are similarly excised with the same or larger gouge (*a*). The inferior facet is excised first and the fragment is removed from the wound. This reveals the articular cartilage of the superior facet which is similarly excised through the subchondral plane, parallel with the plane of the joint (*b*). A piece of autogenous bone graft is then punched into this recess (*c*).

At the distal end of the fusion the facet joints are excised on both sides, but on the concave side the graft is not punched in because further bone may require removal to seat the lower Harrington hook.

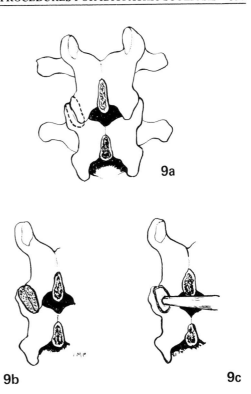

9a

9b   9c

10a&b

Insertion of the upper Harrington distraction hook

The most proximal facet joint on the concave side, which receives the top hook, is cleared of any remaining soft tissue. Gentle traction on the spinous process with Kocher forceps reveals the plane of this joint. A No. 1251* Harrington hook with a sharp forward edge is then inserted into the joint by means of the standard hook clamp and large curved hook driver. The hook should be angled downwards at about 50° as it enters the joint (*a*); otherwise the hook splits the lamina and the hold is weak. The medial edge of the hook should be in line with the lateral edge of the ligamentum flavum, which can just be seen. The hook is brought into a neutral position after the joint is entered and the sharp edge of the hook is gently hammered into a bed in the pedicle (*b*). This hook is removed and replaced with a No. 1253 blunt hook, which is left *in situ*.

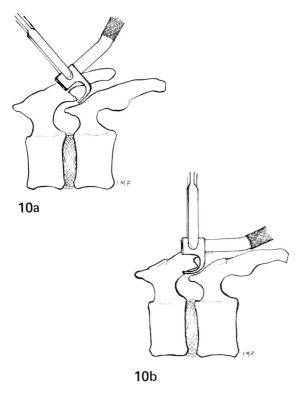

10a

10b

*Numbers refer to catalogue numbers used by Arthrodax-Zimmer U.S.A. of Amersham, Bucks.

11a,b&c

Insertion of the lower Harrington distraction hook

Using a standard fenestration technique, the ligamentum flavum is removed on the concave side just above the distal vertebra. The epidural tissue is gently freed and the lamina which receives the distal hook is carefully trimmed to provide a square bed as shown in *Illustration 6*. The blunt No. 1254 Harrington hook (*a*) is carefully inserted and, if necessary, the lamina trimmed until it has a snug fit, and it is then removed. If the fusion is extending down to the lower lumbar region, in the presence of a lordosis or a thick lamina, a Leatherman hook (No. 6114-01) is useful (*b*). When fusion extends to the pelvis then a Moe sacro-alar hook (No. 6280-02) gives a good purchase (*c*).

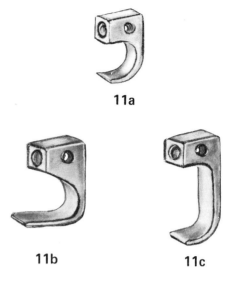

11a

11b   **11c**

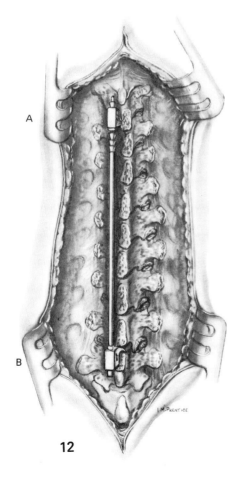

12

Decortication of the laminae and transverse processes

The spinous processes are excised at their bases with an angled bone cutter. The removed bone is fragmented and added to the bone graft already collected.

With the careful use of a large Capener gouge the laminae and transverse processes are then decorticated. The strips of thin bone are left free *in situ* or attached to the transverse process tip.

12

Insertion of Harrington rod

A hook clamp is placed on to the top hook, and the lower hook on a clamp is carefully placed in position. Both hook clamps are supported by an assistant. The distance between the two is measured and a Harrington distraction rod 1 inch (2·5 cm) less than this measurement is chosen. The ratchet end is inserted proximally through the top hook until the collar end has cleared the lower hook. This process requires a gentle side-to-side manoeuvre. The rod is then moved distally to seat the collar end of the lower hook.

13a&b

Distraction of the Harrington rod

The hooks and spine are distracted with the spreaders (*a*). Preferably these should have a gauge attached to measure the distraction force which should not exceed 20–25 kp; After the scoliosis is corrected a 'C' ring washer No. 1273 is placed on the rod, just distal to the top hook, with a 'C' ring clincher (*b*) to prevent the ratchet slipping. A short loop of stainless steel wire twisted around the rod acts just as well.

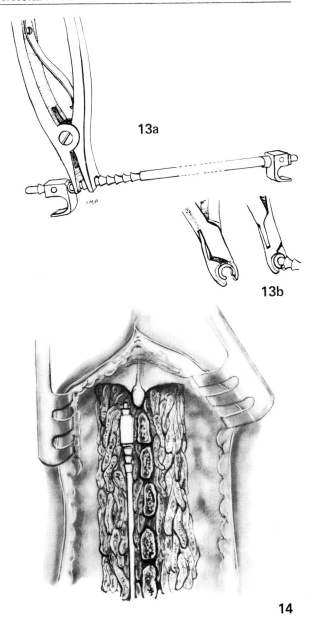

13a

13b

14

14

Addition of autogenous bone chips

The remainder of the cancellous bone graft is laid along the fusion area, the slivers placed longitudinally. After this other bone chips from the spines and iliac bone are added.

Wound closure

During closure it is not necessary to insert suction drainage into the main wound. The muscle and fascial layers are closed. After the subcutaneous fat suture a fine subcuticular continuous suture is used to close the skin and this is supported by Steristrips. This method of skin closure improves the cosmetic appearance of the scar.

POSTOPERATIVE CARE

Patients free of plaster are managed on a firm bed, being 'log rolled' every 2–4 hr from the supine to the lateral 'concave' side-down position. It is important that the trunk is moved in one piece. At 1 week after operation both lateral positions may be used in turning, and the patient may learn to turn himself with the knees and hips flexed. Postoperative x-rays should include anteroposterior and lateral spine views to show both hooks.

During the first 48 hr the patient should be kept in an intensive postoperative ward or intensive care unit. Respiratory physiotherapy including use of the Bird ventilator is important. A fluid balance chart should

be kept and the postoperative haemoglobin noted on the third day. It should be remembered that postoperative blood loss usually equals the amount lost during the operation.

At 2 weeks a holding plaster jacket should be put on, using a Risser or Cotrel plaster table. Patients already in a plaster jacket need to have the cast changed at this stage.

At 3 weeks the patient may be allowed up and a check x-ray taken.

At 3 months the plaster jacket is removed and a Milwaukee brace is applied, which is kept on until 1 year after the operation.

[The illustrations for this Chapter on Surgical Procedures for Idiopathic Scoliosis were drawn by Mrs. I. M. Prentice.]

The Dwyer Anterior Fusion for Scoliosis

M. A. Edgar, M.Chir., F.R.C.S.
Consultant Orthopaedic Surgeon, The Middlesex Hospital, London,
and Royal National Orthopaedic Hospital, London

The operative procedure described below is for a thoracolumbar curve, as shown in *Illustration 3*, and a thoracolumbar approach with division of the diaphragm is used. In lumbar curves where fusion extends proximally to L1 a simple lumbar retroperitoneal approach is adequate.

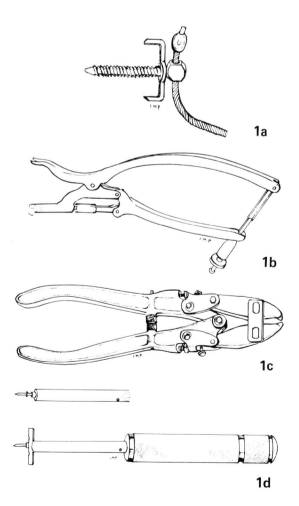

1a

1b

1c

1d

1a-e

Instrumentation

The equipment includes a whole set of cancellous screws with cannulated heads and a set of titanium vertebral plates and titanium multistrand cable. In addition three are titanium end-buttons for the cable (*a*), cable tensioner – Hall-type (*b*), swaging clamp (*c*), introducers for the vertebral plates (*d*), and the screwdriver (*e*).

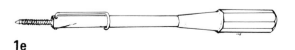

1e

THE OPERATION

2

Position of patient

The patient is placed in the lateral position so that the convexity of the scoliosis is uppermost. The upper arm is positioned forwards on a rest. This stabilizes the patient and rotates the scapula upwards. The apex of the scoliosis is placed over the break in the table, which is then broken to accentuate the convexity of the scoliosis and facilitate removal of the discs. The table is straightened before the compression cable is inserted.

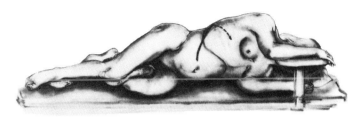

2

3

The incision

With the aid of a pre-operative marker film (*see* page 390) the rib of the highest vertebra in the curve is located. The incision is made along this rib extending posteriorly up to 2 inches (5 cm) from the spine and anteriorly across the costal margin on to the abdomen to the level of the lowest vertebra in the curve. The umbilicus is roughly at the lower border of L3. The extent of the abdominal part of the incision depends on the obliquity of the rib and the level of the rib chosen. In the illustrations the incision is made along the tenth rib.

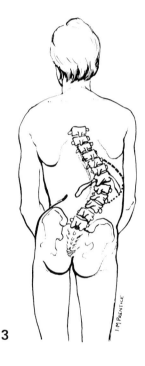

3

4

Exposure of the thoracolumbar spine

The muscles of the chest wall are divided in the line of the incision and the periosteum is reflected off the upper edge of the rib which is left *in situ*. The pleura is incised and the ribs are separated with a self-retaining rib retractor. The lung is collapsed and packed proximally using a moistened saline swab.

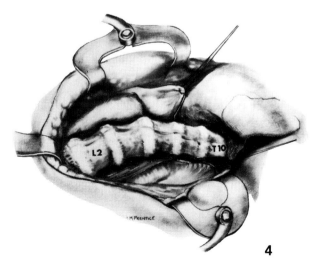

4

The diaphragm is divided along a line about 1 inch (2·5 cm) from its peripheral attachment and the subphrenic extraperitoneal space is entered. Several pairs of stay sutures on either side of this incision help to align the diaphragm correctly during the closure. Anteriorly, as the exposure is developed across the costal margin, the costal cartilage is carefully divided with strong scissors. Using blunt dissection the peritoneum is brought forward off the diaphragm to open the retroperitoneal space further posteriorly.

At this stage the thoracolumbar spine can be palpated. To expose it the following structures from above downwards need to be reflected. The lower mediastinal pleura, the crus of the diaphragm and the psoas origin from the upper lumbar intervertebral discs. Having carefully reflected these structures the segmental intercostal and lumbar vessels need to be diathermied or, if large, carefully ligated to facilitate sufficient reflection of the soft tissues round the vertebral bodies. Division of these vessels is best carried out at the mid-point of the vertebral body so that anastomoses around the intervertebral foramina are not disturbed. Moist saline swabs are used to pack the peritoneum anteriorly and by using soft malleable copper retractors a good exposure of the spine is obtained.

Excision of discs and vertebral end-plates

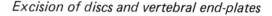

5a

The annulus fibrosus is carefully removed from the disc spaces over the visible part of the circumference using a long-handled scalpel. The discs above and below the vertebrae at the extremes of the fusion are not disturbed. The nucleus pulposus is removed with pituitary rongeurs and the disc space is curetted. The posterior part of the annulus fibrosus is not disturbed, but care is required as this may be thin.

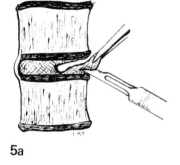

5a

5b&c

The periosteum adjacent to the end-plates is reflected over a few millimetres with a periosteal elevator. This reveals clearly the junction of the cartilage end-plate with the bone. A half-inch osteotome is gently inserted into this plane and the cartilage plate lifted off. It is safer to use a curette to remove the posterior part of the end-plate.

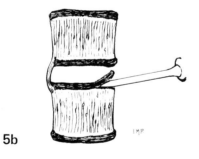

5b

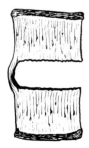

5c

Removal of autogenous bone graft from iliac crest

Through a small incision along the iliac crest below the main incision thin strips of cancellous bone are removed with a Capener gouge. Only a small amount is required and therefore the exposure need not be large.

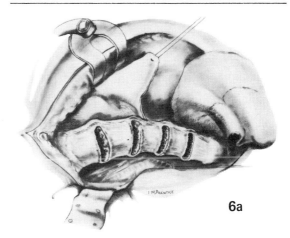

6a

Insertion of Dwyer screws and vertebral plates

6a-c

In the example shown the fusion extends from T10 to L2. The correct size of staple-shaped vertebral plate for each body is determined with a measuring divider. The correct plate is then clamped on to the spiked introducer and tapped into place with a hammer. The spike acts as a starter for the screw. The size of screw for the vertebral body is selected by measuring the depth of the adjacent disc space with a standard depth gauge. The appropriate screw is then inserted with the left index finger tip on the other side of the body. This helps to orientate the direction of the screw. As the screw tightens on to the vertebral plate the tip should just be palpable through the opposite cortex. Care must be taken to ensure that the screw is not directed posteriorly towards the spinal canal. At each end of the fusion where the disc has not been excised the vertebral plate is inserted after a small incision is made into the annulus.

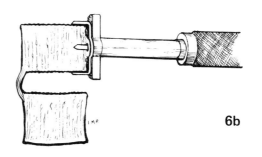

6b

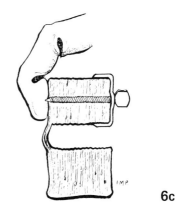

6c

7

It is best to stagger the vertebral plates so that the plate on the apical vertebra which is the most rotated lies most posteriorly. This helps derotation when the cable is tightened.

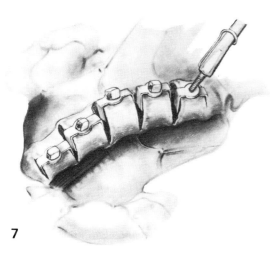

7

*Insertion of compression cable and correction
of curve*

8 a&b

At this point the operating table is straightened in
order to correct the scoliosis as much as possible. A
button is slid on to the cable and swaged on to one
end with the clamp. The cable is threaded through the
cannulated head of the top vertebral screw until
this is against the button. The cable is threaded
through the second screw head. This may be facilitated
by slightly turning the screw head. The tensioning
device is applied to the cable below the second screw.
Before the upper two vertebrae are compressed together, a thin strip of cancellous bone is placed in the
disc space. Excessive compression is avoided at the
first two levels as the top screw may pull out and, if
too much force is used, the curve can be reversed. Before the tensioning device is released the upper two
screw heads are swaged on to the cable with the
swaging clamp.

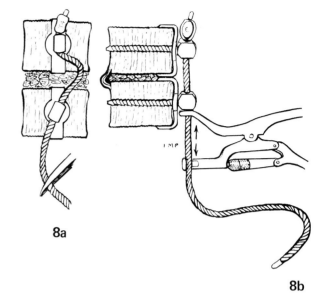

8a

8b

9

The cable is passed through the head of the next
screw and the steps repeated with insertion of bone
graft, compression and swaging. After the bottom
screw head has been swaged on to the cable another
button is threaded on to the cable and swaged as a
safety measure. The cable is then cut flush with the
button. The spinal deformity should now be corrected.

Closure

The pleura, crus and psoas are closed over the fusion
area. The diaphragm is resutured using the stay sutures
to guide the re-alignment. The chest is closed with an
underwater sealed drain to the pleural cavity. The
abdominal and chest walls are closed in layers.

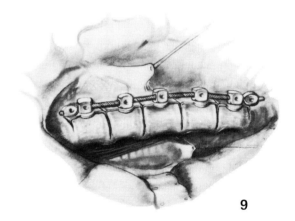

9

POSTOPERATIVE CARE

The Dwyer fixation is rigid enough for the patient to be turned quite safely in an ordinary bed. Postoperative physiotherapy and use of the Bird ventilator is important. The chest drain can usually be removed on the third postoperative day. The patient is best managed in an intensive care unit for the first 48 hr. The fluid balance should be carefully recorded and for the first 2 or 3 days oral intake is limited until any ileus is settled.

Subsequent management is similar to that for the Harrington rod operation (*see* page 391). When the wound is healed at 14 days the patient is put into a plaster body cast and may be safely mobilized straight away. At 3 months the plaster cast is changed for a Milwaukee brace or an Ortholene jacket, and this must be worn until 1 year after operation.

References

Dwyer, A. F. (1973). 'Experience of anterior correction of scoliosis.' *Clin. Orthop.* **93**, 191
Dwyer, A. F. and Schafer, M. F. (1974). Anterior approach to scoliosis.' *J. Bone Jt Surg.* **56B**, 218

[*The illustrations for this Chapter on The Dwyer Anterior Fusion for Scoliosis were drawn by Mrs. I. M. Prentice.*]

Surgical Management of Lumbar Disc Prolapses

Henry V. Crock, M.D., M.S., F.R.C.S., F.R.A.C.S.
Senior Orthopaedic Surgeon, St. Vincent's Hospital,
University of Melbourne

INTRODUCTION

In the English-speaking world the term 'laminectomy' is used commonly to describe any operation for the removal of prolapsed disc tissue. Laminectomy means excision of a lamina and implies its total removal. Properly, this term should be replaced by the phrase: 'operation for the excision of disc fragments', which describes the intent of the procedure for the surgical treatment of disc prolapse in its varying forms. Differing methods of surgical approach will depend on factors such as the size of the spinal canal, the height of the disc space and on the site, size and distribution of the prolapsed disc tissue.

Types of lumbar disc prolapse

The characteristics of prolapses vary with the physical qualities of the affected disc tissue (Crock, 1976). In young persons, discrete small rounded, firm or fluctuant protrusions are found with stretched, but intact annulus fibres covering the prolapse. When these fibres are incised at operation, only a small quantity of disc tissue may escape and be removed, leaving in the disc a defect, which admits neither curettes nor disc rongeurs. The consistency of such discs is often described as rubbery. There are usually some degenerate annular fibres to be found with the extruded nuclear tissue in these cases.

Extrusion of variable quantities of disc tissue (1·1 – 13·5 g) into the spinal canal may be seen when gross degenerative changes have occurred in the disc as a whole. The description of sequestrated disc fragments is then applied. The components of such fragments may include nuclear, annular and end-plate material.

Between these two extremes a variety of pathological changes may be noted. Incomplete sequestration may be associated with marked perineural fibrosis, a finding related to physicochemical changes in the disc (Nachemson, 1969). Calcified nuclear tissue may herniate or calcification may occur in prolapsed tissue and erosion of the dural sac follow (Blikra, 1969).

A sequestrated fragment may migrate to another level from the disc of its origin, leaving a clearly defined oval defect in the posterior annulus. Sequestrated disc tissue may present posterior to the dural sac (Hooper, 1973).

Rarely, disc tissue may prolapse into the vertebral bodies and re-enter the spinal canal, pushing ahead of it a small fragment of vertebral end-plate bone and cartilage. Knowledge of the varying relationships which prolapsed disc tissue may bear to the neural contents of the spinal canal is essential to the understanding of the varied clinical pictures which may present.

In a subrhizal prolapse, the disc fragment lies anterior to the affected nerve root and this usually causes severe pain with objective motor and sensory signs distally in the part of the limb supplied by the compressed nerve root.

1

Prolapses situated between the dural sac and the nerve root sheath — axillary prolapses, or those lying on the outer side of the nerve root sheath — pararhizal prolapses, may produce symptoms of severe sciatica without abnormal objective physical signs. (The illustration shows four types of disc prolapses in the lower lumbar region. On the left side a pararhizal prolapse is shown at the top, below this, migrating sequestrated disc fragments are shown with a small circular annular defect above them. On the right side an axillary prolapse is illustrated at the top and lower down a subrhizal prolapse.)

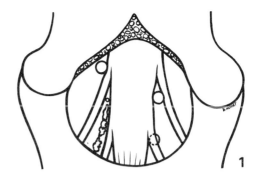

Centrally placed prolapses or a large migrating sequestrated fragment in the spinal canal may give rise to physical signs which vary from day to day and from one leg to the other. Cauda equina claudication with the onset of buttock or leg pains after walking short distances, may also be found (Verbiest, 1955, 1976).

PRE-OPERATIVE

Pre-operative preparation

Full blood examination, including blood grouping and sedimentation rate, should be performed. It is wise to insert an intravenous infusion in all patients before operation for disc disorders, though blood transfusion is rarely indicated.

Pre-operative myelography with a water-soluble medium such as metrizamide (Amipaque) should be performed to confirm the level of the affected disc.

X-rays of the patient's spine should always be available in the operating theatre.

The use of prophylactic chemotherapy may be indicated if there is any antecedent history of serious infection, including previous wound infections.

Anaesthesia

General anaesthesia with muscular relaxation and mechanical ventilation is most commonly employed. Cardiac monitoring is recommended in older patients or whenever it is known that the patient has particular cardiac problems.

2&3

Positioning on the operating table

There are a number of factors which may be critical to the success of this operation, but none is more important than the position in which the patient is placed before the operation commences. A variety of suitable postures is shown in the following illustrations. The most versatile and easily managed is the *prone position*. The supporting sponge rubber U-piece is simply constructed and inexpensive. The right arm is shown dependent and supported on a well-padded arm rest which is suspended below the level of the table. Ulnar neuritis may occur unless the arm is carefully postured in this way. The left arm may rest by the patient's side. The table is angled in the centre. The surgeon's assistant and other observers will have unobstructed views of procedures throughout the course of the operation. The entire range of surgical manoeuvres that may be required for the execution of even the most complex operation, including transdural excision of prolapsed disc tissue, can be accomplished in comfort and without undue restraints on its duration.

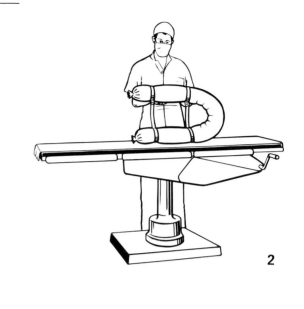

2

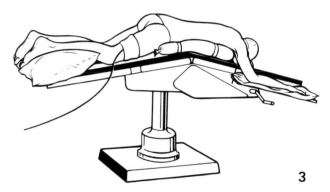

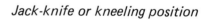

3

4

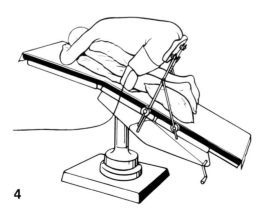

4

Jack-knife or kneeling position

In this position, with the use of a simple frame to support the buttocks excellent operating conditions are provided. Alternatively, the patient may be placed in this position with pillows under the chest so that the abdomen is unsupported. A pillow is placed under the patient's feet and a restraining strap across the legs — though venous obstruction in the lower limbs is then likely to occur. The table is angled. The major objections to the use of this particular posture revolve around the difficulties of setting the patient in position and of dealing with emergencies, which may require the patient to be turned rapidly into a supine position. Particular attention should be paid to the ulnar nerves in this position.

5

Lateral position

The use of this position can be recommended in special circumstances, for example, when the patient is extremely obese or when there are special chest problems which may complicate anaesthesia. Note the pillow between the patient's legs, the restraining strap crossing the iliac crest, the sandbag placed above the dependent iliac crest. The table is angled in the centre. There are objections to the routine use of this position: (*1*) the assistant surgeon is rarely comfortable and has a restricted view of the operation field; (*2*) lighting of the wound area may be difficult; (*3*) haemorrhage control is often more difficult to obtain as is access to the nerve root canal on the dependent side of the spine.

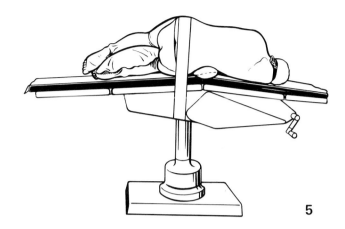

5

Instruments

The recommended essential special instruments and disposable supplies are listed below:

(*1*) Self-retaining retractors.
(*2*) Fine sucker.
(*3*) Bayonet forceps.
(*4*) Long-handled carrier for size 11 or 15 blade scalpel.
(*5*) Watson-Cheyne probe.
(*6*) Nerve root retractor, such as a Scaglietti probe (10 inches — 25 cm — long).
(*7*) A range of bone rongeurs.
(*8*) A range of pituitary type rongeurs, straight, angled outwards at 45° and at 90° with cutting cups of varying dimensions.
(*9*) Hammer.
(*10*) Fine osteotomes and chisels.
(*11*) Ring curettes.
(*12*) 6/0 suture material on fine cutting needles with a fine needle holder.
(*13*) Neurosurgical patties and haemostatic gauze or sponge materials.
(*14*) Bone wax.
(*15*) Bi-polar coagulator.

THE OPERATION

Skin incision

Before the skin incision is made the surgeon should once again inspect the patient's x-rays, paying attention to vertebral anomalies, such as spina bifida occulta and sacralization and noting certain lesions such as spondylolisthesis or isolated disc resorption (Crock, 1976). The level of the planned exposure of the spine should be noted. *Radiographs of the lumbar spine taken in the operating theatre are often of poor quality and cannot, therefore, be relied upon to identify a particular spinal level.*

The skin incision is made in the mid-line or slightly right or left of the spinous processes, extending longitudinally a short distance above and below the vertebral interspace to be explored. It is deepened at once through the subcutaneous fat layer to the level of the lumbodorsal fascia. In extremely obese patients, the depth of the subcutaneous fat layer between the skin and the lumbodorsal aponeurosis over the lumbosacral area, may be 12 cm or more. In such cases this fatty tissue should be carefully handled, avoiding excessive burning with the coagulating diathermy (*see* 'Wound closure', page 414).

Separation of the paraspinal muscles

An incision is made on one side of the tip of a spinous process, using the cutting current diathermy, passed through a suitable blade-shaped end. The incision continues downwards and upwards immediately adjacent to the side of the spinous process parallel to the adjacent interspinous ligaments and then to the sides of the related spinous processes. Bleeding occurs at this stage from posterior branches of the lumbar arteries related to the middle of the side of each spinous process. The muscle mass may be retracted with a closed dissecting forcep placed into the depth of the space, so that the diathermy blade may cut the musculotendinous attachments from the inferior surfaces of the spinous processes and from the interspinous ligaments near their bases. Throughout this procedure the smoke generated by the diathermy cutting tip may be evacuated with the sucker.

The muscle mass is next separated from the outer surface of each lamina using an appropriate 'elevator', such as the Cobb.

Following the use of the muscle elevator which raises the paraspinal muscles laterally to the level of the apophyseal joint capsules, further bleeding may be encountered from posterior branches of the lumbar arteries in the area. This bleeding is readily controlled following the insertion of cotton Raytec swabs (bearing x-ray markers) packed into the depths of the wound along its length.

The same approach is then repeated on the opposite side of the spinous processes until the paraspinal muscle mass has been similarly separated from the roof of the spinal canal. Cotton Raytee swabs are again inserted and the self-retaining retractors of the surgeon's choice then prepared for insertion. Some surgeons favour muscle stripping on one side of the spine only (Finneson, 1973).

Unless the technique described is followed carefully, considerable blood loss may occur, even during this preliminary stage of the approach to the disc prolapse.

The cotton Raytec swabs are removed from the lower end of the wound on either side of the S1 spinous process. Hand-held retractors expose the back of the sacrum allowing the first self-retaining retractor to be inserted and fixed in place. This procedure is repeated at the upper end of the wound and the second self-retaining retractor inserted.

At this stage, cotton Raytec swabs are again packed firmly along one of the paraspinal gutters while attention is focused on the opposite side to identify the lumbosacral junction. Soft-tissue remnants of muscle fibres and fat are then removed from the interspace to be opened. This cleaning-up process can be accomplished rapidly and neatly by using a straight pituitary rongeur with a 4 mm cup, taking off first the muscle remnants from the interspinous ligament and then all the soft tissues from the posterior surface of the ligamentum flavum.

Bleeding is not a problem during these manoeuvres at the lumbosacral junction until the extrasynovial fat pad of the apophyseal joint is removed, if that is necessary. On avulsing this fat pad, quite brisk arterial and venous haemorrhage will occur. The bleeding vessels are readily identified by the use of a sucker and cotton Raytec swab. The vessels are picked up with the bayonet forcep and coagulated with the diathermy. When exposure at the L4-L5 interspace is required following the initial clearing procedure as described above, the pars interarticularis of the fifth lumbar lamina is exposed. The sucker tip may be used as a dissector at this stage, sucking up remnants of fatty tissue. The main stem of the posterior branch of the lumbar artery is found constantly at the middle of the outer edge of the pars interarticularis. From it, arcuate branches pass upwards and downwards towards the capsules of the apophyseal joints. Haemorrhage points are easily identified, though care must be taken not to diathermy the main stem far anterior to the anterior margin of the pars interarticularis. Damage to entrant neural arteries at the intervertebral foramen is thereby avoided. The main stem of the posterior branch of each lumbar artery is accompanied by the corresponding and somewhat larger vein (Crock and Yoshizawa, 1977).

In cases where exposure of both sides of the interspace may be required, the detailed clearing process, just described, is completed on the opposite side.

6 & 7

At this stage, it will be noted that there are some capsular fibres extending medially onto the ligamentum flavum for some distance at its upper margin where it passes beneath the inferior margin of the superior lamina of the interspace. (Note *a* the extension of capsular fibres onto the posterior surface of the ligamentum flavum. The extrasynovial fat pads *b* are showing in an exaggerated form.) These fibres should be removed with a straight pituitary rongeur before opening the ligamentum flavum. Portions of the inferior surface of the superior lamina at the interspace may then require to be excised (using an outward angled rongeur) and in some cases the interspinous ligament may be removed together with portion of the inferior surface of the spinous process at the upper level of the interspace. Some surgeons favour the use of chisels or gauges for this particular manoeuvre. Bone wax may be applied to the cut surface of the cancellous bone.

The ligamentum flavum should then be incised vertically in the mid-line using either a No. 11 or 15 blade scalpel. The cut edge of the ligamentum flavum is picked up with a fine toothed forceps and the incision deepened until either epidural fat or the dura itself is exposed.

The blunt end of the Watson-Cheyne dissector may then be used to widen the opening into the spinal canal. Through the vertical slit in the ligamentum flavum thus created, a small moistened cotton patty is inserted between the ligamentum flavum and the epidural fat using the curved end of the Watson-Cheyne dissector. The ligamentum flavum is then cut in a lateral direction, first at the upper edge of the interspace and later at the lower edge of the interspace, until a flap is raised and turned out laterally.

Even at this early stage of the opening of the spinal canal, the presence of a large prolapse can be suspected when difficulty is experienced during the insertion of the patty or patties, particularly when efforts are made to push them further laterally under the ligamentum flavum as the flap is enlarged.

When the ligamentum flavum has been turned laterally as a flap to the level of the apophyseal joint, a fourth incision is then most commonly made in it, again in a vertical direction to excise the flap.

Following this initial opening into the spinal canal proper, the surgeon must then identify certain landmarks. The Watson-Cheyne probe is the most valuable instrument for this purpose. Either the blunt or curved end may be inserted depending on the size of the protrusion at the affected level. If the prolapse is small, then the blunt end may be inserted laterally so that the pedicle on the inferior side of the intervertebral disc space may be palpated. The regional nerve root is then palpated. Moving upwards, the posterior surface of the disc may be felt and the disposition of a prolapse assessed.

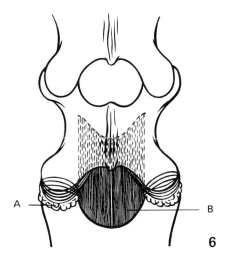

6

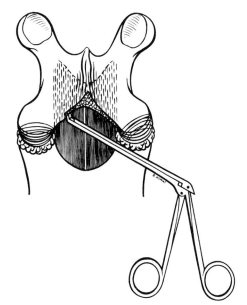

7

Wider exposure may be required and this is usually most easily achieved with a 45° outward angled rongeur. Assuming, for example, that it is necessary to remove more of the outer edge of the ligamentum flavum, then the sucker with a moistened patty on its tip may be used to retract the dura and nerve roots towards the mid-line, while the rongeur is inserted beneath the edge of the ligamentum flavum under direct vision. Depending on the size of the prolapse, it may or may not be possible to insert the angled rongeur. If attempts are made to force the foot-plate of the rongeur between the ligamentum flavum and the nerve root which is being pressed backwards by a large disc prolapse, then the root may be bruised or crushed. On occasions, even a thin rongeur cannot be inserted. The interspace will need to be enlarged either superiorly or inferiorly or in both directions until sufficient space has been created to allow identification of the nerve root as it traverses the interspace.

8

When the prolapse is large and subrhizal at the L5-S1 level for example, then enlargement of the interspace may be necessary by removal of part of the superior border of the lamina of S1, commencing initially in the mid-line and passing laterally. It may be necessary to perform a decompression of the S1 nerve root canal by removing the medial portion of the S1 facet flush with the inner margin of the S1 pedicle. The illustration shows a fourth lumbar vertebra from behind. On the right side of the specimen the fifth lumbar nerve root canal has been unroofed and the inner margin of the pedicle is shown. In the operation of nerve root canal decompression, the apex of the facet also needs to be removed.

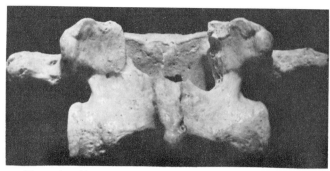

(Reproduced by courtesy of J. B. Lippincott Co. from *Clinical Orthopaedics and Related Research*, Vol. 115, 1976)   **8**

9 & 10

During the more complicated manoeuvres of this type, haemorrhage from the external vertebral venous plexus surrounding the nerve root and lateral to it may occur. Such haemorrhage is usually not troublesome when the patient is in the prone position. On occasions, however, the external vertebral venous plexus may be distended and brisk venous haemorrhage may occur following damage to some of the radicular branches of this system of veins. (*Illustration 9* shows the detailed anatomy of the anterior internal vertebral venous plexus in the lumbar region. The cut edge of the dural sac is retracted slightly towards the mid-line. Note the large radicular vein which emerges from the dural sac medial to the nerve root.) Venous haemorrhage is always readily controlled with the gentle use of a patty and sucker as illustrated. Occasionally, bleeding from one of the large venous radicles can be troublesome and it may be necessary to identify this using the sucker and a patty. The bleeding point or several points are grasped with the bayonet forceps and coagulated with low-voltage or bipolar coagulating currents.

At other times, bleeding from several points of the plexiform system of veins can be controlled by light packing of a haemostatic substance held in place with a moistened patty.

It should be possible to obtain good exposure of the field and bleeding should be minimal before any attempt is made to retract the nerve root for the final exposure of prolapsed disc material.

For the sake of clarity and brevity, special points of technique will be described in relation to individual types of disc prolapse.

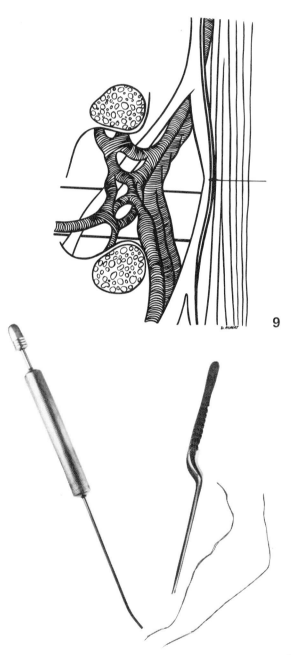

9

10

SMALL SUBRHIZAL PROLAPSE

11

Partial excision of the ligamentum flavum on one side will afford satsifactory access to the canal. Initially, identification of the landmarks of pedicle, disc and affected nerve root is made using the sucker and patty as a medial retractor and the blunt end of the Watson-Cheyne dissector in the lateral part of the canal. (The photograph is a dissection of the lower lumbar spine in an adult and shows some of the relations of the lumbar nerve roots. Note especially the origins of the nerve root sleeves from the dural sac and the course of the nerve roots in relation to the pedicles.)

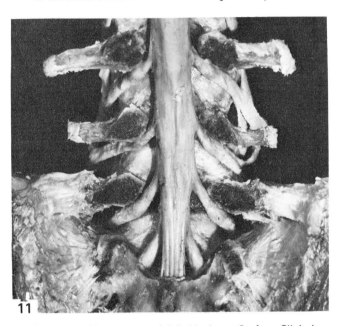

11

(Reproduced by courtesy of J. B. Lippincott Co. from *Clinical Orthopaedics and Related Research,* Vol. 115, 1976)

Blunt dissection will separate the epidural fat and the nerve root can usually be easily retracted medially. The discrete rounded prolapse with intact annular fibres is then outlined and a suitable nerve root retractor inserted. The surgeon may use the sucker with a moist patty on its tip as a retractor laterally in the interspace while the assistant holds the nerve root medially. In a dry field it should then be possible to incise the annular fibres over the prolapse in a cruciate fashion using a No. 11 or 15 blade scalpel. The prolapsed tissue then begins to emerge spontaneously and it may be picked out with a straight pituitary rongeur of appropriate dimension varying from 1 to 4 mm bite.

Only a small volume of disc tissue can be removed in such cases and curettage of the interspace is not recommended.

LARGE SUBRHIZAL PROLAPSE

In such cases, adequate exposure on the side of the prolapse is essential. Technical details for the enlargement both superiorly and inferiorly have been outlined above. Identification of the affected root may be a problem, because in such circumstances the root is often flattened and its lateral margin not easily identified. It may be of the same colour as the disc prolapse beneath it.

It is essential under such circumstances to identify the nerve root sleeve at its junction with the dura above or to identify the main stem of the nerve root at the level of the inferior pedicle. By either method, with the use of an appropriate nerve root dissector, the outer edge of the nerve root can be identified and retracted medially. Very fine straight and curved pituitary rongeurs will be required in such a case to remove the first of the fragment of prolapsed tissue, possibly through a minute incision in intact annular fibres. Only after the removal of initial fragments with small instruments, will it become possible to complete the dissection and retraction of the nerve root medially from the bulk of the prolapse.

12

As the tension on the nerve root is released so can it be more easily retracted. The opening in the annular fibres may be enlarged under vision and rongeurs of increasing cup size inserted for removal of free disc fragments from the interspace. The disposition of the instruments during removal of prolapsed disc tissues is shown. The sucker with a patty on the end of it may be used as a retractor held by the surgeon in his left hand while, with the rongeur in his right hand the fragments are lifted out from the interspace.

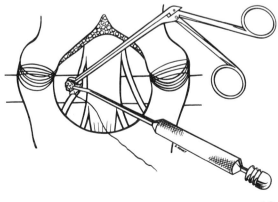

12

13

It is in such cases that quite large amounts of disc material may be removed and the risk of penetration of rongeurs deep into the interspace with the possibility of damage to intra-abdominal structures is high. The use of ring curettes is recommended in such cases for curettage of loose disc fragments and vertebral end-plate material. When large amounts of disc material have been removed, of the order of several grams of tissue, then it is wise to perform a root canal decompression on both sides of the interspace (*see Illustration 9*), completing removal of ligamentum flavum far laterally and removing the inner margins of the superior articular facet of the inferior vertebra at the interspace on each side. In addition, with angled rongeurs it may be necessary to remove the apices of both the superior facets on the inferior side of the interspace. Excision of the whole facet joint in the course of this operation should be avoided.

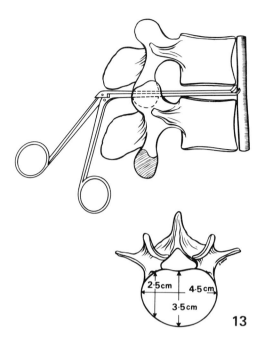

13

THE MANAGEMENT OF SEQUESTRATED DISC FRAGMENTS

The finding of free fragments of disc tissue in the spinal canal may pose specific problems at operation. These problems relate, more than anything else, to the site of origin of the disc tissue. If, for example, free fragments of disc tissue are found at the lumbosacral level, yet the posterior annular fibres of the L5-S1 disc space are found to be normal, then exploration of the higher interspace is essential. In these circumstances careful palpation of the L5-S1 disc with the blunt end of the Watson-Cheyne dissector beneath the dural sac towards the mid-line, will be necessary before it can be safely assumed that the disc tissue has not arisen from that interspace.

If in other circumstances the L4-5 interspace has been exposed and a rather adherent nerve root retracted from the back of the disc to reveal a circumscribed rounded defect in the annulus, then free sequestrated disc material may be found at the lower interspace.

CENTRAL DISC PROLAPSE

The presence of a central disc prolapse is usually, though not always, suspected in the early stages of opening of the spinal canal. For example, the canal may be opened on one side and the nerve root which comes into view cannot be retracted towards the mid-line, though the disc beneath it and lateral to it appears normal. In such a case, digital palpation of the dural sac is essential and will lead the surgeon to establish this diagnosis.

In such a case, wide exposure is required even involving excision of the whole of the spinous process and the arch of the lamina on the superior side of the interspace.

In these circumstances, careful attention is paid to the removal of the laminal arch leaving intact the pars interarticularis on each side. Once adequate exposure of the spinal canal has been achieved, the surgeon may determine the size of the central disc prolapse by careful digital palpation. He should then prepare to open the dura in the mid-line assuming that he has been unable to gain access to the disc on either side of the interspace.

TRANSDURAL APPROACH TO CENTRAL DISC PROLAPSE

Having determined to remove the fragments by a transdural approach, then the special instruments listed above must be available, especially the fine sutures and needle holders which will be required to repair the dural opening. In addition, 3 inch long lintine strips with attached threads should be available as these may need to be placed along each edge of the dural sac to prevent seepage of blood into the subarachnoid space after the dura has been opened.

The dural vessels in the mid-line may be coagulated over the length of the proposed dural incision using very low voltage coagulating current. This done, the dura is incised with a No. 15 blade scalpel and a protective probe introduced near the top of the incision. This is followed downwards progressively as the full length of the dural incision is made.

At a later stage, any uncontrolled forward movement with a rongeur introduces the added risk of major vessel injury or gut injury on the anterior vertebral margin of the interspace.

Bearing these hazards in mind, the actual process of removal of disc tissue is easily and rapidly accomplished by the transdural root following separate anterior incision of the dura and the posterior longitudinal ligament over the disc space. It is likely, however, that the prolapse will have emerged on one side of this ligament.

Depending on the volume of disc material that can be removed with straight or angled pituitary rongeurs of varying sizes, so the question of curettage of the disc space may arise. If large quantities of disc material can be easily removed, it is wise to use a ring curette to clear other remnants.

Although some authors recommend closure of the anterior layer of the dural sac following this procedure, this is not always necessary. However, careful closure of the posterior layer should be obtained using a continuous 6/0 dural stitch. The retaining sutures which were earlier inserted, are used to retract the dura in the final stages of closure and care is taken at all times to avoid transfixion of any of the cauda equina filaments in the closing suture.

14

Cerebrospinal fluid is allowed to escape. It should be aspirated from the wound, but at all times the sucker should now be covered with patty. An inexperienced surgeon or an inexperienced assistant may from any point onwards in this operation inflict irreversible damage on filaments of the cauda equina. Remembering that the vessels of the cauda equina are minute, then only smooth rounded instruments (as shown) should be used to retract the filaments from the mid-line laterally on each side. At no stage should an unguarded sucker be placed within the dural sac itself or a whole nerve root may be avulsed up the sucker.

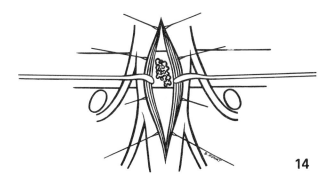

14

In cases of this type, especially when many fragments of intervertebral disc tissue have been removed from the interspace, it is wise to perform a bilateral nerve root canal decompression to complete the procedure. This involves excision of the upper edge of the inferior lamina together with the over-hanging border of the superior articular process of the interspace and excision of the whole of the ligamentum flavum laterally at the intervertebral foramen level, together with the tip of the superior articular process. This dissection is carried out on both sides and is best done by using 45° outward angled pituitary rongeurs of appropriate sizes.

DISC PROLAPSES ASSOCIATED WITH OTHER SPECIAL PROBLEMS

Disc prolapse associated with spinal canal stenosis

This situation should be recognized pre-operatively in most instances, especially if myelography has been performed. The disc prolapses found in these cases are often small. It is essential to perform an adequate spinal canal or nerve root canal decompression on both sides in such cases.

Nerve root and other anomalies

Associated anomalies of nerve roots or of the blood vessels associated with nerve roots, especially arterial anomalies (Crock and Yoshizawa, 1977): recognition of nerve root or of vascular anomalies requires excellent technique of exposure. The nerve root which sometimes arises from the dural sac at right angles passing directly laterally through the intervertebral foramen across the posterior surface of the disc, may easily be mistaken for a prolapse at operation. It may therefore be incised, excised or avulsed in error.

Isolated disc resorption

Unilateral sciatica in cases of isolated disc resorption (Crock, 1976) is not common. The most important part of the surgery for this condition is the nerve root canal decompression and foramenotomy which can usually be performed with preservation of the laminal arch. The disc prolapse in such instances is usually a small fragment of vertebral end-plate cartilage situated subrhizally. It may be adherent to the under-surface of the nerve root requiring careful dissection, especially as the root may be flattened in these circumstances.

Disc prolapse in association with spondylolisthesis

Disc prolapse may occur at the level of a spondylolisthesis or above it. Excision of the prolapsed disc fragments is essential, but questions of complete spinal canal and nerve root canal decompression including removal of the loose lamina, together with decisions on the use of spinal fusion techniques may all arise.

Upper lumbar disc prolapses

They may occur in the L1-2 L2-3 area in associati with the conus medullaris in some cases. Operatic in this area carry hazards of spinal cord injury a.. retraction of the dural sac must be performed with great care at all times. Similarly, the introduction of large jawed pituitary rongeurs or large ring curettes may be hazardous.

Preserving the bony canal

In the past it has been common practice to remove either half of one side of a lamina or to cut a narrow channel between two disc spaces across one half of a lamina in the course of seeking out otherwise elusive disc prolapses. This interference with the roofing apparatus of the spinal canal is to be avoided, particularly in cases with spinal canal or nerve root canal stenosis. Exploration of an intervertebral disc space can be accurately and competently performed through a limited exposure, carried out along the lines recommended above. If no lesion is found at one level, due to error, then it is better to look at the next level upwards or downwards from the primary exploration without disturbing the integrity of the lamina.

Wound closure

Suction drainage may be used, though following leakage of cerebrospinal fluid or opening of the dura for transdural disc excision, suction drainage should be avoided.

Dural tears are most likely to occur in complicated cases, for example where there is associated spinal canal stenosis and opening of the canal proves difficult, or again in the course of separating an adherent root from a disc prolapse. These defects should be identified carefully and repaired with fine sutures.

Undue haste, poor haemorrhage control and careless handling of rongeurs or root retractors may lead to serious dural injuries. Indeed, dural tears may be inflicted even before the ligamentum flavum has been opened if rongeurs 'slip' into the spinal canal.

Careful attention to wound closure is important. Deep sutures may be placed in the muscle layer, but these should be tied only to the point of approximation of the muscle masses in the mid-line. Most attention should be focused on tight closure of the lumbodorsal fascia with interrupted sutures.

In extremely obese patients, it is wise to use subcuticular plain catgut or Dexon sutures tied carefully to avoid crushing the fatty tissue. Excessive use of diathermy in the fatty layer and rough handling of this tissue will result in the leakage of liquefied fat from the wound. Infection in this layer may subsequently become troublesome.

The skin is closed with interrupted nylon sutures.

References

Blikra, J. (1969). 'Intradural herniated lumbar disc.' *J. Neurosurg.* **31,** 676

Crock, H. V. (1976). 'Traumatic disc injury'. In *Vinken and Bruyn's Handbook of Clinical Neurology.* Amsterdam: North Holland Publishing Co

Crock, H. V. and Yoshizawa, H. (1977). *The Blood Supply of the Vertebral Column and Spinal Cord in Man.* New York: Springer Verlag

Finneson, B. E. (1973). *Low Back Pain.* Philadelphia: J. B. Lippincott Co.

Hooper, J. (1973). 'Low back pain and manipulation.' *Med. J. Aust.* **1,** 549

Nachemson, A. (1969). 'Intradiscal measurements of pH in patients with lumbar rhizopathies.' *Acta orthop. scand.* **40,** 23

Verbiest, H. (1955). 'Further experience of the pathological influence of a developmental narrowness of the bony lumbar vertebral canal.' *J. Bone Jt Surg.* **37B,** 576

Verbiest, H. (1976). *Neurogenic Intermittent Claudication.* Amsterdam: North-Holland Publishing Co.

[*The illustrations for this Chapter on Surgical Management of Lumbar Disc Prolapses were drawn by Mr. D. Howat.*]

Direct Repair of the Bony Defect in Spondylolisthesis

J. E. Buck, F.R.C.S.(Eng.), F.R.C.S.(Ed.)
Consultant Orthopaedic Surgeon, Greenwich and Bexley Area Health Authority

PRE - OPERATIVE

Indications

The patient must have sufficient disability to warrant the domestic and occupational disturbance involved — this means 2 months off light or sedentary work and 3 or 4 months off heavy work or sport. A progressive slip on serial x-rays is a positive indication.

Contra-indications

A slip of more than 3 or 4 mm, or an obvious derangement of the intervertebral disc space, are both contra-indications, as are also a neurological defect or a marked sciatic element in the symptoms.

Object

The operation aims to fix the fracture site or defect with screws as shown while a cancellous inlay/onlay graft restores bony continuity.

Preparation

The skin is cleaned and shaved in the usual way.

Position of patient

The patient is prone and flexed over a Wilson frame or other device to minimize abdominal pressure.

THE OPERATION

The incision

Any spinal approach may be used which will show the whole lamina, the joint above, the base of the transverse process and the iliac crest donor site.

1

Identification of the defect

After separating the muscles from the sides of the spine and the back of the laminae a rugine is passed upwards and laterally over the lamina towards the superior facet and comes to lie in the defect immediately below that facet. Moving the spinous process with a Pennybacker nibbler will confirm the position of the false joint and the fibrous tissue comprising it may then be freely removed with the nibbler, exposing the back of the pedicle and the base of the transverse process.

Retraction during this stage is done with a long-bladed Travers and exposure is assisted by a Hohmann spike or narrow bone lever the tip of which is placed above or below the transverse process.

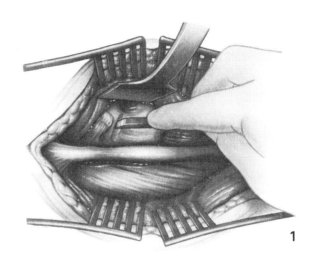

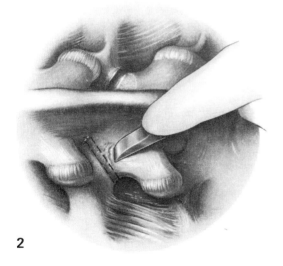

2

Preparation of the graft area

The defect and adjacent surfaces must now be thoroughly cleaned of all fibrous tissue and sclerotic bone and a small and very sharp periosteal elevator is essential (Adson's —straight or curved). A high-speed burr makes the work easy but within the defect a narrow angled nibbler (Cushing's) is usually necessary.

3&4

Placing the screws

The inferior edge of the lamina is squared off with a nibbler and a 7/64 or 3 mm drill is entered between the cortical plates and directed visually towards the defect. A long drill — at least 15 cm — is required, otherwise the drill chuck fouls the lower end of the wound or the sacral spine and the drill will not lie in the correct line. The drill must be seen to cross the defect and there is then about 1 cm of bone available before the drill is felt to pass out into the foramen above the defect but the screw must be short enough not to do this or it may irritate the nerve in that foramen. When both sides are drilled the introduction of the screws at once abolishes the instability of the lamina as well as the characteristic lateral mobility of the vertebra above. If the drill appears at all likely to split the lamina a 2 mm drill and Hick's screws must be substituted.

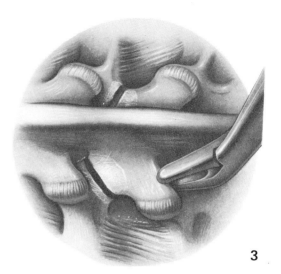

3

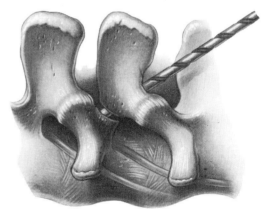

4

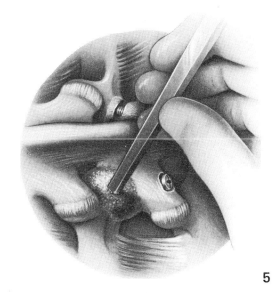

5

5,6&7

The graft

Small cancellous grafts are taken from the iliac crest and packed into the defect and around it on the posterior and lateral aspects. Care must be taken not to push grafts through the defect into the underlying foramen.

If there is a spina bifida a third screw may be entered transversely and supported with a suitable bone graft but the area must be prepared like the other graft sites.

Wound closure is in the usual layers with vacuum drainage which is removed in 24 hr or when drainage stops.

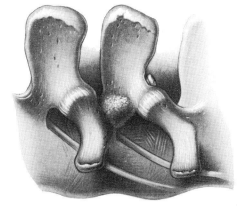

6

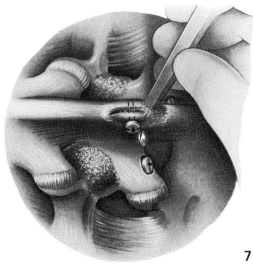

7

POSTOPERATIVE CARE

The patient is mobilized on the second or third day and in the case of narrow or unilateral defects a corset gives adequate protection. With wide or multiple defects a plaster or Glassona jacket is required for the first 6—8 weeks.

8, 9 & 10

Minimum immobilization time is 8 weeks and a few have required double this but control x-rays at 8 and 12 weeks will guide in this matter — three views are required: anteroposterior, lateral or oblique.

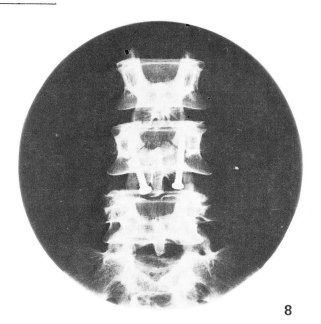

8

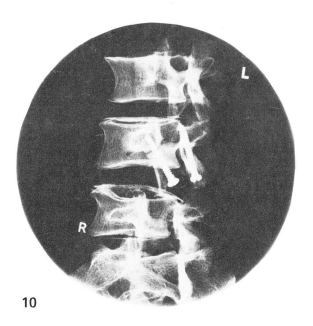

10

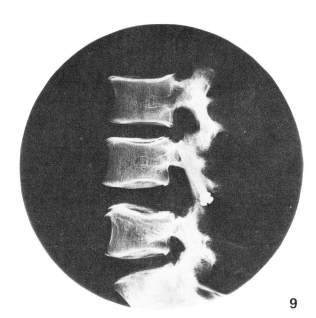

9

[*The illustrations for this Chapter on Direct Repair of the Bony Defect in Spondylolisthesis were drawn by Mr. M. J. Courtney.*]

Intertransverse Fusion for Spondylolisthesis and Lumbar Instability

E. O'Gorman Kirwan, F.R.C.S.(Eng.), F.R.C.S.(Ed.)
Consultant Orthopaedic Surgeon, University College Hospital and
Royal National Orthopaedic Hospital, London

GENERAL PRINCIPLES

Spondylolisthesis is a mechanical derangement which has a number of very different aetiological types.

Surgery may be required to:

(*1*) relieve the symptoms caused by compression of the neural elements on the spinal canal (decompression);

(*2*) relieve the pain of instability (arthrodesis); or

(*3*) a combination of both.

If there are no neural compressive symptoms the dorsal mid-line muscles may be preserved and an intertransverse fusion performed by splitting the erector spinae muscles bilaterally in their lateral two-thirds.

Conversely, if a combined procedure of decompression and fusion is required, a mid-line approach with extensive muscle retraction as far as the tips of the transverse processes will be required.

THE OPERATIONS

INTERTRANSVERSE FUSION WITHOUT DECOMPRESSION

1a&b

Skin incisions

Two curved vertical incisions extending across the posterior iliac crest and about 3 inches (7·5 cm) from the mid-line are normally used (*a*).

A transverse skin incision just below the iliac crest produces a more cosmetic scar and can be used if the patient is not very large or the extent of the fusion is limited (*b*).

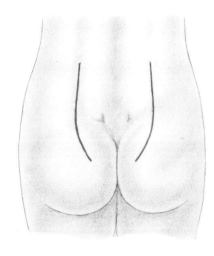

1a

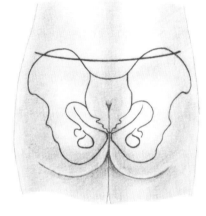

1b

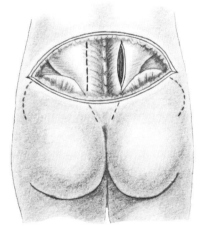

2

2

Division of dorsolumbar fascia

The dorsolumbar fascia is split vertically in its lateral two-thirds and the erector spinae muscles are split in the same plane.

3

Stripping of soft tissues

The wound is deepened until the transverse processes, upper surface of the ala of the sacrum and facet joints are exposed.

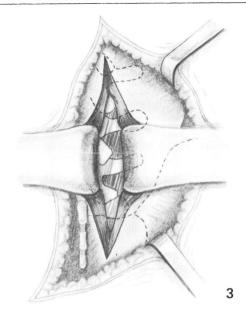

3

4

Clearing of articular surfaces

The joint surfaces should be excised with a small osteotome.

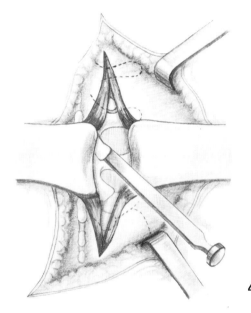

4

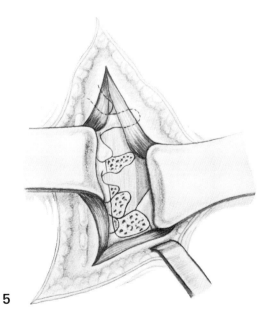

5

5

Decortication

Meticulous decortication of the upper surface of the sacrum, the lateral aspect of the articular facets and the transverse processes should be done using a gouge and nibbler.

6

Grafting

Cancellous slivers taken from the posterior iliac crest are packed into the area.

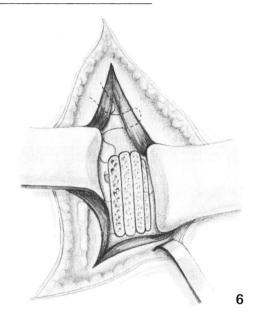

6

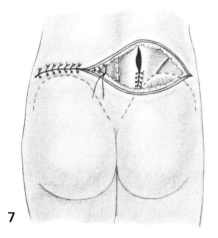

7

7

Wound closure

Interrupted sutures to dorsolumbar fascia, subcutaneous fat and skin are inserted.

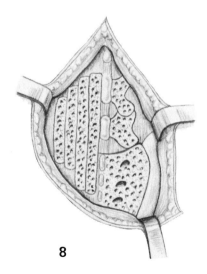

8

INTERTRANSVERSE FUSION WITH DECOMPRESSION

8

Through a curved mid-line incision the sacrospinalis muscle is reflected from each side of the sacrum, exposing the alae lateral to the articular facets. The muscle is retracted manually on each side. After decompression of the spine the outer side of the superior articular processes of L4 and L5 are exposed and decorticated. Cancellous grafts are placed in the lateral gutter lying on the transverse processes and ala of the sacrum.

[The illustrations for this Chapter on Intertransverse Fusion for Spondylolisthesis and Lumbar Instability were drawn by Mrs. A. Barrett.]

Lateral Fusion of the Lumbar Spine

E. W. O. Adkins, F.R.C.S.
Consultant Orthopaedic Surgeon, Derbyshire Royal Infirmary and
Derby City Hospital

PRE - OPERATIVE

Indications

This procedure is suitable for all cases of intervertebral fusion in the lower lumbar spine. It is particularly applicable to cases requiring preliminary exploration of the spine by laminectomy. Such cases fall mainly into the following two categories:

(*1*) *Spondylolisthesis.* The loose lamina must be removed and the adjacent disc and nerve roots explored and dealt with as necessary. Lateral arthrodesis allows single-space fusion of the unstable segment of the spine.

(*2*) *Backache* due to spondylosis and degenerative lesions of the discs. Many such cases will give a history of root pain, and exploration of the spinal canal to deal with any involvement of the nerve roots, e.g. by decompression or posterior rhizotomy, is essential.

THE OPERATION

1

The incision

The patient is placed in the lateral position with the legs flexed in front of the body. A sandbag is positioned under the flank to keep the lumbar spine straight.

The operation is performed through a mid-line incision extending from L3 to S2 spinous processes.

After preparation of the beds for the grafts, a second incision for removal of a suitable length of graft is made along the iliac crest.

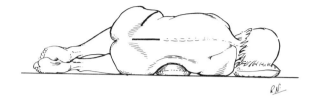

1

2

Exploration of spinal canal

The spinal muscles are dissected from the spinous processes and laminae and retracted laterally by a Balfour retractor. In cases of spondylolisthesis the loose lamina is excised completely as far forward as the pseudarthrosis in the pars interarticularis. In other cases a hemilaminectomy or occasionally a total laminectomy is performed to allow exploration of the discs and nerve roots.

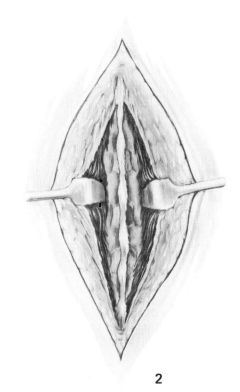

2

3

Exposure of transverse processes

The skin and subcutaneous tissues are dissected from the spinal muscles and reflected laterally as far as the posterior iliac spines. The erector spinae is then divided transversely at the level of the upper border of the ala of the sacrum, freed by sharp dissection from the interfacetal joints and transverse processes and retracted upwards. Meticulous cleaning of the bones is not necessary, but the adjacent margins of the transverse processes must be clearly defined.

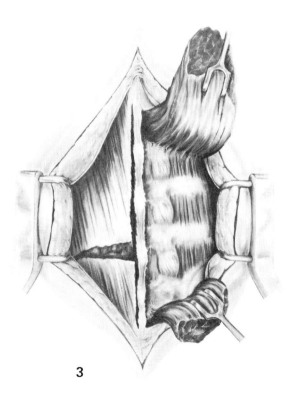

3

4

Preparation of graft beds

A slot is cut in the upper border of the sacrum immediately lateral to the sacral facet. This is done by making two parallel cuts with an osteotome and prizing out the intervening bone with a gouge. Shallow grooves are then cut in the edges of the transverse processes, which must be handled with care as they are easily broken. The best instrument for this is an extra large Citelli type forceps.

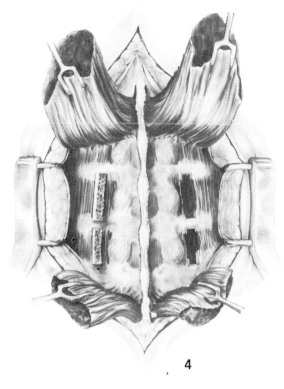

4

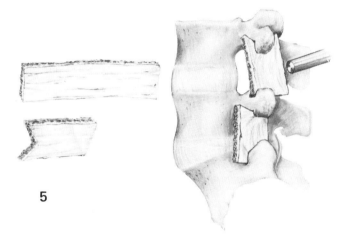

5

5&6

Cutting and insertion of grafts

The length of graft required is determined by opening a Luc forceps in the prepared bed of each space to be grafted. The iliac crest is exposed through the second incision and the required length of bone, 0·5–0·75 inch wide, cut from the crest. The individual grafts are cut to length and shaped as shown. Note the oblique cut at the lower end of the grafts. One point of the upper end is inserted in front of the lower border of the transverse process and the lower end then punched into position. The oblique cut of this end ensures that the graft becomes firmly impacted as it is punched home.

Closure of wound

The ends of the erector spinae are drawn together with a mattress suture and their aponeuroses sutured across the mid-line. The wound is drained by vacuum suction.

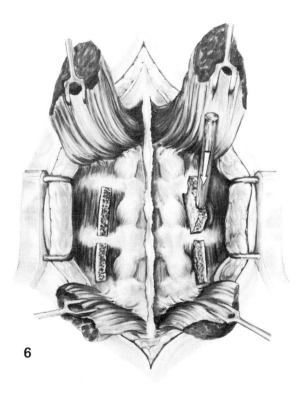

6

POSTOPERATIVE CARE

The patient is transferred from the operating table to the posterior shell of a previously prepared plaster bed, turning as necessary, for 2 weeks. At the end of this period a jacket-spica, including one thigh as far as the knee, is applied and the patient mobilized. If the grafts have been firmly impacted in position, 6 weeks' immobilization is probably adequate. However, if their stability is doubtful, 12 weeks is advisable.

[*The illustrations for this Chapter on Lateral Fusion of the Lumbar Spine were drawn by Mr. R. A. H. Neave.*]

Posterior Lumbar Spinal Fusion

E. O'Gorman Kirwan, F.R.C.S.(Eng.), F.R.C.S.(Ed.)
Consultant Orthopaedic Surgeon, University College Hospital and
Royal National Orthopaedic Hospital, London

PRE - OPERATIVE

Indications and contra-indications

The posterior elements must be intact, thereby excluding lytic spondylolisthesis with a defect in the pars interarticularis or when extensive laminectomies have been performed.

The advantage of this technique is that it facilitates combined exposure of the neural canal and subsequent removal of discs or facetectomy with arthrodesis in one exposure and thereby preserves the segmental neurovascular supply to the dorsal musculature. It can also provide internal fixation with consequent earlier mobilization and comfort to the patient and does not necessarily require a brace or plaster-of-Paris.

Pre-operative preparation

No special measures are necessary.

Anaesthesia

General anaesthetic with intratracheal intubation is essential. Blood transfusion may be necessary.

Position on table

The patient is placed in the prone position on a spinal support which allows the abdomen to hang freely in order to prevent pressure on the intra-abdominal veins. The anterosuperior spines should be over the break in the table to allow flexion and extension under vision.

THE OPERATION

1

The incision

The skin incision extends from above the third lumbar spine to the first sacral spine and then curves to one side, producing a flap in order to facilitate exposure of the posterior iliac crest.

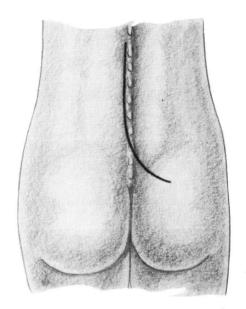

1

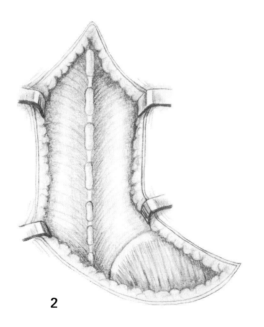

2

2

Exposure of iliac donor site

The flap consisting of the skin and superficial fascia is elevated, exposing the donor crest; care must be taken to avoid damage to the structurally important dorso-lumbar fascia at its insertion into the iliac crest.

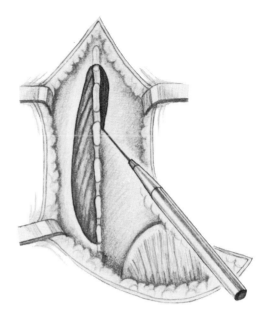

3

3&4

Stripping of muscles

The fascia is divided in the mid-line on either side of the spinous processes using cutting diathermy. The muscles are elevated and stripped from the spinous processes, laminae and articular facets using a Cobb's elevator and not an osteotome, in order to avoid damage to the articular facet capsules at higher levels.

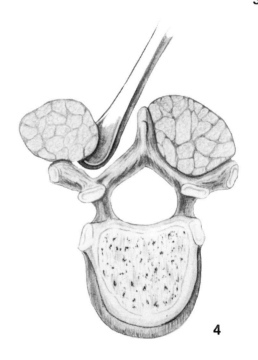

4

5&6

Decortication of laminae

Further dissection is needed to clear soft tissues from the laminae, spinous processes and capsule of the articular facets. The bone is then decorticated using a Capener gouge.

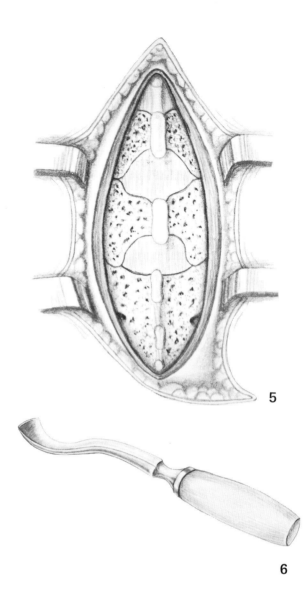

5

6

7

Insertion of screws

Holes are drilled into the laminae of the vertebra above using a hand drill; the drill, $\frac{1}{8}$ inch in diameter, is directed at an angle varying with the segmental level so as to lie in bone and avoid damage to the nerve roots.

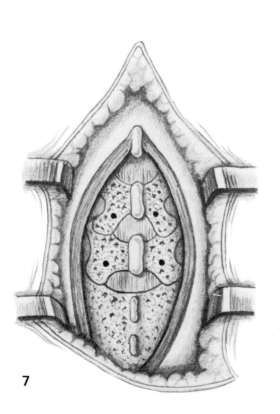

7

8

Direction of screws

The screws must travel from the vertebra above, across the joint and enter the pedicle and body of the vertebra below.

Angle and length of screw
L4—L5   10—15° degrees from mid-line
                   30° upwards from horizontal
                   Length 1·25—1·75 inches (3—4·5 cm)
Lumbosacral   30° outwards from mid-line
level   30° upwards from horizontal
                   Length 1·5—2 inches (4—5 cm)

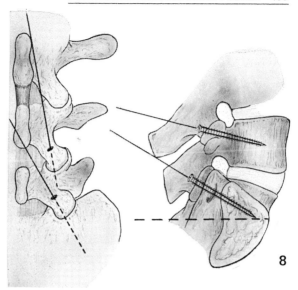

8

9

Removal of bone from the ilium

Bone must be taken from the outer table of the iliac crest, avoiding any damage to the insertion of the dorsolumbar fascia. The gluteal fascia and gluteus maximus are elevated from the outer table and graft taken as cancellous slivers after removal of the cortical lid. The gluteus maximus and fascia are then re-sutured to the iliac crest.

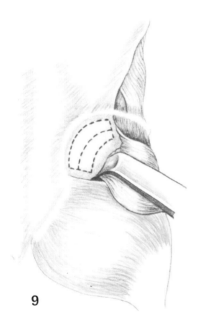

9

10

Insertion of graft

The slivers are placed on the decorticated laminae and chips inserted around them.

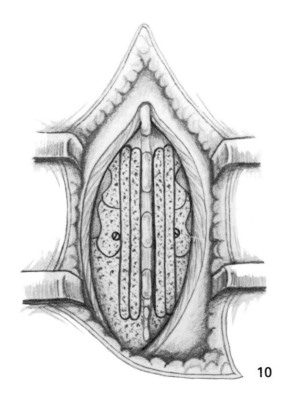

10

11

Suture of dorsolumbar fascia

The dorsolumbar fascia is sutured across the mid-line, replacing the muscles in their correct position. Closure of the wound is completed with interrupted subcutaneous and skin drainage.

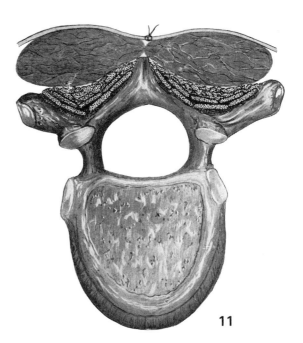

11

12

Drainage of wound

A vacuum drain is inserted into the donor site and crosses the mid-line deep to the superficial fascia.

POSTOPERATIVE CARE

A gauze and wool dressing is applied and the patient is nursed in an ordinary bed. The drain is removed after 48 hr.

The patient is mobilized out of bed when muscle control has returned. The patient should be able to turn freely in bed and do extension, abdominal and straight leg raising exercises before being allowed to walk. This is usually accomplished within 5–10 days.

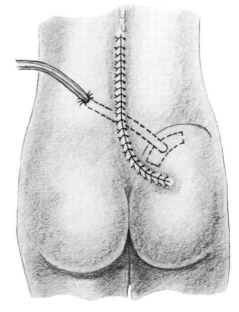

12

[*The illustrations for this Chapter on Posterior Lumbar Spinal Fusion were drawn by Mrs. A. Barrett and Mr. F. Price.*]

Anterior Interbody Fusion for Spondylolisthesis (Transperitoneal Approach)

Douglas Freebody, M.B., B.S., F.R.C.S.(Eng.), F.R.C.S.(Ed.)
Consultant Orthopaedic Surgeon, Kingston Group of Hospitals

INTRODUCTION

Stabilization of the loose lumbar vertebra will restore the normal weight-bearing function of the spine through the vertebral bodies and thus prevent soft tissue and ligamentous strain and nerve root irritation. Stabilization is provided by *interbody fusion.*

PRE-OPERATIVE

Indications

(1) Recurrent and persistent backache due to instability.

(2) Development of nerve root irritation.

(3) Radiological evidence of increasing 'slip' of the vertebra.

(4) Degenerative changes occurring in the intervening disc.

(5) The effect of possible future pregnancies.

(6) Intolerance to wearing a belt and to restriction in the adolescent.

Contra-indications

(1) When the patient has had multiple abdominal operations (with or without peritonitis) or has symptoms suggesting adhesions. In such cases the retroperitoneal approach may be considered.

(2) When there is evidence of root pressure (disc prolapse). The patient must be free of sciatic pain as the result of bed rest before anterior fusion is attempted.

(3) In females on the contraceptive pill. This should be stopped for at least 2—3 months before operation.

(4) In cases in which there is excessive forward displacement the operation will be more difficult, and the technique will have to be modified to suit the case.

X-ray examination

The degree of slip and the condition of the disc are assessed. Persistence of sciatica after rest may require myelography. In major slips particular attention must be paid to L4-L5; the presence of a retrospondylolisthesis at this level will necessitate its inclusion in the fusion.

Pre-operative preparation

A posterior plaster bed is made, and to correct the excessive lumbar lordosis so frequently seen, a pad of Gamgee tissue, 7·8 cm thick and just less than the width of the patient's pelvis, is placed under the patient's abdomen. This posterior shell is later mounted on a light metal frame, which can be easily secured to the operating table. The patient must become acclimatized to living in the bed by spending 5—7 days in it before operation to ensure that it is comfortable. An anterior shell can then be made for turning. During the 48 hr before operation the patient is encouraged to walk about to improve circulation, but must only rest in the bed. Attention to bowel and bladder function in the bed is essential. A rectal wash-out is given on the morning of operation and prior to going to the theatre an indwelling catheter is inserted into the bladder.

Anaesthesia

Hypotensive anaesthesia reduces the bleeding from cancellous bone very considerably — a digital systolic pressure of 60 mmHg is ideal.

THE OPERATION

1

Taking the graft from the left iliac crest

The patient is positioned for the removal of the graft by placing a large sandbag under the left buttock to lift the crest off the bed. An elliptical incision is made below the iliac crest, and the attachment of tensor fascii and the glutei are reflected from the ileum. A graft, 2 inches (5 cm) long and $7/8$ inch (22 mm) wide, is cut from below the crest as a window or trap-door, using an osteotome or power saw. This leaves the attachment of the oblique abdominal muscles undisturbed. The wound is closed with a Redivac drain.

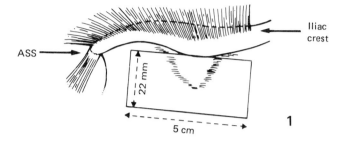

Abdominal approach

The patient is repositioned in the plaster bed. Having secured the bed to the table, it is adjusted to a 30° Trendelenburg tilt. The abdomen is draped and opened through a left paramedian incision. The viscera are retracted and packed off, and an abdominal retractor is then inserted. The sacral promontory is displayed and the bifurcation identified.

2

Infiltration of posterior peritoneum

The areolar tissue behind the posterior peritoneum is infiltrated with about 40 ml of a solution of 1 : 200,000 adrenaline in normal saline. The peritoneum is incised to the right of the mid-line. The areolar tissue is swept aside laterally revealing the *presacral* plexus, which crosses the left common iliac vessels and courses downwards and medially across the pelvis. The middle sacral vessels are identified, divided and ligated. *Diathermy must not be used over the sacral promontory* because of possible damage to the plexus.

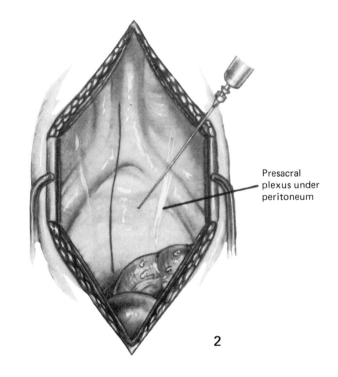

Presacral plexus under peritoneum

3 & 4

Exposure of the lumbosacral joint

The common iliac vessels are mobilized and retracted by rubber-covered pin retractors inserted into L5. The lumbosacral disc is displayed and a triradiate incision is made over the disc and the lower border of L5. Three curtains, consisting of longitudinal ligament and a thin layer of annulus, are elevated and retracted. The annulus is separated from the bony margin with a scalpel, followed by blunt dissection with a sharpened Bristow's bone elevator. The disc is then removed together with the vertebral plates. All disc nuclear material must be removed back to the posterior annulus.

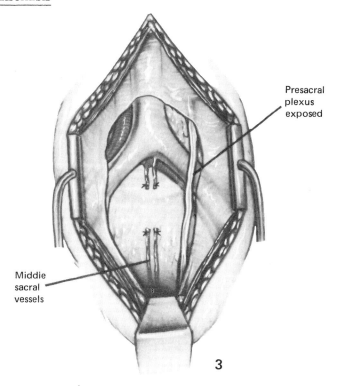

Presacral plexus exposed

Middle sacral vessels

3

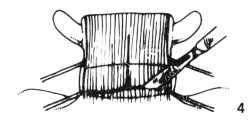

4

5

Preparation of the recesses for the graft

A block of bone $^7/_8$ inch (22 mm) wide and $^1/_3$ inch (8 mm) in height, is cut from the lower border of L5. Then, using a special angled osteotome, a recess extending upwards for about 13 mm is cut into the cancellous bone of the upper part of the vertebra. A dowel hole of equal size as the recess and about 1 $^3/_4$ inch (20 mm) deep is cut in the top of the sacrum. The anterior margin of the sacrum is carefully preserved. Any projecting portions of the sclerosed vertebral plate remaining are reduced by using a special bone rasp, thus allowing the graft to sink back against the posterior wall.

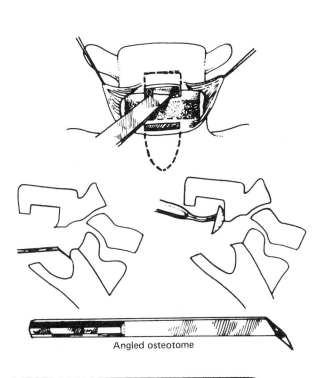

Angled osteotome

5 Bone rasp

6

Trimming of the block graft

The graft is fashioned from the bone and measures $7/8$ inch (22 mm) in width and $1\,1/2 - 1\,3/4$ inches— (38—44 mm) in length. It is shaped to a point at its lower end. The posterior surface is scored by vertical saw cuts to open up the cancellous bone.

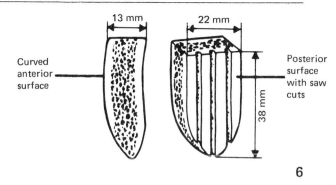

6

7

Insertion of the block graft

The joint space has to be prized open with bone levers to allow the pointed end of the graft to be inserted into the dowel hole in the sacrum. The graft is then driven home until its upper end is level with the margin of the recess cut in L5. By placing the rectangular punch over the front of the graft it can be driven back into the body of L5. When the bone levers are withdrawn the undercut recess will slide over the top of the graft, locking it in the cancellous bed.

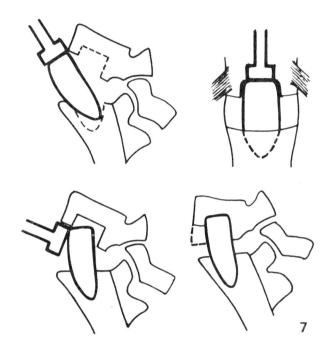

7

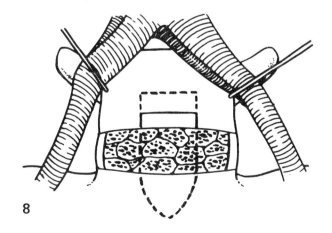

8

8

Packing of remaining joint space

Any remaining space between the vertebrae is then packed with chips.

9

Closure

The curtains are sutured, closing the space. This prevents the displacement of the bone chips and also helps to control bleeding from cancellous bone. The pin retractors are removed, followed by suture of the posterior peritoneum. The abdomen is closed.

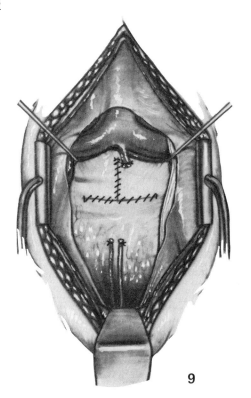

9

POSTOPERATIVE CARE

Before the patient leaves the theatre, the anaesthetist passes a nasogastric tube into the stomach through which hourly aspirations are made of any gastric fluid that may collect. Aspiration is continued until normal bowel sounds are restored. Oral fluids are restricted during the first 12 hr and then gradually increased to 60 ml (this increase is controlled by the amount of aspirate). The body fluids are maintained by intravenous drip during the first 48 hr. The nasogastric tube can be removed at this stage. A flatus tube is passed should abdominal distension develop. A rectal suppository is given on the third day and the catheter is removed at the same time. Breathing exercises are given routinely and leg movements are encouraged.

The patient is nursed in the plaster bed for 4–6 weeks, depending on the degree of slip present. An x-ray is taken with the patient in the anterior shell at the end of the third week to check the position of the graft. A plaster cast of the patient is made for preparation of the polythene jacket, which the patient will wear day and night for 3 months. This is followed by a further 3–4 months in a lumbosacral belt.

Avoidance of possible complications

(*1*) Bleeding into the areolar tissue is controlled by infiltrating this layer with adrenaline in saline. Haemorrhage from cancellous bone is easily controlled by packing the cavity with ribbon gauze soaked in normal saline.

(*2*) *Ileus* is avoided by the use of the nasogastric tube, restricted fluids and hourly aspirations.

(*3*) *Thrombosis.* The patient is encouraged to move his legs before and after operation. Anticoagulants are only given when there has been excessive handling or retraction of the main vessels. Any patient who has been on the contraceptive pill should be given anticoagulants until ambulant.

(*4*) In the event of *fracture* of the *graft* or development of *non-fusion* the anterior approach should not be repeated because of fibrosis over the promontory; a posterolateral approach with bone grafting using cancellous chips will ensure fusion anteriorly and posteriorly.

(*5*) Return of sciatica after successful fusion can be due to a 'moving' loose lamina, especially if the slip has been considerable. These cases respond well to removal of the loose lamina.

[*The illustrations for this Chapter on Anterior Interbody Fusion for Spondylolisthesis (Transperitoneal Approach) were drawn by Mr. G. Lyth.*]